OXFORD MEDICAL PUBLICATIONS
THE PLACE OF BIRTH

THE PLACE OF BIRTH

A study of the environment in which
birth takes place with special
reference to home confinements

EDITED BY SHEILA KITZINGER
AND JOHN A. DAVIS

1978

OXFORD UNIVERSITY PRESS
OXFORD   NEW YORK   TORONTO

Oxford University Press, Walton Street, Oxford OX2 6DP

OXFORD LONDON GLASGOW
NEW YORK TORONTO MELBOURNE WELLINGTON
CAPE TOWN IBADAN NAIROBI DAR ES SALAAM LUSAKA
KUALA LUMPUR SINGAPORE JAKARTA HONG KONG TOKYO
DELHI BOMBAY CALCUTTA MADRAS KARACHI

British Library Cataloguing in Publication Data

The place of birth.—(Oxford medical publications).
  1. Childbirth
  I. Kitzinger, Sheila II. Davis, John Allen
  III. Series
  618.4   RG652   77–30067

  ISBN 0–19–261125–9

*Filmset by Northumberland Press Ltd,
Gateshead, Tyne & Wear
and printed in Great Britain by
Richard Clay (The Chaucer Press) Ltd, Bungay, Suffolk*

Preface

Before it was carried out, the integration of the personal and public health services seemed to be a reasonable and economical measure calculated to avoid duplication and to make better use of limited resources, but it has led in practice to situations in which individual choice in what are often very private matters tends to be overruled in aid of what is held to be the greatest good for the greatest number.

Giving birth is one such situation; and the result has been a central policy dictated to some extent by the wish to improve statistics as opposed to meeting individual needs. No one would deny that each infant and particularly every maternal death is a tragedy to be prevented if at all possible, nor that modern obstetric care, which was developed in the hospital setting, has been at least partly responsible for the dramatic decrease in both maternal and perinatal mortality over the past half century. But it is not necessarily perverse to question whether our present priority should be to reach minimum figures for perinatal mortality at any price when this includes giving up things which free human beings have often felt to be more important than their own survival—such as freedom to live their own lives their own way and to make individual choices in line with their own sense of values.

Observation of the animal kingdom makes it clear that reproduction is, in many species, an activity which for a time takes a family out of the herd in an assertion that its particular set of genes and its own way of relating to the environment have survival value beyond a single generation; and the medical profession is, or ought to be, concerned with the biological roots of our being which often contain stronger imperatives than our present collective values take account of.

This book arose from discussion between obstetricians, paediatricians, psychiatrists, psychotherapists, statisticians, sociologists, midwives, and general practitioners who, at the invitation of the National Childbirth Trust, and with funds kindly made available by it, took part in a number of meetings held at its headquarters in London. The authors have made no attempt to speak with one voice nor to describe a method to which all doctors and their patients should conform; that was not their purpose. They represent many shades of opinion though all were in some way concerned about the direction that modern obstetrics appeared to be taking under the impetus of advances in technology and the increasing bureaucracy involved with medical care. The editors do not advocate home delivery for all women; but they have come to question the received opinion that the findings of the 1958 perinatal mortality survey have established for all time that home delivery is much less safe than hospital delivery for all classes of mother and baby—findings which have been used to reinforce the belief of obstetricians that hospital birth is *a priori* safer. A hundred years ago the opposite view could have been held on better evidence and there is no reason to believe that social conditions or medical knowledge and skill are static. It may be that the psychological need for professionals to be in charge creates situations in which intervention becomes necessary by interrupting natural rhythms and taking away from women the feeling that they are in control of their own bodies. We question therefore the policy whereby many women are being deprived of the right and opportunity to give birth to their babies in their own homes (when they want to do so) on the grounds that this represents for them an unacceptable risk. What the order of this risk is; what the evidence on which it is estimated; how far it is inherent in home delivery and avoidable in hospital delivery; and whether government, acting on the advice of the obstetric establishment, has the duty or right to dictate to women and their attendants what risks they should or should not take, rather than letting them judge the evidence for themselves, the editors will be content to let their readers decide. However, what is certain is that once the personal midwifery services have been dismantled there can in present economic circumstances be little chance of their resurrection, with the consequence that there will be no choice in future. It could also be that, once granted a monopoly, hospitals will be pushed by the need for economy into providing a more highly centralized and impersonal service at the very moment when the decline in the birth-rate gives it the opportunity to provide a more personal and selective service to the great benefit of the next generation—a generation which because it will be smaller in numbers will need to have the very best personal qualities to carry the burdens that will fall upon it. Such a centralizing policy might involve booking all women into large units with all technical facilities laid on (at least, Unions permitting, from nine till five, five days a week) with induction for the dilatory, anaesthesia for the frightened, early discharge usually on the bottle for the majority of babies, and special care for the rest. This might result in the lowest mortality for the least expenditure but it will not necessarily bring about the greatest happiness and fulfilment for the large body of women who choose motherhood as the best expression of their values and on whose devotion the preservation of our present caring culture depends.

However, there may be another way: really good antenatal care for all, achieved as in France and Finland by paying maternity benefits in the clinics (which could be made more easily accessible, private, personal, and convenient for those attending them); the development of a technology which would enable the physician accoucheur to pick out, before and during labour, those foetuses at risk and the admission of their mothers to a hospital staffed and equipped to cope humanely and efficiently with the small proportion of abnormal births 24 hours a day, 7 days a week; and home delivery for those who wish it when the evidence suggests that no risks unacceptable to the woman concerned and her chosen attendants are being taken. Such a plan would also include the training of general practitioner obstetricians or domiciliary obstetricians in the skills needed for 'standing by' the corps of domiciliary midwives and being prepared to deal with whatever unexpected emergencies that may arise (Curzon and Mountrose 1976). This medical attendant would need a considerable knowledge of perinatal medicine but would necessarily leave major intervention procedures to the hospital into which all women or babies requiring them would be diverted or transferred.

The immediate introduction of such a system is of course no more feasible now than was universal hospital delivery 20 years ago; but it is something towards which we could be working and which in the 1980s might alleviate the separation of family, mother, and baby at birth which the present system inevitably entails and the price of which could be, in a significant minority, emotional handicaps just as crippling and expensive as physical ones. Even Sir John Peel was prevailed upon to deliver Her Majesty the Queen at home; and her choice is one that in a civilized society which puts first thing first— and successful reproduction is the *sine qua non* for biological and cultural survival—should also be available for her subjects with the same degree of safety. Women are territorial mammals and for them no place can be as comfortable emotionally as their own home if they have made one. Body functions, as we all know from our own experience, are dependent on ease of mind; and ease of mind is more effective than technology in promoting normal parturition and lactation (Holt *et al.* 1977). What can happen to obstetrics when women's feelings are disregarded is well described in Ian Young's book *The private life of Islam* (1974).

A further topical consideration is that since hospital-based private midwifery is to be phased out, and since private clinics will never command the round-the-clock resources that a large district general hospital can provide— and which are what is said to make hospital safer than home—it would seem that the choice for those unlikely to need the resources of the hospital, and wishing in a very personal matter for personal service, will have to be delivery at home, where at least the patient is on her own territory and in charge. The inadequate nursing-home is the worst of all options.

The evidence in the chapters that follow suggests that the imposition of nearly 100 per cent hospital delivery has not brought about all the benefits once thought *a priori* likely to follow, and has had disadvantages not foreseen when adequate care was a life-and-death matter. It represented the logical outcome of a service based on the abnormal and designed mainly to cope with the negative aspects of childbirth. Perhaps a concentration on the positive aspects might not only suit the customer better but in the long run also serve the legitimate aspirations of the profession and the Ministry. British obstetrics has always been distinguished among other specialties by a commendable effort to audit its results. The simplest figures to collect and the most important to act on relate to mortality; but it should be possible also to collect data on morbidity and on customer satisfaction, which are different but not unimportant facets.

The editors believe that the evidence marshalled in subsequent chapters makes it clear that for some responsible women, and for some responsible and well-trained doctors and midwives, home delivery could become a reasonable choice; and if so it should be kept open if a demand exists. To provide such a service would be the first step towards a society dominated not as at present by the providers of services, but by the consumer, who in a free society ought to call the tune. It is not always right for the professional to refuse to share responsibility except on his own ground and terms, and it is not always right for government to make the best of conditions as they find them rather than to attempt to improve them. Homes fit for babies to be born in and the old to die in are slogans to be put alongside homes for heroes to live in—for living involves being born and dying within a loving community such as most families still comprise. We hope that every member of every Community Health Council and Obstetric Health Care Planning Team will read our book and that it will not be dismissed unread by those who determine central policies as special pleading on the part of middle-class women who 'don't know how well-off they are'. We acknowledge the great achievements of the obstetric specialty in making childbirth safer and less of an ordeal; but as on any long climb, the attainment of one summit is what makes the next one visible. The question is whether for obstetrics the way ahead lies in humanizing the hospital or making the home safe.

J.A.D.
S.K.

March 1977

References

Curzen, P. and Mountrose, U. M. (1976). 'The general practitioners role in the management of labour.' *British Medical Journal*, iv, 1433–4.

Holt, J., McLennan, A. H., and Carrie, L. (1977). 'Lumbar epidural analgesia in labour: relation to fetal malposition and instrumental delivery.' *British Medical Journal* i, 14–16.

Young, I. (1974). *The private life of Islam*. A. Lane, London.

Acknowledgements

The editors are grateful for discussion with Professor Neville Butler, Dr. Dermot McCarthy, Dr. Lawrence Goldie, Mrs. Susan Clayton, Dr. Christine Cooper, Dr. Keith Hudson, Dr. Mary Lindsay, Lady Micklethwait, Dr. Pat Russell, Mrs. Ruth Stone, Dr. Theresa Watts, and Mrs. Audrey Wise MP. The book would never have seen the light of day had not Mrs. Audrey Macefield assisted in putting it together and typing the final version. Chapter 3 is adapted from an article first published by Dr. Chalmers in *Paediatrics* **58**, 308–12 (1976).

Joel Richman and W. O. Goldthorp wish to acknowledge the stimulating discussion Jim Lord, Boris Allen, and John Phillips provided when writing Chapter 10. They would also like to thank Margaret Stacey for commenting on the typescript. The authors are responsible for the final presentation.

In various places, use has been made of the Report on Confidential Enquiries, for which the editors are indebted to the Controller of Her Majesty's Stationery Office.

Contents

Antenatal care and the choice of place of birth

Antenatal care is the keystone of good obstetrics. It is also the basis on which sound advice can be given to an expectant mother as to where she should choose to have her baby.

In this chapter an obstetrician describes the type of antenatal care which is most effective, and suggests the factors to be considered by the doctor and the woman in his or her care in deciding whether a home confinement is feasible with that particular pregnancy. It is against this background that the material in other chapters needs to be evaluated.

The pattern of care the expectant mother is to receive should be mapped out with her at the time of the antenatal booking examination. Whether this is undertaken by the family practitioner obstetrician or hospital obstetrician depends upon locally agreed obstetric policy. At the booking examination an attempt is made to give the mother a full clinical investigation so that a base is established from which to foresee as many as possible of the abnormalities which may occur during pregnancy or labour. The aim is a full review of the mother and unborn child in medical, obstetric, psychological, and sociological terms. With this information the doctor can discuss with the mother arrangements for antenatal care and confinement. The options are discussed in Chapter 8.

This chapter deals with the identification at booking and during later pregnancy of mothers and babies at risk, and the principles of antenatal care for those planning a home confinement. High-risk cases include those with inherent risks which are identifiable at booking, and those with risks which become identifiable later in pregnancy.

Risks identifiable at booking

It is now almost universal practice for high-risk factors identifiable at booking to be considered as indications for hospital confinement. A typical list of these would include the following:

a primigravidae over 30 years of age;
b multigravidae
   (i)   over 35 years of age;
   (ii) gravidae 4;

c social class IV and V;
d disorders of maternal growth, including small stature and gross obesity;
e medical disorders;
f rhesus and other forms of iso-immunization;
g previous operations on the uterus;
h previous third-stage abnormality;
i bad obstetric history;
j previous low-birthweight babies.

But these are guidelines rather than hard and fast rules, and should be interpreted in the light of all information relating to each individual mother and her environment.

Age and parity

The overall influence of age and parity on maternal mortality, directly due to complications of pregnancy, labour, and the puerperium is seen in Table 1.1, taken from the *Report on Confidential Enquiries into Maternal Deaths in England and Wales 1970–72* (Arthure, Tomkinson, Organe, Lewis, Adelstein, and Weatherall, 1975). The table covers all maternities, whether confined in hospital, at home, or in another institution. Thus the risk of maternal death in pregnancy for mothers having their first four babies generally increases with age, independently of parity. The Dutch experience is similar (Stolte, Bout, and Janssens 1972).

Table 1.1 Death-rates per million maternities by age and parity

| Age | Parity | | | | |
	1	2	3	4	5+
Under 20	101·4	23·2	—	—	—
20–24	121·0	57·7	141·7	146·9	206·4
25–29	134·3	92·7	65·9	141·2	357·3
30–34	169·5	101·9	208·8	196·1	434·9
35–39	487·0	361·8	336·4	583·3	511·1
40+	785·5	536·7	975·9	615·4	1127·7

Of more immediate concern to mothers when considering venue for confinement are considerations relating to perinatal mortality and morbidity. In 1975 there were some 200 perinatal infant deaths for every maternal death (and many handicapped survivors; there are indeed about 20 babies born with cerebral palsy alone for every maternal death (Wynn and Wynn 1976)). The influence of maternal age and parity is shown in Tables 1.2 and 2.3, taken from *British Births 1970* (Chamberlain, Chamberlain, Howlett, and Claireaux 1975). This perinatal mortality survey is based on a nationwide sample of all births which occurred during 1 week in that year. In both tables perinatal mortality shows a U-shaped pattern for age and parity; high at low ages and for first pregnancy, low in the 20s and for second and third pregnancy, and rising at higher ages and parity.

The difficulty of interpreting from statistics the prognosis for an indi-

Table 1.2 Age of mothers according to outcome —all singletons

Age	Total	Perinatal mortality per 1000 total births
Under 20	1 647	28·6
20–24	5 961	18·0
25–29	5 136	19·3
30–34	2 533	20·9
35 +	1 435	35·7
not known	103	29·1
Total	16 815	21·4

Table 1.3 Parity of mothers according to outcome —all singletons

Parity	Total	Perinatal mortality per 1000 total births
0†	6 312	23·2
1	5 361	15·9
2, 3	3 962	23·0
4 +	1 180	32·3
Total	16 815	21·4

† May include some where parity not known

vidual can be demonstrated by the following. First, in regard to age: analysis of data from the 1958 perinatal mortality survey showed that after allowance had been made for their relatively adverse parity and social class distribution, perinatal mortality in the late teenage group was lower than at any other age period (Feldstein and Butler 1965). Secondly, in regard to parity: data relating to the multipara whose previous pregnancies were successful are not yet available. However, unpublished observations from the 1958 British Perinatal Mortality Survey show that mothers having their fifth pregnancy *whose four previous pregnancies and labours have been normal* are not a high-risk group, provided they are not 'elderly' (Butler, 1977).

Social class

The striking association between socio-economic status and perinatal mortality has been known for many years. Table 1.4 from the 1970 births

Table 1.4 Social class distribution according to outcome —all singletons

Social class	Total	Perinatal mortality rates
1	800	7·5
2	1 837	15·8
3	9 027	19·6
4	2 338	26·5
5	1 014	27·6
Armed forces	380	26·4
Students	83	—
Other	7	—
Unsupported motherst	1 235	37·4
Ill-defined and not known	94	—
Total	16 815	21·4

† Includes single, widowed, divorced, and separated mothers

survey shows the social class distribution of mothers with singleton pregnancies and the outcomes. This social-class classification by the Office of Population, Censuses and Surveys can indicate only broad groups with varying standards of living and must be interpreted with caution. In one area, 'skilled workers' may mean workers in heavy industrial plants living in physically old and unhealthy urban conditions, whereas in another area they may be predominantly those in light industry living in a healthy physical setting (Illsley and Kincaid 1969). Social class *per se* is not the determinant: for example, it has been demonstrated that the influence of social class on low birthweight can be 'explained' by other factors such as smoking, the degree of pre-eclamptic toxaemia, and the height and parity of the mother (Butler 1974). Perinatal mortality rates show considerable regional variation, with a clear fall from the North of Britain to the South. The regional differences are paralleled by differences in health, physique, reproduction habits, and environment of the mothers (Baird and Thomson 1969). Regional studies examined longitudinally show that the perinatal mortality of social class 5 remains twice that of social class 1 in any given population.

Maternal height

There is a close association between maternal height and perinatal mortality; the shorter the mother the higher the mortality rate. The most probable

Table 1.5 Maternal height —singletons

Maternal height	Total	Perinatal mortality per 1000 total births
Less than 1·58 m	3 958	25·3
1·58–1·64 m	7 313	21·9
1·65+ m	5 372	17·2
Not known	172	46·5†
Total	16 815	21·4

† This group is likely to be biased by mothers who did not attend for antenatal care and whose heights were not recorded

reason is that many mothers in the lower income group fail to reach the full stature of which they are genetically capable, due to their having been brought up in an unsatisfactory environment and on inferior diets. On the other hand, the majority of mothers in the upper income group will have experienced an environment capable of sustaining optimum growth. That the higher perinatal mortality rate in short mothers is not confined to deaths from mechanical causes—disproportion between size of baby and maternal pelvis—supports the opinion that many cases of short mothers are due to interference with normal growth and development (Baird and Thomson 1969).

The arbitrary dividing line between normal and short mothers used in most clinics is 1·52 m. All short mothers should be booked initially for hospital confinement. A previous normal obstetric history does not preclude difficult labour in future because later-born children are usually bigger. However, if the otherwise well-developed and well-nourished short mother has an uneventful pregnancy and no problem of engagement of head near term, she could well be reconsidered for confinement at home.

Previous third-stage abnormality

The *Report of Confidential Enquiries into Maternal Deaths in England and Wales 1970–72* reveals that four mothers delivered at home died from post-partum haemorrhage (Arthure *et al.* 1975). These account for a quarter of the deaths from post-partum haemorrhage in the triennium. The case histories show there were avoidable factors in three of the four, with refusal by mother to accept the need for a hospital confinement being one.

A history of post-partum haemorrhage or retention of the placenta is a contra-indication to home confinement because of the likelihood of recurrence in a future pregnancy. This hazard remains even after one or more intervening pregnancies with a normal third stage of labour. Mothers who have had third-stage trouble should be suspected of being capable of a repeat performance.

Previous low-birthweight babies

The outcome of pregnancy is related to the length of gestation and it has long been recognized that pre-term onset of labour is *the greatest single cause of perinatal mortality*. Identification of this risk at booking is usually not possible. Past performance is some guide. As the condition tends to recur in subsequent pregnancies, a previous second trimester abortion or pre-term labour is one predictor. In some of these cases there may be cervical incompetence resulting from previous injury to the cervix. A new problem results from the implementation of the 1967 Abortion Act. A significant number of mothers who have had their pregnancies terminated ask that their family practitioner should not be informed and may not admit their termination during a subsequent pregnancy which is thus jeopardized. The overall foetal loss in this group is high, with second trimester abortions and pre-term deliveries predominating (Richardson and Dixon 1976).

Probably one third of low-birthweight babies are not, in fact premature but are mature babies who have retarded intrauterine growth. Taking both of these groups together, babies weighing 2·5 kg or less make up 6 per cent of live births and account for two thirds of all perinatal deaths. Amongst the survivors there is an increased incidence of physical and intellectual deficits. During antenatal care particular attention should be paid to the recognition of retardation of foetal growth so that these pregnancies may have the benefit of care in good obstetric and neonatal units.

Comment

As already stated, all circumstances relating to a mother and her environment must be taken into consideration when making plans for antenatal care and confinement. Inevitably there are grey areas such as the primigravidae aged 30-plus and the multigravidae aged 35-plus who desire home confinement. There are added risks with increasing age, but hospital antenatal care and confinement does not guarantee the lowest possible perinatal mortality and morbidity (see Chapter 4). The 1970 births survey shows that despite the increase in the proportion of mothers confined in hospital, perinatal mortality rates have declined least among the 'at-risk' groups, as far as age is concerned (Chamberlain *et al.* 1975). So in addition to the variables already described, the family practitioner needs to take account of the current state of obstetrics and neonatology in a particular hospital. Standards vary between hospitals, and within a particular hospital from time to time (see Chapter 5).

Risks identifiable later in pregnancy

If home confinement has been selected, antenatal care is conducted by the family practitioner and the midwife working together. To avoid tiresome travel near term, some examinations should be conducted in the mother's home. That the initial decision regarding booking for home confinement is provisional must be clearly understood by all concerned, because it may be altered if a situation arises which renders home confinement less safe than confinement in a maternity hospital. Some risks identifiable during subsequent examinations and which are easy to detect include pre-eclamptic toxaemia, ante-partum haemorrhage, and malpresentations. Others, such as foetal growth retardation, present more difficulty. Practically all can be detected if mothers attend regularly and their advisers are meticulous in the conduct of the examinations. At each visit the mother's record must be to hand so that the results of previous observations and tests are available for comparison. The observations include (a) enquiry about general health, (b) body weight, (c) blood-pressure, (d) urine examination, (e) haemoglobin examination, (f) uterine size, (g) activity of the foetus, (h) volume of amniotic fluid, (i) presentation of the foetus.

General health

Although pregnancy and childbearing are normal events to doctors and midwives, for the individual mother the experience is unique and to most women, mysterious. At every antenatal visit the mother should be given the opportunity to ask questions. Extra time should be allocated to those, usually the less sophisticated, who do not ask questions. They may not do so for fear of being considered stupid or a nuisance.

Many mothers fear they will have an abnormal baby. The role of the midwife is crucial here because it is to the understanding midwife the woman may first tell her fears. In hospital clinics the mother may be over-awed and may see different staff at each visit, but these hindrances to relationships do not prevail where the mother is being cared for by her own family practitioner and midwife.

Maternal weight gain

Weighing is frequently carried out in a careless manner that renders it use-less. For weight-recording the mother should wear a standard gown. The 1972 U.S. Collaborative Perinatal Study indicates that a maternal weight gain of 9–14 kg is optimal with respect to the lowest rates of perinatal mortality and delivery of low-birthweight infants (Niswander and Gordon 1972). The practice of putting the above-average-weight mother on a reducing diet at the very time she needs to be well fed for the sake of her child is misguided. Attempts to reduce excessive maternal weight gain by dietary means not only impair foetal growth but result in a persistent size deficit in the children (Blumenthal 1976).

Blood-pressure

Some disorders of pregnancy are symptomless and the most common is pre-eclamptic toxaemia, the ultimate cause of which is not known. A confirmed rise in blood-pressure is usually the earliest sign. It is for this reason that blood-pressure recordings at every antenatal visit are mandatory. The reports on confidential enquiries into maternal deaths show there has been a remarkable fall over the past 20 years in maternal mortality from toxaemia of pregnancy including eclampsia. In the triennium 1970–2, when death occurred, poor antenatal care and infrequent visits by the mother were to be found in two thirds of all cases of toxaemia, and in three quarters of those in which fits occurred (Arthure *et al.* 1975). The reduction in maternal mortality from toxaemias of pregnancy is to a substantial degree a consequence of vigilance in antenatal care. Mothers who do not keep ante-natal appointments are automatically at risk. Thus, those who undertake their antenatal care must devise effective means of keeping in contact with such mothers.

Examination of urine

In addition to routine chemical examination, in many clinics a mid-stream or clean-catch specimen of urine is routinely submitted to a bacterial count. This is done in the belief that significant bacteruria is a forerunner of frank renal infection in pregnancy and a cause of pre-term labour (Wren 1970). This needs to be substantiated in further studies, but meanwhile efforts should be made routinely to test urine bacteriologically, to make sure mothers are not harbouring unsuspected infection. Do-It-Yourself kits are available for this purpose.

Haemoglobin estimation

Haemoglobin estimations are required at booking and at regular intervals throughout pregnancy because significant anaemia may be present without obvious clinical signs. This is particularly so in mothers of non-Caucasian origin. Haemoglobin levels persisting below 12·6 g in spite of iron and folate supplement warrant special investigation (Steingold 1966).

Uterine size

The size of the uterus is assessed at each visit. By convention, this is recorded by comparing it to the size expected in a normal pregnancy at a particular gestational age. What is more important is to note *the rate of increase* in uterine size and for this purpose serial observations by one examiner are necessary. Because of inter-observer variation a series of observations by different examiners are necessarily less helpful here. The examiner needs to consider both the size of the foetus and the volume of the amniotic fluid because each contribute to the growth of the uterus and abnormality of either will alter the growth trajectory. A much neglected test is the measurement of abdominal girth at the level of the umbilicus. Static and falling maternal weight and abdominal girth in late pregnancy are associated with an increased incidence of retardation of foetal growth, and also foetal distress in labour whatever the baby's weight (Elder, Burton, Gordon, Hawkins, and McClure Browne 1970).

Foetal activity

More can be learned from palpation of the uterus, provided it is performed without hurry. While the hands are resting on the abdomen the examiner will detect foetal movement. If the foetus is apparently resting, a little indentation may provoke movement. The mother will be aware of such movement and this is the best time to ask her about foetal activity. Normal foetal movements are associated with a good outcome and can thus be reassuring. In cases of disturbed foetal well-being spontaneous movements decrease, and they cease some 12–48 hours before death resulting from chronic foetal growth retardation. Provided one bears in mind that after the foetal head is engaged gross foetal activity is much reduced, the 12-hour daily foetal movement count is an easily applied method of checking foetal well-being and may be a better predictor of foetal asphyxia and impending intra-uterine death than the expensive placental function tests in current use (Pearson and Weaver 1976).

Volume of amniotic fluid

During palpation of the uterus the examiner should try to assess the volume of amniotic fluid and classify this as average, excessive, or diminished. When the foetal head or a limb is palpated between two finger-tips, in the presence of a normal volume of amniotic fluid a characteristic sensation is imparted to the examining fingers. If the amniotic fluid volume is excessive, the uterus will feel tense and cystic. If the amniotic fluid volume is markedly reduced there is a characteristic doughy sensation. Near term the foetal kidneys excrete about 500 ml of dilute urine per day. This is the principal source of amniotic fluid and it is reduced in cases of severe growth retardation in the third trimester.

Engagement of the foetal head near term
With a normal cephalic presentation the ability of the head to engage should be checked. If there are doubts about this the mother should be examined when standing up. As she assumes the erect position the head will often descend and engage. If doubts remain referral for assessment by a consultant obstetrician is indicated.

Comment
In this section emphasis has been placed on those components of ordinary care which can have a positive effect on perinatal well-being. When maternal disorders, or doubts about the normality of foetal growth and development arise, such cases should be referred to a consultant obstetrician. Antepartum death during the later weeks of pregnancy remains an unresolved problem. The hopes that more intensive antenatal care in hospitals would reduce these foetal deaths have not yet been fulfilled. In particular the availability of foetal cephalometry and maternal urinary oestriol measurements has not increased prevention of these still births (Beard 1976). A comparison of the work and results of two obstetric teams in the city of Cardiff over a 5-year period failed to demonstrate any advantage of a policy characterized by a wider use of induction of labour and antepartum monitoring with serial foetal cephalometry and maternal urinary oestriol measurements (Chalmers, Lawson, and Turnbull 1976). A very high incidence of induction (for example, over 40 per cent of all births in England and Wales in 1974 (Yellowlees 1976) is possible only if amniocentesis is used to check foetal lung maturity or X-rays performed to check the foetal skeletal development. These procedures are not without risk.

Pre-term spontaneous delivery of normally developing children continues to outweigh all other causes of early neonatal death. Vaginal bleeding in the second trimester increases the likelihood of this disorder. Whatever the booking arrangements, mothers who go into pre-term labour should be transferred without delay to the maternity hospital containing the regional intensive-care baby unit. The best incubator for transport to an intensive-care baby unit is the mother's uterus.

Non-predictable risks arising in labour

How good are the screening procedures whose purpose is to divert all high-risk pregnancies to the hospital service? Ideally, tests of these would require controlled experimentation but this is not feasible. However, the limited information as yet available from the 1970 births survey suggests that selection of cases for home confinement at that time was satisfactory. Out of a total of 16 815 births, 2077 took place at home and the perinatal mortality rate amongst these was 4·3 per 1000 births (Chamberlain *et al.* 1975). But no matter how good the screening procedures, some problems are bound to arise occasionally when mothers have domiciliary confinements. Some of the more serious of these require comment.

Cord prolapse

The complication of prolapse of the umbilical cord continues to take nearly as heavy a toll of normal healthy babies as it has always done. Even if the known causes of risk—any conditions which interfere with the close application of the presenting part to the lower uterine segment and the brim of the pelvis—are removed, there remains an incidence of about 1 in 2000 in the supposedly normal case. When this occurs in early labour in hospital, the baby may be rescued by Caesarean section. Such babies almost invariably die if confined any appreciable distance from an ever-ready operating theatre. This is one of the unavoidable risks in cases properly booked for home confinement.

Post-partum haemorrhage

The possibility of post-partum haemorrhage has to be accepted when carefully selected mothers are delivered in their own homes. The tragedy of death from post-partum haemorrhage can be avoided only if confinements take place in areas staffed by efficient obstetric flying squads. Experience has shown it is dangerous to transfer a mother to hospital with the placenta undelivered; it usually is safer for the flying squad to resuscitate the mother if she is shocked and to remove the placenta in her home. For this reason an anaesthetist is a member of the team.

Foetal distress and birth asphyxia

When foetal distress arises the obstetric flying squad, which includes a neonatologist, is called. Whether completion of confinement takes place at home or in hospital is a matter for clinical judgement. Inevitably, some babies will have difficulty in establishing respiration. More lives are lost in the first 5 minutes of extra-uterine life than during the following 50 years. It is for this reason that the family practitioner should be present at the time of delivery. (Chapter 9 describes his role at that time.) Prolonged birth asphyxia is invariably preceded by foetal distress. For the early detection of foetal asphyxia during labour continuous foetal heart-rate recording may be required. If this opinion is substantiated, domiciliary midwives should then adopt the new technique of monitoring and thus augment the excellent surveillance provided by the uninterrupted attendance of one midwife throughout labour (hospitals, with few exceptions, do not provide the latter; in fact, the most common cause of complaint is that of being left alone during labour (Ferster 1977)).

The 1970 births survey investigated the incidence of respiratory depression at birth according to the place of birth. The incidence in those delivered in consultant beds in National Health Service hospitals was over five times higher than for those delivered at home (Chamberlain *et al.* 1975). The authors suggest 'this might indicate a good usage of selection of cases for hospital delivery under consultant care', but do not provide the necessary data. Since the majority of cases in consultant units would not have had the accepted risk factors, it might also indicate the hazards to the foetus resulting from widespread use of induction of labour and consequent increased use of narcotics and anaesthetics.

Conclusion

The current debate on British obstetric practice is well reviewed by Chalmers (1976). The assumptions underlying the goal of 100 per cent hospital confinements (see Huntingford, Chapter 16 of this book) are being questioned both by the public and professional workers. As a result of a strike by hospital ancillary personnel in Tameside, Greater Manchester, in 1973, many mothers who had been booked for hospital confinement were obliged to have their babies at home. This provided an opportunity to evaluate some mothers' attitude to domiciliary confinement (Goldthorp and Richman 1974). Although the survey contained an obvious bias—it was conducted by local authority midwives who had a vested interest in continuing domiciliary confinements—it revealed that the majority of mothers preferred home confinements. The mother's subjective experience of labour, whether difficult or easy, was not the critical factor in her decision concerning the venue of a future birth.

Because the birth of a child is a family event many mothers consider home is the proper place to have their babies. Home could be the *right* place if they are in the category of low risk and remain normal throughout pregnancy. The decision as to whether birth is to be in hospital or at home should always take into full account the mother's wishes. However, it should be explained to her that if she is in the category of high risk the facilities of a good obstetric and neonatal unit should be available to her and her baby.

Only on a foundation of good antenatal care can the right choice be made.

References

Arthure, H., Tomkinson, J., Organe, G., Lewis, E. M., Adelstein, A. M., and Weatherall, J. A. C. (1975). *Report on Confidential Enquiries into Maternal Deaths in England and Wales, 1970–1972*, pp. 23, 111, and 134. H.M.S.O., London.

Baird, D. and Thomson, A. M. (1969). *Perinatal Problems* (eds. N. R. Butler and E. D. Alberman), pp. 18, 253, 257, and 282. Churchill Livingstone, Edinburgh and London.

Beard, R. W. (1976). *Prevention of handicap through antenatal care* (eds. A. C. Turnbull and F. P. Woodford), p. 169. Excerpta Medica, North Holland.

Blumenthal, I. (1976). 'Diet and diuretics in pregnancy and subsequent growth of offspring'. *British Medical Journal* ii, 733.

Butler, N. R. (1974). *Size at Birth*, p. 63. Excerpta Medica, North Holland.

Butler, N. R. (1977). Personal communication.

Chalmers, I. (1976). British debate on obstetric practice. *Paediatrics* **58**, 308.

Chalmers, I., Lawson, J. C., and Turnbull, A. C. (1976). 'Evaluation of different approaches to obstetric care: Part II'. *British Journal of Obstetrics and Gynaecology* **83**, 921.

Chamberlain, R., Chamberlain, G., Howlett, B., and Claireaux, A. (1975). *British Births 1970*, pp. 20, 21, 23, 26, and 114. Heinemann, London.

Elder, M. G., Burton, E. R., Gordon, H., Hawkins, D. F., and McClure Browne, J. C. (1970). 'Maternal weight and girth changes in late pregnancy and the diagnosis of placental insufficiency'. *Journal of Obstetrics and Gynaecology of the British Commonwealth* **77**, 481.

Feldstein, M. S. and Butler, N. R. (1965). 'Analysis of factors affecting perinatal mortality. A multivariate statistical approach'. *British Journal of Preventive and Social Medicine* **19**, 128.

Ferster, G. (1977). Personal communication.

Goldthorp, W. O. and Richman, J. (1974). 'Maternal attitudes to unintended home confinement'. *Practitioner* **212**, 845.

Illsley, R. and Kincaid, J. C. (1969). *Perinatal Problems* (eds. N. R. Butler and E. D. Alberman), p. 32. Churchill Livingstone, Edinburgh and London.

Niswander, K. R. and Gordon, M. (1972). *The Women and their Pregnancies*, p. 126. Saunders, London.

Pearson, J. F. and Weaver, J. B. (1976). 'Fetal activity and fetal wellbeing: an evaluation'. *British Medical Journal* i, 1305.

Richardson, J. A. and Dixon, G. (1976). 'Effects of legal termination on subsequent pregnancy'. *British Medical Journal* i, 1303.

Steingold, L. (1966). In *Recent Advances in Obstetrics*, 11th edn. (eds. J. Stallworthy and G. Bourne) p. 101. Churchill, London.

Stolte, L. A. M., Bout, J., and Janssens, J. (1972). 'Age and parity in relation to maternal death and non-obstetrical death in the Netherlands'. *European Journal of Obstetrics and Gynecology* **2**, 11.

Wren, B. G. (1970). 'Subclinical renal infection and prematurity'. *Obstetrical and Gynaecological Survey* **25**, 1045.

Wynn, M. and Wynn, A. (1976). *Prevention of Handicap of Perinatal Origin*, p. 2. Foundation for Education and Research in Childbearing, London.

Yellowlees, H. (1976). *On the state of the public health for 1975*, p. 60. H.M.S.O., London.

Policies for maternity care in England and Wales: too fast and too far?

The latest figures for perinatal mortality, analysed and commented on in detail in which home and hospital confinements are compared are usually those of Professor Neville Butler's perinatal mortality survey of 1958, when 46 per cent of births took place in consultant units, 20 per cent in general practitioner units, 34 per cent at home, and there was evidence of inadequate selection and poor antenatal care. Yet obstetrics and, perhaps above all, antenatal care, have changed considerably since that date (Chapter 1 of this book), and there is a strong case for having a fresh look both at the 1958 perinatal mortality statistics and for analysing figures for subsequent years.

In 1958 a woman booked for home delivery attended antenatal clinics on average less often than one receiving hospital care and there was often late diagnosis of complications, and less follow-up. Even so, the statistics did not demonstrate higher perinatal mortality at home, and the Butler report did not attempt to indict home confinements. What it did do was to examine certain complications in women who should not have been selected for birth at home. The report demonstrated that even then there were at least 25 per cent of 'low-risk' women who had a perinatal mortality as low as 1 per cent.

At present the average perinatal mortality of healthy mothers who have already had one or two babies and normal pregnancies and deliveries is approximately one third that which it was in 1958. We can conclude, then, that there is a larger percentage for whom pregnancy will be straightforward and uncomplicated.

In this chapter Professor Ashford examines regional statistics of perinatal mortality, comparing the outcome in consultant units, general practitioner units, and in home confinements. He asks whether in fact we have more hospital confinements than we need, and whether there is any contribution to safety for mothers who do not appear to require these special obstetric services to have their babies in hospital.

Introduction

During the past two decades fundamental changes have taken place in the pattern of maternity care in England and Wales. Over the same period there has been a steady decline in maternal, perinatal, neonatal, and infant mortality. Although it is widely accepted that the outcome of delivery re-flects many factors in addition to the circumstances of the current pregnancy, there is a natural tendency to interpret these parallel trends as evidence of a causal relationship. This argument is sometimes extended even further to embrace each separate aspect of change, the conclusion being reached that the way in which the maternity services have developed represented virtually the best that could have been achieved, given the limits upon finance and other resources to which the National Health Service (NHS) has been subject.

Even if the reduction in mortality is regarded as a major criterion of the success of the maternity services, evidence from both within and outside the country suggests that the current position is less satisfactory than might appear at first sight. First, there are the large variations in measures of infant survival such as perinatal mortality between different geographical areas and between different sections of the community, which in relative terms have not diminished over the past 20 years. Secondly, international comparisons indicate that England and Wales have fallen behind in the 'league tables' of perinatal mortality and that more has been achieved in many other European countries (see Richards, this book, Table 5.1). Furthermore, there is a growing realization that since survival of mother and child has become the general rule, greater emphasis should be given to other criteria, including the preferences and reaction of the mother and her whole family to the pregnancy, the delivery, and the post-natal period.

In terms of the development of policies for the provision of medical care, the maternity services have several unique advantages. The population for whom a service must be provided is clearly defined, the general requirements of each member of this population are very similar, objective indicators of outcome exist, and accurate information about some of these indicators is available for defined geographical areas from the vital statistics system. In addition, the birth-rate has fallen substantially and pressure on resources has declined, so providing the opportunity for the NHS to consider a wider range of options. This being so, it is timely to review the progress which has been made and to pose the question as to whether better use might be made of the opportunities which are now available. Two main classes of evidence will be considered. First, there is the information available on a national basis which inevitably tends to be imprecise and non-specific. Secondly, there are the results of more detailed local studies, which allow the practical implications of various policy options to be explored in the context of the provision and management of specific services.

The options in maternity care

The first stage in the delivery of maternity care is the confirmation of pregnancy, which under the NHS is normally carried out by the general practitioner (GP). At this time, an initial decision is made as to whether the GP should undertake responsibility for antenatal care or whether the patient should be referred to a consultant unit (CU) for assessment and/or continuing care during the pregnancy. In the event, some mothers receive antenatal care solely from the GP, some remain under the surveillance of the CU after the initial referral, and the remainder receive care both from the CU and the GP either as a result of deliberate policy or because of events taking place during the pregnancy. Thus, the options in terms of antenatal care concern the relative roles of the CU and the GP, the frequency and timing of antenatal contacts with the patient, and the content of the care which is received.

A second main aspect of the provision of maternity care is the selection of the place of delivery. An initial booking is normally made soon after pregnancy, but many patients are eventually delivered elsewhere than at the place at which they were booked, either as a result of an obstetric emergency or for other reasons. The available places of delivery belong to three main classes, CUs, general practitioner units (GPUs), or home. A small minority of patients are delivered at private (non-NHS) nursing homes. Over many years a policy has been developed of selecting potential 'high-risk' cases for CU care, on the very reasonable assumption that the more intensive facilities should be reserved for those who need them most. However, because of the uncertainties inherent in the process of gestation and delivery, the assessment of the actual risk can be made with complete accuracy only after the mother has been delivered. Thus, whilst more than one standard of care exists within the system, there must always be a chance that a 'high-risk' case will not be identified at a sufficiently early stage. The possibility of mistakes of this kind must be balanced against both the beneficial effects of the alternative, less intensive, regimes and also the adverse effects of exposure to 'high-technology' hospital care of mothers whose delivery is without complication (Richards, this book). In addition to specific medical requirements, hospital confinement in both main types of NHS institution provides an essential service when home confinement is ruled out by adverse social or environmental conditions.

Following delivery in hospital, the period of post-natal stay reflects pressure on resources as much as purely clinical considerations. Although there is evidence that for deliveries without significant complication lengths of stay as short as 48 hours produce no adverse clinical effects, average lengths of post-natal stay of 7 days or more are by no means uncommon in the NHS. Following discharge from hospital, further care is provided by the domiciliary midwifery service. Reduction in length of stay tends to transfer post-natal care from the hospital to the domiciliary midwifery staff, but provides an effective means of bringing the supply of hospital resources into balance with the demand. Indeed, by the standards of other similar countries, the average lengths of post-natal stay are relatively long and there exists a large potential reserve capacity in terms of hospital maternity beds within NHS institutions. Thus, given an adequate domiciliary service, the reduction of the length of post-natal stay offers the possibility of making more intensive use of hospital facilities and thus provides a further option in the running of the maternity services.

Trends in place of confinement

The only information generally available concerning place of confinement
is that contained in the annual returns made by each local authority (or Area
Health Authority) to central government (LHS 27/1 returns). Two categories
only are employed—home or private nursing home on the one hand and
NHS institution on the other. No distinction is made between different
grades of institution: the term covers both the large, well-equipped CU and
the small remote GPU where the facilities are little better than those found

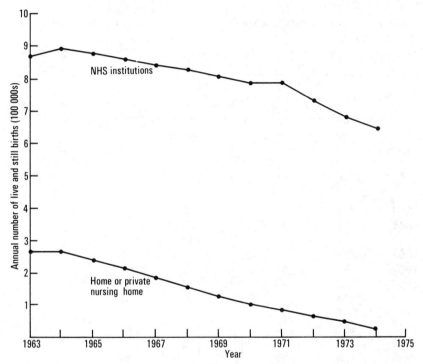

Fig. 2.1 Trends in place of confinement, England and Wales, 1963–74. (Source:
LHS 27 × 1 returns.)

in the average home. The format of the LHS 27/1 return last changed in
1963 and the numbers of deliveries in England and Wales in the two
categories of place of confinement during the period 1963–74 are shown in
Fig. 2.1. The total number of births reached a peak of 890 000 in 1964 and
has since declined steadily as time has passed, apart from a brief period of
stability in 1972 and 1973. The numbers of live and still births delivered at
home or in private nursing homes has dropped even more sharply, from
about 270 000 in 1963 to 28 000 in 1974. This represents a fall in the proportion of births taking place other than at NHS institutions, from just under
1 in 3 in 1963 to less than 1 in 20 in 1974.

The LHS 27/1 data also throw some light upon the effectiveness of the selection of high-risk cases for hospital care. To the extent that high risk is associated with low birthweight, this policy has met with increasing success, since the proportion of live and still births weighing 2·5 kg or less delivered at home or in private nursing home has declined from 17·5 per cent in 1963 to 2·9 per cent in 1974, the annual figures being substantially lower than those for all birthweights in each successive year. The proportion of the low-weight live births delivered at home and subsequently transferred to hospital has remained stable at about one quarter over the whole period.

Table 2.1 Secular trends in place of confinement. Extreme values in the regions of England and Wales.
Births at home or in private nursing homes: rate per 1000 live and still births.

| | Type of Local Authority | | | |
| | County Boroughs | | Others | |
Year	Highest	Lowest	Highest	Lowest
1963	393	190	392	167
1964	374	176	381	142
1965	412	193	362	116
1966	376	174	332	101
1967	353	155	309	80
1968	323	134	278	66
1969	300	116	245	64
1970	271	87	210	51
1971	242	59	178	43
1972	206	41	147	31
1973	168	19	107	20

Prior to reorganization of local government in 1974, local authorities could be classified in terms of whether or not they were county boroughs. By definition county boroughs cover the more urban parts of the country and the other local authorities are less densely populated. The local authorities can also be further sub-divided on a regional basis, using the 11 standard regions employed by the Registrar General prior to 1965. The extent of the variation in home confinement rate between different parts of the country may be assessed in terms of the maximum and minimum rates for each type of local authority within each region. The results obtained are summarized in Table 2.1 which indicates that for both types of local authority there were considerable variations at any given time. In the county boroughs in 1963 the maximum and minimum rates were respectively 393 and 190. Both sets of figures declined steadily with time, but by 1973 the range was still as large as 168–19. The results for the other local authorities show a similar pattern of variation. The highest home confinement rates for both types of local authority were reported in the Eastern region. In the county boroughs the lowest rates were recorded in London and the South East (1963–9) and South Wales (1970–4). The lowest rates for the other local authorities all refer to the Central and North Wales region.

It is an unfortunate deficiency of the way in which statistical information about births is recorded that no evidence is generally available about what proportion of the births in NHS institutions took place in CUs and what proportion in GPUs situated close to or remote from CUs. There are known to be wide geographical variations in the balance between CU and GPU beds in different parts of the country. On the whole, greater emphasis is given to GPUs in the less densely populated districts, presumably in an attempt to limit the distance a mother must travel to obtain a hospital confinement. A special study carried out of some 50 000 births taking place in the South West of England in 1965 showed that some 43 per cent were delivered at CUs, 28 per cent at GPUs, 26 per cent at home, and 1·5 per cent in private nursing homes. Since that time, the total number of births has fallen by one fifth. Coupled with the great reduction in the proportion of births at home, deliveries have tended to be concentrated at the CUs.

Table 2.2 shows the distribution of place of confinement in the 10 local authorities in the South West of England in 1965. There are substantial differences in the proportions of home confinements and in the proportion of hospital confinements in CUs, even within this fairly homogeneous region. This set of data also provides some information about the selection of high-risk cases for particular places of delivery. The proportions of low-weight (taken in this case as 5 lb 9 oz or less, to ameliorate the effects of digit preference in recording birthweight)) births in the various local authorities are shown in Table 2.3. The results for CU deliveries fall into two main groups. Devon, Exeter, and Somerset, with the lowest proportions of CU confinements, have the highest proportions of low-weight births. Although the CU confinement rates in the remaining local authorities vary from 40 to 75 per cent, the proportions of low-weight births are effectively constant and are contained within the range 114–123 per 1000. The proportions of low-weight births at the GPUs and home are considerably lower than at the CUs, which is consistent with the declared policy of selecting high-risk cases for CU delivery. For the home deliveries, the proportion of low-weight births tends to be high in local authorities in which the home confinement rate is relatively high and vice versa.

The 1965 data have also been analysed in terms of maternal characteristics. The results show only a slight association between social class and place of confinement, but a general tendency for the CUs to concentrate upon high-parity deliveries at the expense of the GPUs. The position as regards maternal age was inconsistent, in that in local authorities with the lower proportions of CU confinements the younger mothers were under-represented in the CUs. For example, the lowest overall rates of CU confinement of 31 and 32 per cent were reported for Exeter and Devon, where the corresponding rates for mothers of 19 years of age or less were 26 and 24 per cent respectively. In contrast, Gloucester City and Cheltenham had the highest overall rates of CU confinement of 66 and 75 per cent, with rates of 77 and 86 per cent respectively for the youngest group of mothers. For mothers of more than 35 years of age there was a marked trend towards CU confinements at the expense of the GPUs and home. As might be anticipated on general grounds, the majority of unmarried mothers were delivered in the CUs. In general, however, potential high-risk mothers (risk being predicted in terms of parity, maternal age, social class, or legitimacy) were being delivered in substantial numbers in each of the three main types of place of confinement.

Trends in the outcome of care

In the circumstances prevailing in England and Wales during recent years, maternal mortality has been extremely low and the great majority of infant deaths have occurred before the end of the first week of life (Huntingford, this book). It follows that the most relevant single indicator of the outcome of care is perinatal mortality, comprising the total of still births and deaths following live birth within the first 7 days of life. By aggregating these two separate components of mortality, difficulties associated with the differentiation between still birth and death following live birth within the first few minutes of life are avoided. Trends in perinatal mortality in England and Wales during the period 1963–4 are summarized in Fig. 2.2, on the basis of data derived from the LHS 27/1 returns and the Registrar General's annual statistical reviews. Over the whole period, there has been a general tendency for perinatal mortality to fall uniformly with time, the level achieved in 1974 being only two thirds of that prevailing at the beginning of the period. Reference to Fig. 2.2 shows that in any given year perinatal mortality was substantially higher in the county boroughs than in the other local authorities. Within each type of local authority there is a general tendency for perinatal mortality to fall with time at a fairly steady rate, which is virtually the same for both types.

In addition to the overall mortality levels, the range of variation of mortality rates between different parts of England and Wales provides a relevant indicator of the success of the maternity services in achieving an equally high standard throughout the country. The county boroughs and other local authorities were therefore sub-divided in terms of the 11 standard regions used by the Registrar General prior to 1965 and the perinatal mortality rate was calculated for each region and type of local authority separately in each

Table 2.2 South West of England —1965
Distribution of births (percentage) in terms of place of delivery and local authority

| Place of delivery | Local authority | | | | | | | | | | |
	Devon	Cornwall	Somerset	Gloucestershire	Exeter	Plymouth	Bath	Bristol	Gloucester City	Cheltenham	All
CU	32	40	31	45	31	49	43	62	66	75	43
GPU	38	23	47	28	46	15	35†	14	1	0	27
Home	28	33	22	26	22	36	14	22	33	24	26
Other	2	4	0	1	1	0	8	2	0	1	4

‡ Mixed GPU/CU

Table 2.3 South West of England —1965
Low weight (5 lb 9 oz or less) births in terms of place of confinement and local authority: Rate per 1000 live and still births

| Place of delivery | Local authority | | | | | | | | | | |
	Devon	Cornwall	Somerset	Gloucestershire	Exeter	Plymouth	Bath	Bristol	Gloucester City	Cheltenham	All
CU	150	120	138	118	154	123	116	114	118	120	119
GPU	44	35	40	40	47	41	62†	41	—	—	36
Home	27	38	41	36	42	38	16	30	55	29	30
All	74	70	69	74	80	81	77	84	97	99	73

‡ Mixed GPU/CU

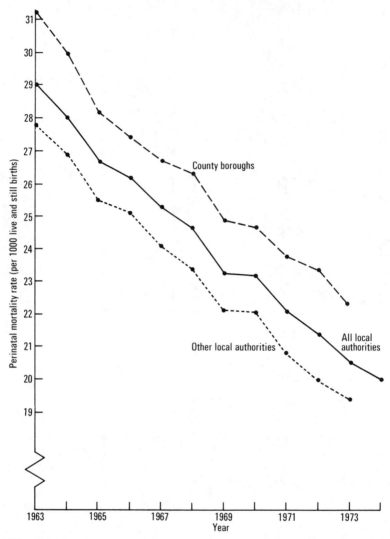

Fig. 2.2 Trends in perinatal mortality, England and Wales, 1963–74. (Source: LHS 27 × 1 returns.)

successive year. The results obtained are summarized in Table 2.4, which shows the highest and lowest rates for each category. In 1963 the perinatal mortality rates for the county boroughs varied from 35·7 to 26·7 per 1000. Both maximum and minimum rates declined year by year and the range in 1973 was from 26·7 to 19·1 per 1000. Thus, the performance of the best region in 1963 was equivalent to that of the worst region in 1973. Furthermore, when the maximum rate is expressed as a proportion of the minimum

Table 2.4 Secular trends in perinatal mortality
Extreme values in the regions of England and Wales: rate per 1000 live and still births

| | Type of local authority | | | |
| | County Boroughs | | Others | |
Year	Highest	Lowest	Highest	Lowest
1963	35·7	26·7	36·3	25·0
1964	33·8	25·2	34·1	23·4
1965	33·0	23·6	32·0	21·2
1966	31·5	23·9	31·0	22·5
1967	31·2	23·4	29·3	20·7
1968	32·0	21·4	30·4	20·5
1969	30·5	18·8	28·2	18·5
1970	29·2	21·6	27·2	19·0
1971	29·6	20·0	24·1	16·7
1972	26·3	18·0	23·2	15·1
1973	26·7	19·1	22·0	17·4

the differences between the highest and the lowest rates has tended to increase over the years. Amongst the county boroughs, almost all the highest rates were reported for the North West and almost all the lowest rates for the South, the South East, and the South West. The perinatal mortality rates for the other local authorities varied from 36·3 to 25·0 per 1000 in 1963 and from 22·0 to 17·4 per 1000 in 1973. For this type of local authority the highest result in any one year is about one and a half times as great as the lowest. In the other local authorities the majority of the highest rates were reported for South Wales and all the lowest rates were reported for the South, South East, and South West.

It is generally accepted that of the wide variety of factors which may affect the outcome of pregnancy, maturity (as represented by period of gestation and pattern of growth) is dominant. The most reliable single indicator of maturity, and the only measure which is available for births in England and Wales, is birthweight. The general form of the perinatal mortality–birthweight relation is illustrated in Fig. 2.3, which refers to some 50 000 births in the South West of England during 1965. These results have been plotted on the non-uniform 'probit' scale commonly used in connection with biological assay. On this scale, perinatal mortality falls uniformly with age, reaching a minimum at about 3·5 kg. The range of variation of perinatal mortality with birthweight is extremely wide and for this reason it is often

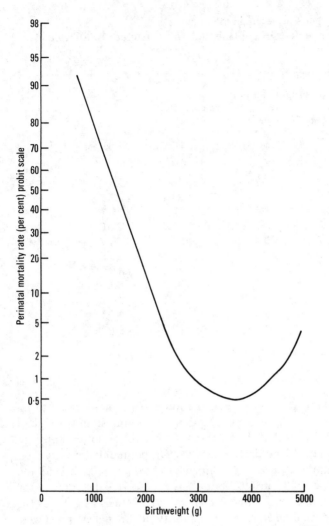

Fig. 2.3 Perinatal mortality and birthweight in South West of England 1965.

useful to sub-divide the observations into two groups—below 2·501 kg and above 2·500 kg.

The trends in perinatal mortality amongst the low-weight births (below 2·501 kg) in England and Wales during the period 1963–74 are sum-marized in Fig. 2.4 and the corresponding data for the higher weight (above 2·500 kg) births are given in Fig. 2.5. In each graph the trends are shown separately for the county boroughs and the other local authorities. Reference to Fig. 2.4 shows that amongst the low-weight births (which account for about 7 per cent of the total of live and still births but more than 50 per

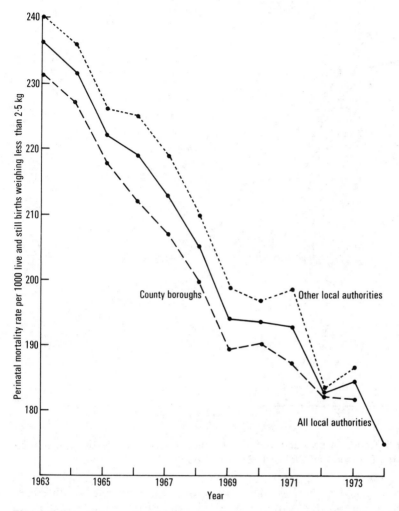

Fig. 2.4 Trends in perinatal mortality for low-weight births by type of local authority, England and Wales, 1963–74. (Source: LHS 27 × 1 returns.)

cent of the perinatal deaths) perinatal mortality has tended to fall with time, although at a decreasing rate. There was a definite hesitation during the period 1969–71 and a slight increase between 1972 and 1973. Mortality in the county boroughs was lower than in the other local authorities for almost the whole of the period, although since 1971 the differences are less marked than in the earlier years. The perinatal mortality rates for the higher-weight births show a general tendency to decrease with time, although the absolute levels are very much lower than for the low-weight births. In contrast to the low-weight births, the rates for the county boroughs have been

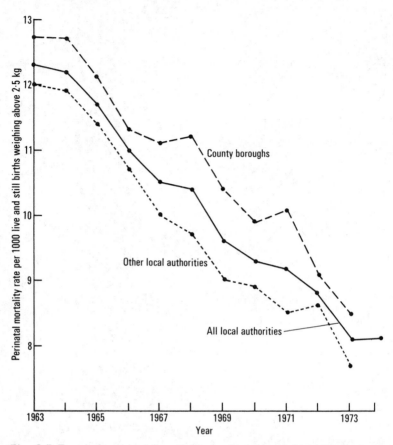

Fig. 2.5 Trends in perinatal mortality for higher-weight births by type of local authority, England and Wales, 1963–74. (Source: LHS 27 × 1 returns.)

consistently higher than for the other local authorities, but the difference tended to increase during the latter part of the 1960s and subsequently to decrease towards the end of the period under review.

The LHS 27/1 returns also provide information about the time of death amongst the low-weight births. Table 2.5 compares the average rates of still birth, first-day death, death between 24 hours and 7 days, and death between 8 and 28 days in England and Wales over the three-year periods 1963–5, 1967–9, and 1971–3. Still-birth rates have fallen in all except the lowest birthweight group. In contrast, death-rates in the first day of life have fallen in the below 1·001 kg and 1·001–1·500 kg groups, but show no consistent trend in the 1·501–2·000 kg and 2·001–2·250 kg groups. However, when still births and first-day deaths are taken together, there have been reductions in mortality in all birthweight groups. Mortality between 24 hours and 7 days increased between 1963–5 and 1967–9 in the two lowest birthweight groups, but fell consistently over the remainder of the range. Rates

Table 2.5 Secular trends in mortality–birthweight relationship in England and Wales, 1963–5, 1967–9, 1971–3.
Rate per 1000 live and still births

Mortality grade	Birthweight (kg)					
	Below 1·001	1·001– 1·500	1·501– 2·000	2·001– 2·250	2·251– 2·500	Below 2·501
1 Stillbirths	405	366	183	75·2	41·6	129
	389	336	157	66·4	34·5	112
	400	314	142	57·6	28·4	101
2 Death within 24 h	387	195	72·4	27·2	13·1	67·5
	383	189	65·8	24·0	10·4	61·2
	363	187	66·5	24·7	10·3	58·6
3 Death between 24 h and 7 days	103	94·6	49·3	21·8	11·2	34·1
	108	95·6	44·3	17·7	8·9	30·9
	98·4	86·0	40·0	15·7	8·1	27·5
4 Death between 8 and 28 days	13·3	16·5	7·7	6·1	4·3	7·0
	16·6	15·6	9·9	6·2	4·3	7·2
	14·7	19·2	9·5	5·4	4·4	7·5
1 + 2	793	561	255	102	54·6	197
	772	525	223	90·4	44·9	173
	763	501	208	82·3	38·7	160
1 + 2 + 3 (perinatal mortality)	896	656	304	124	65·8	231
	880	621	268	108	53·9	204
	861	587	248	98·0	46·8	187
1 + 2 + 3 + 4 (overall mortality)	909	672	312	130	70·1	237
	897	636	277	114	58·1	211
	876	606	258	103	51·2	195

The first, second, and third figures in each cell refer respectively to the rates for 1963–5, 1967–9 and 1971–3 of death between 7 and 28 days show no consistent trend. These results point to a general reduction in mortality over the period which was small amongst the below 1·501 kg birthweight groups, but becomes more pronounced in both proportional and absolute terms as birthweight increases. There is also evidence of the postponement of death, particularly in infants of very low birthweight.

Within a population the overall perinatal mortality rate reflects the distribution of birthweight: on average, a population with a relatively high proportion of low-weight births will tend to have a relatively high overall perinatal mortality rate and vice versa. The proportions of low-weight births in the county boroughs and other local authorities of England and Wales between 1963 and 1974 are shown in Table 2.6. When both types of local

Table 2.6 Secular trends in the proportions of births weighing less than 2·5 kg in England and Wales, 1963–74
Rate per 1000 live and still births

| Year | Type of local authority | | |
	County Boroughs (including London)	Others	All
1963	84·2	68·8	74·6
1964	80·8	67·2	72·2
1965	78·0	65·7	71·2
1966	80·4	67·2	73·2
1967	80·0	67·3	73·0
1968	80·4	68·4	73·9
1969	81·0	68·8	74·3
1970	82·2	69·9	75·4
1971	77·3	64·8	70·3
1972	82·1	65·0	70·3
1973	78·9	64·9	70·9
1974	—	—	70·5

authorities are taken together the results show no consistent pattern. Following a steady fall in the proportion of low-weight births during the first 3 years, the trend reversed in 1966 and there was a marked, although somewhat erratic, increase over the next 5 years, the peak of 75·4 per 1000 being reached in 1970. This was followed by a sharp fall to 70·3 per 1000 in 1971 and a similar level was reported for the remaining 3 years under review. The proportion of low-weight births in the county boroughs was substantially higher than in the remaining, less urban, local authorities throughout the period. The county boroughs and the other local authorities separately show the same trends as the combined data and in particular the sharp fall between 1970 and 1971. This latter sudden reversal is present when the two types of local authority are further sub-divided on a regional basis and clearly represents a phenomenon which affected the whole country.

The significance of the steady decrease in overall perinatal mortality (see Fig. 2.2) during the period 1963–74 must be assessed in the context of these changes in birthweight distribution. Progress between 1965 and 1970 took place against a background of an increasing proportion of low-weight births. Overall perinatal mortality continued to fall at a steady rate until 1974, but there is no evidence of any specific effect of the more favourable birthweight distribution since 1970. At the mortality rates prevailing in 1970, the change in the proportion of low-weight births between 1970 and 1971 would in itself be expected to produce a fall in perinatal mortality rate of about 1·2 per 1000. The actual decrease was in fact 1·1 per 1000 which suggests that there was no significant improvement in perinatal mortality for a given birthweight between these 2 years.

Place of confinement and outcome

When facilities of different standards are available to a population, the selection of cases in terms of potential risk must produce differences in case-mix between the various places of confinement. Furthermore, the extent of such differences may reflect the relative provision of different types of care, as illustrated in Tables 2.2 and 2.3. This means that direct comparison of the hazard associated with the various places of confinement is valid only if due account is taken of differences in case-mix. Table 2.7 shows the perinatal mortality rates in the three main types of place of confinement for the local authorities in the South West of England in 1965. The overall mortality rate was substantially higher in the CUs than in the GPUs, which in turn was the same as for home deliveries. These differences reflect to some extent the adverse birthweight distribution at the CUs, but even when allowance is made for this factor, mortality is consistently higher in the CUs for all birthweights above about 1·5 kg. The perinatal mortality rates for the separate places of confinement show greater variation than the overall rates in the local authorities. As might be expected on general grounds, mortality amongst the CU confinements tends to be relatively high in local authorities where the proportion of such confinements is relatively low and vice versa. However, there is no consistent relationship of this type for home confinements. Nor does the overall perinatal mortality in a local authority reflect the distribution of cases amongst the various places of confinement.

Further information about the risk associated with the various places of confinement is provided by special studies carried out in three geographical areas in 1970 (Ferster and Pethybridge 1974). The results are summarized

Table 2.7 South West of England —1965
Perinatal mortality in terms of place of confinement and local authority: Rate per 1000 live and still births

Place of delivery	Local authority										All
	Devon	Cornwall	Somerset	Gloucestershire	Exeter	Plymouth	Bath	Bristol	Gloucester City	Cheltenham	
CU	52	55	51	39	69	40	57	42	37	31	45
GPU	10	9	15	4	8	7	9‡	5	—	—	10
Home	14	12	13	10	6	4	5	8	7	0	10
All	24	29	24	22	27	22	28	29	26	24	25

‡ Mixed GPU/CU

Table 2.8 Some statistics on the outcome of maternity care in three HMC Areas, 1970

Place of confinement		Deliveries		Perinatal mortality	Deliveries with intervention per cent	Average length of stay in hospital	
		Number	Per cent			Intervention	
						No	Yes
HMC1 South West England							
CU	City	1501	41	48·6	57	6·8	10·5
GPU1	City	911 ⎫		3·3	14	5·1	6·3
GPU2	Rural	98 ⎪		10·2	3	6·4	6·0
GPU3	Rural	356 ⎬ 46		11·2	47	4·6	6·4
GPU4	Rural	270 ⎪		14·7	15	7·1	7·0
GPU5	Rural	90 ⎭		11·1	16	7·2	8·9
Domiciliary	City	211 ⎫ 13		4·7	2	—	—
Domiciliary	County	254 ⎭		0	‡	—	—
HMC2 East Midlands							
CU	City	1655	51	36·7	46	6·4	8·9
GPU1	City	514 ⎫ 22		3·9	10	7·6	8·8
GPU2	Rural	193 ⎭		5·2	6	6·8	6·9
Domiciliary	City	279 ⎫ 27		3·6	3	—	—
Domiciliary	County	617 ⎭		‡	‡	—	—
HMC3 North West England							
CU	City	2642	78	35·5	39	7·4	10·0
GPU	City	395	11	10·1	3	8·0	6·3
Domiciliary	City	345	10	8·7	2	—	—

† Rate per 1000 live and still births
‡ Unknown

in Table 2.8, which shows that a distinction was made between GPUs situated remote from and close to the corresponding CU. The results in the three areas show a very consistent pattern. The highest perinatal mortality rates are found in the CUs, reflecting the adverse case-mix. The rates for deliveries in the city GPUs and at home in each district are in close agreement. However, mortality in the rural GPUs is higher than in the corresponding city GPUs and in HMC (Hospital Management Committee) area HMC1 the difference is statistically significant.

In this particular study each delivery was classified in terms of whether or not any form of intervention took place. The interventions cover a wide range of procedures from surgical or medical induction to emergency

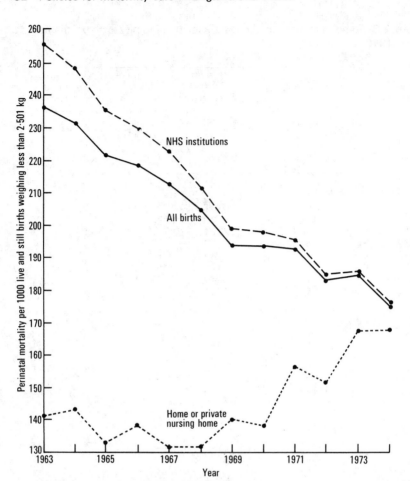

Fig. 2.6 Trends in perinatal mortality for low-weight births by place of confinement, England and Wales, 1963–74.

Caesarian operations. As might be expected on general grounds, the percentage of CU interventions increases as the proportion of CU deliveries in the district decreases. It is interesting that the proportion of interventions in GPUs in HMC1 was at the same general level as in the CUs, although the GPU interventions probably involved less extreme procedures than those in the CUs.

It is unfortunate that there is no general source of information about the perinatal mortality associated with particular types of place of confinement in England and Wales. The only relevant information is that derived from the LHS 27/1 returns, which refers only to the low-weight births. Fig. 2.6 shows the trends in perinatal mortality between 1963 and 1974 for births weighing less than 2·501 kg in NHS institutions on the one hand and home or private nursing homes on the other. As the proportion of institutional confinements has increased year by year, the perinatal mortality rate for institutions has approached that for all births ever more closely. Mortality for institutional confinements has fallen faster than the rate for all births as a result of the progressive dilution of the case-mix. For births taking place at home or in private nursing homes, the mortality rate remained effectively constant and much lower than that for institutional births up to 1968. Since that date, the rate has tended to increase and by 1974 was only slightly less than the average for all births. This may result from a deterioration of the domiciliary services as the home confinement rate has decreased or possibly there have been adverse changes in the characteristics of the mothers delivered at home.

Further insight into the performance of the maternity care system can be obtained by comparing the perinatal mortality and institutional confinement rates amongst the 160–70 local authorities existing in England and Wales prior to the 1974 reorganization of the structure of local government. In any given year, both quantities show a high degree of variation and the question can be posed as to whether, on average, local authorities with relatively high rates of institutional confinement tend to have relatively high or relatively low perinatal mortality rates. A regression analysis was therefore carried out of perinatal mortality on hospital confinement rates for the various local authorities in each successive year between 1956 and 1973 (Fryer and Ashford 1972). In each of the first 12 years of this period, the local authorities with *above* average institutional confinement rates tended to have *below* average perinatal mortality. The strength of this relation decreased year by year whilst the institutional confinement rate rose from 656 to 778 per 1000 live and still births. However, following the further increases in the proportion of institutional confinements in 1968 and 1969 the trend was reversed, the local authorities with the *above* average institutional confinement rates also having *above* average perinatal mortality. As the institutional confinement rate increased still further between 1970 and 1973 the association with mortality became progressively more tenuous, probably as a result of the steady reduction of the variability of institutional confinement rates between the local authorities. Separate analyses were also carried out for the above-2·500 kg and below-2·501 kg birthweight groups. Higher hospital confinement rates amongst the low-weight births were associated with lower perinatal mortality rates amongst the low-weight births for most of the period. However, the pattern noted in the results for all birthweights was also present for the higher-weight births, which suggests that the changes relate largely to this part of the spectrum of birthweights.

Observational data of this kind can never provide absolute proof of a causal relationship, but these results do suggest that increases in hospital confinement rates after 1967 were counter-productive in terms of obtaining further reductions in mortality. This conclusion is supported by the trends in the mortality rates for home and private nursing homes noted in Fig. 26. Indeed, the analysis by Ashford and Riley (1975) of variations in perinatal mortality between the local authorities in the South West of England and the West Midlands indicates that many characteristics of local authorities and their populations are more closely associated with perinatal mortality than hospital confinement rates.

Antenatal care

Although there is a tendency to concentrate upon the delivery as a key factor, the provision of antenatal care is an important (and perhaps a more important) issue. There is little quantitative data about patterns of antenatal care on a general basis and it is necessary to rely upon specific studies of particular local services in order to obtain relevant quantitative information about this most important topic. A penetrating study of the antenatal care system has been carried out by Ferster and Jenkins (1976) in three districts in the North, the North West, and the South West of England covering in all some 6000 mothers delivered during the calendar year May 1972–April 1973. At the very least, the results provide a snapshot of the way in which antenatal care is delivered in different parts of the country and confirm the great diversity of existing practices.

The first step in the delivery of antenatal care is the confirmation of pregnancy. In both the North and the South West about half the mothers delivered in the CU had paid their first antenatal visit to their GP by the seventh week of gestation and virtually all by the sixteenth week. The higher social class mothers tended to make the initial visit to their GP several weeks earlier than those from the lower social classes, but there was little difference in the distributions of time of first GP visit in terms of whether or not the subsequent delivery resulted in a perinatal death. These results suggest that the process of initial confirmation of pregnancy with the GP is satisfactory in that in most cases a regime of antenatal care is instituted reasonably early in the pregnancy.

Marked differences were found in the use made of the CU for antenatal care. For example, in the North, some three quarters of the mothers delivered in the CU had paid at least one visit to the CU (a teaching hospital) by the eighteenth week of gestation and nine tenths had at least one antenatal visit before delivery. The position in the South West was very different. Amongst the deliveries which did not result in perinatal death, only one third had visited the CU for antenatal care by the eighteenth week of gestation and just over one quarter of the mothers eventually delivered in the CU had no previous antenatal care there. Amongst the CU deliveries which did result in perinatal death, less than one tenth had visited the CU by the eighteenth week and only one third had made an antenatal visit prior to delivery. There was no appreciable difference between the social classes in the pattern of CU antenatal care received in the North, but in the South

West the higher social classes tended to obtain antenatal care at the CU in greater numbers and at an earlier stage than the lower social classes. The evidence also suggests that women of higher social class attend for antenatal care more often than the average in their particular district. On this basis, the coordination between the GP and the CU could be substantially improved in some areas and the high proportion of perinatal deaths at the South Western CU with no record of antenatal care at that CU is particularly significant. The higher social classes appear to obtain an above average level of care, although perhaps their need is less than that of the remainder of the population.

These uncertainties about the use of the CU emphasize the need to ensure an appropriate balance between the antenatal care provided by the GPs and in the CUs. Mothers in the three districts were classified in terms of 'potential high risk', using a system based upon parity, maternal age, social class, and marital status which reflects conventional obstetric wisdom. When judged in terms of outcome, the proportion of perinatal deaths amongst CU deliveries was actually *lower* for the 'potential high-risk' mothers than amongst the remainder of the population in two of the districts, and the corresponding mortality rates were equal in the third. Furthermore, although the classification of potential high risk could have been made in all cases at the initial antenatal visit to the GP, there was no evidence that early referral to the CU occurred either amongst the potential high-risk patients or indeed amongst mothers whose delivery resulted in perinatal death. In summary, intensive antenatal resources in the CU do not appear to be applied effectively when the mothers are classified in terms of either potential high risk or of actual risk.

The consumption of resources in the CU was measured in terms of intervention at delivery and length of post-natal stay. It was found that patients receiving antenatal care at the CU for the first time late in the pregnancy or not at all tended to require more resources than those seen at the CU earlier in pregnancy. This may indicate that early CU antenatal care tended to reduce the need for intensive care at the time of delivery and subsequently. Alternatively, the CU antenatal care is being concentrated upon the wrong section of the population. Whatever the explanation, the allocation of resources for antenatal care would appear to be inefficient.

Economic issues

Within the NHS there is no general quantitative information about the resource implications or costs of alternative regimes during the antenatal, delivery, and post-natal periods. However, estimates of the NHS costs of maternity care from the confirmation of pregnancy to 6 weeks after delivery have been made by Ferster and Pethybridge (1973). The results obtained in three districts in 1970 are summarized in Table 2.9. A consistent feature of these results is that the domiciliary deliveries were comparable in cost

Table 2.9 Cost estimated (£) of maternity care in three HMC areas, 1970

Place of confinement	Intervention at delivery	Insti-tutional† (3)	Local authority (ante/ post-natal care)‡ (4)	GP supplemental maternity fee (5)	Total (6)
HMC1 South West England					
	No	56	15	8·40 A/N§ 3·25 P/N 11·65 Total	83
CU					
	Yes	95	8	8·40 A/N 3·25 P/N 11·65 Total	115
City GPU	No	43	25	19·90	88
	Yes	57	18	19·90	95
Rural GPUs	No	65–105	14–18	19·90	103–127
	Yes	18–122	10–16	19·90	112–152
(City and County)	No	—	50–79	19·90	70–99
HMC2 East Midlands					
	No	67	19	8·40 A/N 3·25 P/N 11·65 Total	98
CU					
	Yes	103	12	8·40 A/N 3·25 P/N 11·65 Total	127
City GPU	No	91	14	19·90	125
	Yes	114	12	19·90	146
Rural GPU	No	138	16	19·90	174
	Yes	156	16	19·90	192
(City and County	No	—	58	19·90	77

HMC3 North West England					
City CU	No	82	20	8·40 A/N 3·25 P/N 11·65 Total	114
	Yes	129	13	8·40 A/N 3·25 P/N 11·65 Total	154
City GPU	No	96	17	19·90	133
	Yes	87	23	19·90	130
City domiciliary	No	—	60	19·90	80

† Estimates to nearest £
‡ These costs exclude maternity benefits and grants provided by the DHSS
§ A/N = antenatal; P/N = post-natal

to the cheapest of the hospitals in each area and very much lower than the most expensive. In each case, there was considerable surplus capacity in the domiciliary service as a result of the fact that the number of such deliveries had been run down faster than the available staff. If the staffing levels had been in balance with the work-load, the overall costs of home deliveries would have been considerably lower. A further and somewhat surprising observation is the cost per delivery in the GPUs, and particularly the rural GPUs, which was up to twice as high for non-intervention deliveries as in the corresponding CUs. This underlines the paradox that the less intensive form of institutional care was substantially more expensive per delivery.

Various studies have been carried out of alternative policies for the provision of maternity care in particular local situations, using some of the techniques of operational research (Ashford, Ferster, and Pethybridge 1973; Ashford and Hunt 1975). These exercises point conclusively to the fact that, given the birth-rate prevailing in 1970, reductions in the cost of a local maternity service of up to 25 per cent can be achieved by closing small GPUs and by expanding domiciliary deliveries to about 30 per cent of the total, without increasing the levels of perinatal or neonatal mortality. With the subsequent reductions in birth-rate, the excess capacity within the maternity services is now even greater and the range of possible policies even wider.

As part of the economic studies, the costs to the family of maternity care were assessed in one of the geographical areas by means of a retrospective enquiry based upon personal interview covering 334 families. The direct maternity costs to the family of those items which vary between different places of delivery are summarized in Table 2.10. This table covers travel to antenatal clinics, travel to visit the GP, baby-sitting during antenatal checks and classes and hospital confinement, travel during the hospital confinement, travel of a visiting helper, domestic help, personal items for the mother, household items, and extra heating and laundry. A distinction has been made in Table 2.10 between the cost of 'household' items (such as redecoration and washing machines) and all other costs, the former being considered separately since they include 'durables' which may be used after the pregnancy and by other members of the family.

Table 2.10 Direct (monetary) family cost by 1970 stream of care for maternity cases using a city's institutions

1970 stream of care	Sample (per cent)	Total cost minus household cost (£)			Household cost (£)		
		Average	Standard deviation	Range	Average	Standard deviation	Range
Home confinement	18	17	8	0–40	11	26	0–126
GPU, <8-day stay	22	20	11	0–76	17	33	0–120
CU, <8-day stay	9	18	14	0–72	22	34	0–120
GPU, ⩾8-day stay	18	10	5	0–22	17	32	0–150
CU, >8-day stay	23	15	10	0–67	21	36	0–148
GPU transfers to CU for confinement	10	19	19	0–98	14	25	0–95

The results show significant differences between the different places of confinement, but the costs of home confinement are certainly not greater than those for the shorter hospital stays. (Hospital inpatient stays of 8 days or more reflect for the most part intervention during delivery.) There were significant variations in costs in terms of the parity of the birth (as expected) but not in terms of social class. As part of this enquiry the reactions of the mothers to their recent pregnancy were studied. Most mothers were concerned that their maternity care, and particularly the delivery, should result in the minimum disruption to the family. The most common cause of complaint was that of being left alone during labour.

Comment

The way in which the NHS maternity services have developed during the past two decades can be summed up as an unhappy combination of over-reaction to a declared policy and under-reaction to changing circumstances. The Committee of Enquiry into the cost of the National Health Service (a continuing pre-occupation of successive governments) under the Chairman-ship of Mr. C. W. Guillebaud, which presented its report in November 1955 (Ministry of Health 1956) recommended that the organization of the maternity services should be reviewed at an early date. As a direct result, the Cranbrook Committee was set up in 1956 and produced its report in 1959 (Ministry of Health 1959). Although it accepted that the then existing tri-partite system must continue for some time to come, the Committee recommended that there should be a clearer definition of the responsibilities of the respective bodies providing the different parts of the service and greater coordination and cooperation between them. The Committee also recommended that provision should be made over the country as a whole for a sufficient number of maternity beds to allow for an average of 70 per cent of institutional confinements, on the assumption that the normal period of stay after delivery would be 10 days. Additional maternity beds to achieve this end were provided during the 1960s, but in the meantime clinical practice changed and the average length of post-natal stay fell to well below the assumed level. In the event, the institutional confinement rate was about 60 per cent in 1958, reached the Cranbrook target in 1965 and, in the absence of any restriction on hospital resources, has continued to increase until at the present time home confinement survives only as an exceptional procedure. Policies were again reviewed in the Peel Report (Department of Health and Social Security 1970) which accepted the changes which had been made in the interim period to the pattern of care. The greater part of the growth in hospital maternity beds during the 1960s took place in GPUs, many of which are remote from hospitals with consultant obstetric and paediatric cover and lack basic facilities. The unwisdom of promoting isolated hospital care of this kind was eventually appreciated and more recent policies envisage the provision of GP maternity beds in close proximity to CUs.

Concurrent with these increases in hospital resources and reductions in the average length of post-natal stay has come a steady decline in the birth-rate and in the total number of deliveries. Thus, increased hospital resources have been available for decreased numbers of deliveries, so much so that even with the virtual elimination of home confinements, the surplus of hos-pital maternity resources has increased year by year. For obvious reasons, the excess has tended to be manifested most clearly in the GPUs, with the result that most GPUs have been grossly under-used during recent years. This under-occupation has tended to increase the cost per delivery of GPU confinements to levels which are greatly in excess of the average for CUs, which may be incomparably better staffed and equipped. Although some small cost penalty might be justified in the interests of involving the GP more closely in hospital care or in providing a more local service for the patient, the size of the differential in favour of the CU over many of the existing GPUs is too great to be justified in rational terms even if there were no general pressure on public resources. In addition to hospital beds, the fall in the number of births has led to an excess of midwifery staff, and particularly of those skilled in domiciliary care. Indeed, the great reduction in home confinements has in any event presented a challenge to those responsible for providing a satisfactory role for domiciliary midwives.

The size of the current surplus of resources for maternity care has been assessed by the author and his collaborators in the context of the provision of an efficient service in individual health care Districts which collectively cover about one tenth of the population of England and Wales. In most of the Districts examined in detail the existing CUs could cope with the current birth-rate and many would have a substantial margin given the existing and fairly generous average lengths of post-natal stay. In only a small proportion of Districts has there been any specific reaction on the part of the managers of the NHS and the characteristic situation is for GPUs to be running at well below one half of their total capacity and CUs at below three quarters. On a national scale central government made no specific request to the NHS for a review of the provision of resources for maternity care until 1976.

In spite of the surplus of staff and facilities, the recent evidence about the delivery of antenatal care described above suggests that there is room for improvement in some Districts. The specialized antenatal care available only at CUs is not apparently being concentrated upon the cases which would be classed as potential high risk according to the currently accepted criteria or indeed according to the outcome of delivery. Initial assessment is by the GP in most cases, but some mothers who are eventually delivered in the CU either have no CU antenatal care or are referred to the CU very late in the pregnancy. It is unfortunate that the 1974 reorganization of the NHS does not in itself ensure greater cooperation in clinical matters between the GP and the consultant obstetrician. The improvement of coordination and the attainment of greater uniformity of criteria for selection for CU antenatal care and delivery will not be achieved without deliberate and persistent effort. The community midwife is in a position to play a decisive role in this respect, a role which would probably be assisted by a standard screening procedure carried out at the CU. In so far as some of the mothers who have the greatest need for antenatal care do not appear to be making the fullest use of the available services, the payment of social security maternity benefits as an integral part of the health care programme on the lines currently being followed in Finland and France might be helpful. However, the patient should not be asked to bear the whole of the responsibility for any existing deficiencies in the antenatal care programme and there is clearly room for improved coordination within the health services.

As far as the performance of the maternity services is concerned, the statistical evidence is generally encouraging, in the sense that as measured by reductions in perinatal mortality progress is being maintained. However, the continuing and very substantial gaps between the best and the worst in the system suggest that the distribution of resources could be improved. There is also a very strong indication that new measures may be required to ensure that greater equality of access to services is achieved. In terms of the allocation of existing services, there is evidence that more attention given to the higher-weight births might produce worthwhile benefits, particularly in the more urban parts of the country. Progress in terms of the survival of very low-weight births has been slow and a deliberate decision to emphasize the more mundane preventive aspects of antenatal care would probably lead to a better use of resources. Analysis of the trends in mortality and the pattern of confinement suggests that, given the standards achieved in 1967–8, a proportion of home deliveries of about 25 per cent would produce at least as low a level of perinatal mortality as is at present obtained with a much smaller home confinement rate. Small GPUs remote from CUs seem to involve risks to the infant (and possibly also to the mother) which are not present in central GPUs or more particularly in CUs.

On this basis, there are several possible directions in which policies could develop. Perhaps the simplest and most clear-cut would be to nominate the CU as the specific focus of all maternity care. The CU would be responsible for both initial assessment and monitoring and antenatal care, which could be provided by the CU working in conjunction with the GP and the community midwife. All deliveries would take place in the CU and the length of post-natal stay would be regulated according to pressure upon resources. Given the existing surplus, provision could be made in this way to cope with any likely future increase in the birth-rate. Maternity beds in GPUs would be available for reallocation to other specialties and would in many cases be particularly suitable for use for the care of the elderly in close proximity to their own home. Very substantial cost savings for maternity care would be expected and difficulties over the coordination of care would be reduced. On general grounds, it is unlikely that there would be any disadvantage in terms of outcome and some improvements in indicators such as perinatal mortality might be expected. The concentration of responsibility in this way would also be likely to make any attempts to reallocate resources to Districts or to population groups with an adverse record in matters such as perinatal mortality more fruitful. The obvious disadvantage would be, of course, to diminish the role of the GP in maternity care. At the same time, the choices available to the mother in terms of antenatal care or place of delivery would be greatly diminished.

A second and rather more complicated alternative would be to make provision for a proportion of home deliveries. Past experience suggests that a level of at least one quarter of all deliveries would be required to maintain a viable service and that the outcome could be at least as good as is obtained with the present system. A policy of this kind would free resources in the CU and, when the necessary adjustments in staffing and hospital management had been made, would produce a further reduction in the total cost of maternity care in the District. The GP could retain some responsibility for maternity care, even if the CU were to be given formal responsibility for ante-natal assessment. The community midwife would also have additional and appropriate responsibilities. Finally, and perhaps most importantly, choice would be restored to the mother and her family.

Given the present and probable future demands upon the resources for the NHS, the existing policy for the delivery of maternity care is not defensible. Although the existence of the GPU does provide some choice for the patient in terms of hospital care, the expense is completely out of step with the benefit. Changes must be made and other and more cost-effective means must be found of bringing the GP closer to hospital medicine if this is considered to be a desirable objective. The provision by the NHS of free transport services for the patient and her visitors might help to reduce the very natural resistance of the populations of country districts to the removal of maternity services from their local area. The reallocation of such rural maternity beds to the elderly might also appeal to local opinion as a more logical and acceptable use of resources.

Changes of the type envisaged would lead to very substantial savings, which would probably be of the order of one quarter of the current total costs of the NHS maternity services. Even if only part of such savings were to be retained for maternity care, very large sums of money would be available to direct towards those parts of the system which are in greatest need of improvement. There are several obvious candidates for change. First is the improvement of the effectiveness of antenatal care, which could best be achieved by a clearer definition of responsibilities and by closer coordination of the different agencies involved. Secondly, more deliberate attempts should be made to bring the standards of those parts of the population currently at the greatest disadvantage closer to the average level. This would involve the direction of resources both towards particular geographical areas, such as the cities and metropolitan districts, and towards particular groups within populations, such as the lower social classes and unmarried mothers. The statistical evidence suggests that the greatest room for improvement exists in the care of higher-weight births and that the excessive concentration of clinical effort upon immature infants may be misplaced. It does not necessarily follow that the required changes can be achieved solely or even mainly by improvements in medical care. Other non-medical activities may prove to be more effective, but any such improvements in education, nutrition, or general life patterns could best be centred upon the antenatal care programmes provided by the NHS. Finally, the main obstacle to the development of more cost-effective policies is the absence of reliable statistical information. Only when such information is available will it be possible to ensure that the service provided is properly adjusted to the constantly changing needs and aspirations of the population which the NHS is intended to serve.

References

Ashford, J. R. and Hunt, R. G. (1975). In *Measuring for Management: quantitative methods in health service management* (ed. G. McLachlan), p. 79. Oxford University Press for the Nuffield Provincial Hospitals Trust.

—— and Riley, V. C. (1975). In *Measuring for management: quantitative methods in health service management* (ed. G. McLachlan), p. 53. Oxford University Press for the Nuffield Provincial Hospitals Trust.

——, Ferster, G., and Pethybridge, R. J. (1973). *Community Medicine* **129**, 309–17.

Department of Health and Social Security Welsh Office, Central Health Services Council (1970). *Domiciliary midwifery and maternity bed needs*. Report of a sub-committee of the Standing Maternity and Midwifery Advisory Committee (Peel Report). H.M.S.O., London.

Ferster, G. and Jenkins, D. M. (1976). *The Lancet*, 727–9.

—— and Pethybridge, R. J. (1973). *The Hospital and Health Services Review*, 243–7.

—— and —— (1974). *The Hospital and Health Services Review*, 82–6.

Fryer, J. G. and Ashford, J. R. (1972). *British Journal of Preventive and Social Medicine* **26**, 1–9.

Ministry of Health (1956). *Report of the Committee of Enquiry into the Cost of the National Health Service (Guillebaud Committee)*. Cmd. 9663. H.M.S.O., London.

—— (1959). *Report of the Maternity Services Committee (Cranbrook Report)*. H.M.S.O., London.

Implications of the current debate on obstetric practice

Evaluation of innovative obstetric techniques, some of which may themselves introduce new hazards in childbirth, and all of which are more likely to be used in hospital than at home, is inconsistent and disorganized. The new technology of obstetrics has led to discussion involving not only obstetricians and paediatricians, but also the public, and has become a matter of general concern. This chapter looks at the unfolding of this dialogue and makes a case for experimental studies before different obstetric practices can be effectively evaluated.

Development and innovation in the management of childbirth over the last 10 years has taken place at an unparalleled rate. Care during pregnancy has been extended and elaborated to include assessment of foetal well-being by placental function tests and serial ultrasound cephalometry. Early recognition of chromosomal, biochemical, and neural tube abnormalities in the foetus has become possible. Efficient pharmacological control of labour with oxytocin and prostaglandins has increased the scope for induction and augmentation of labour, and this in turn has prompted the development of techniques to assess the gestational age and functional maturity of the foetus more accurately than previously. Because labour itself poses a particular threat to the safety of both mother and baby, policies of universal hospital confinement have been promoted, and, in many maternity units, the use of partography, cardiotocography, foetal scalp blood sampling, and lumbar epidural block has become routine. In spite of the scientific connotations of these developments, there have been few systematic attempts to evaluate their effects. The relative contributions of these various changes to reduced perinatal and maternal mortality rates, if any, is unknown.

The variety of obstetric practice in Britain allows one to assume that there are some obstetricians and midwives who have had misgivings about some of these developments. However, these doubts have only recently been expressed in the literature. In the past, academic challenge has come from disciplines often regarded as peripheral to obstetrics, such as sociology and psychology (Kitzinger 1971; Stacey 1972; Walker 1972; Bardon 1973). However, it was 'consumer' organizations, notably the Patients' Association and the Association for Improvements in the Maternity Services, which were to play the key role in promoting an active debate which continues today. The debate gathered momentum following a report by the Oxford Consumer

Group in early 1974: a public opinion survey of the health services found more adverse comments about the maternity services than any other branch of the National Health Service (Robinson 1974). It is particularly interesting that the report related to a city with a new maternity hospital, relatively favourable staffing levels, and one of the lowest perinatal mortality rates in the United Kingdom. The public debate stimulated by this report focused particularly on the widened use of induction of labour.

By mid-1974 public discussion was developing at an extremely rapid rate. Over the months that followed, most of the major national daily and Sunday newspapers carried articles and correspondence discussing current obstetric practice. The broadcasting media and local newspapers were also quick to reflect the obvious public interest in the increased use of induction. Eventually Parliament joined the debate, first through written questions and answers, and later through questions put by Members on the floor of the House. Reacting to obvious public concern and aware of the dearth of relevant facts, the Department of Health and Social Security commissioned a national survey of experiences during childbirth from the Institute for Social Studies in Medical Care.

Although the media continued to concentrate on induced labour, it became clear that the underlying debate was concerned with more fundamental aspects of the maternity services. As in a similar, if less intense, controversy 15 years earlier (Morris 1960, Ministry of Health 1961), the quality of human relations and the effectiveness of communications in obstetric practice emerged as key issues. The perceived shortcomings of the hospital maternity services in these respects prompted some to adopt a confrontational approach. One group, for example, stated, 'Women should be informed about all aspects of childbirth and they should have the positive right to choose what happens to them whenever this is possible' (Swansea Women and Health Group 1974). Others were concerned to create the opportunities to identify common ground and foster mutual understanding between the various participants in the debate (*The Guardian*, 1974). Others, concerned that the vigorous implementation of a policy of universal hospital confinement contributed to unsatisfactory relationships between women and their attendants in childbirth, formed pressure groups to ensure that the option of domiciliary confinement was kept open.† The National Childbirth Trust convened a multidisciplinary study group to examine the implications of restricting provision for domiciliary delivery and to reconsider the evidence on which the policy of universal hospital confinement was based.

Obstetrician/gynaecologists are particularly vulnerable to lay criticism compared with their colleagues in other branches of medicine. Lay comment on the management of pregnancy, whether for antenatal care, delivery, or possible therapeutic abortion, reflects the fact that pregnancy is an event of considerable emotional and cultural significance which has usually been

† For example the founding of the Society to Support Home Confinements in Durham.

seen as a normal, physiological process. Pregnant women are therefore less willing to adopt the role of a sick patient in which doctors, throughout their training, have been tacitly encouraged to see their clients. Literature critical of the tendency of modern obstetrics to force pregnancy and childbirth into a medical model (bearing titles such as *The cultural warping of childbirth*, *Immaculate deception*, and *The trap of medicalised motherhood*), echo Illich's thesis that the very philosophy of modern medicine is 'anti-health' (Illich 1974).

The response of medical professionals to this public challenge varied. About 6 months after the emergence of public discussion, overt debate within the profession itself was ushered in by an editorial in *The Lancet* (1974) entitled, 'A time to be born'. The editorial pointed out that 'maternal *cris de coeur* were no longer completely muffled by the paternalism of traditional ante-natal care' and that 'anyone was free to join the argument concerning induction on grounds of social or medical convenience'. It ended by stating that 'until unequivocal evidence is available, the public is right in continuing to question medical practices of doubtful validity that are based on convenience'. The subsequent participation by some obstetricians in public discussions and multidisciplinary groups reflected the spirit of *The Lancet* editorial, and in a few instances obstetricians were responsible for organizing such meetings.†

In contrast, a television programme on induction prompted a rather more cautionary leading article in the *British Medical Journal* (1975). The article referred to 'vociferous press compaigns arguing that women are being dealt with unfairly by a conservative profession' and continued '... with such a background there is clearly a risk that the programme could persuade some viewers that the medical advice they had been given had been out-of-date, or part of an experiment, or in some other way wrong; and a television producer who achieves that result is surely taking on himself the role that Stanley Baldwin attributed to the harlot—power without responsibility.' This charge of 'self-appointed and self-taught experts' exercising power without responsibility was repudiated in subsequent correspondence from three television producers, including one who had been congratulated by the leading article for having done a 'first class job of health education' (Massey and Bates 1975; Reid 1975).

Medical lack of confidence in lay judgement was demonstrated further in an interesting exchange of correspondence in *The Lancet* (Robinson 1975). The chairman of the Patients' Association contributed a well-documented critique of a research report on elective induction of labour. This prompted an obstetrician to remark that the letter had been written with 'a degree

---

† For example, a public meeting was called by the obstetricians at Upton Hospital, Slough, on 11 December 1974; a meeting of the Open Section of the Royal Society of Medicine on 10 April 1975; and the co-sponsorship of the Seminar on Human Relations in Obstetric Practice by Professor Melville Kerr and Professor Margaret Stacey at Warwick University in October 1975

of scholarship which made it plain that it was prepared by a doctor with an extensive knowledge of the literature'. This accusation was denied by the author of the critique, who pointed out that one did not need to be a doctor to acquire an extensive knowledge of the literature but simply 'a good library and a curiosity acquired by reading over 800 letters from women about induced births'.

It is difficult to assess the prevalence within the profession of these contrasting attitudes to lay comment. The composition of the Royal College of Obstetricians and Gynaecologists' study group on the management of labour may give some indication of feeling in mid-1975. The group was comprised of 31 doctors, 2 physiologists, 2 midwives, a woman journalist, and the President of the National Childbirth Trust (Beard, Brudenell, Dunn, and Fairweather 1976). A further indication might be the response rate to a survey of attitudes to induced labour conducted by the Institute for Social Studies in Medical Care funded by the Department of Health and Social Security. The final response rates in 1976 among representative samples of recently delivered women, hospital midwives, and consultant obstetricians were 91 per cent, 81 per cent, and 58 per cent respectively (Cartwright 1976, personal communication). However, the lower response rate among obstetricians is possibly partly or wholly explained by the fact that they were approached by postal questionnaire whereas the other two groups were interviewed directly.

But in attempting to assess the profession's response to public criticism it would be easy to forget the fact that obstetricians in general, and British obstetricians in particular, have made greater efforts to monitor the quality of their work than most other specialities within medical practice. The work of Dugald Baird and his colleagues in Aberdeen was pioneering in this respect. The national perinatal mortality surveys of 1946, 1958, and 1970, together with the triennial reports on Confidential Enquiries into Maternal Deaths (H.M.S.O.), are evidence of willingness on the part of clinicians to monitor the outcome of pregnancy.

Indeed the reaction of obstetricians to the situation created by the public debate compares well with, for example, the silence with which cardiologists have greeted the challenging results of a trial comparing home with hospital management of acute myocardial infarction (Mather, Morgan, Pearson, et al. 1976). By contrast, the Royal College of Obstetricians and Gynaecologists published a report early in 1976 (Beard, Brudenell, Dunn, and Fairweather 1976) which not only illustrated just how divided medical opinion was on some aspects of perinatal management but also included some contribution from representatives of women using the maternity services. The fact that research in the field of pregnancy and childbirth has become the fastest-growing sub-speciality within British medical sociology must also imply at least some measure of growth in collaboration between obstetricians and sociologists.

In contrast to a view of pregnancy and labour which stresses the cultural, social, and emotional importance of these processes which are often considered to be purely physiological, it is their potential for rapid and catastrophic departure from normality which remains the overriding concern of obstetricians. Rare though such occurrences may be, they are harrowing experiences for all those involved. In the face of uncertainties concerning the prediction of such events, it is perhaps understandable that modern obstetrics has become characterized by multiphasic screening procedures designed to facilitate intervention to preempt the development of serious complications in either mother or child. It has been suggested elsewhere that 'it is hardly surprising that obstetricians should have seized with delight upon the ability to determine the point of onset of labour themselves by the use of intravenous medication' faced with the 'disturbing uncertainties' in accurately predicting the onset of spontaneous labour (Maclean 1975). What does seem to have happened is that there has been a tendency to redefine the limits within which a pregnancy should be deemed physiological. Although this rather arbitrary recategorizing process is often not explicit, it appears that an increasing proportion of pregnant women are seen as 'abnormal' or 'at increased risk'. The divided opinion within the profession concerning the management of pregnancy and childbirth is a reflection of differing definitions of normality.

The division within the medical profession concerning the management of pregnancy is also an expression of the general lack of satisfactory information concerning the effects of the various interventions which characterize modern obstetrics. With the active incorporation of biochemistry and electronics into their speciality, obstetricians have achieved a scientific respectability which their colleagues in other branches of medicine sometimes denied them in the past. But much of the claim that modern obstetrics, and current medical practice as a whole, is scientific rests on incidental features of similarity between scientific research and present-day medical practice. Clinicians may be involved in scientific ('pure') research but the separation between this work and clinical intervention is not bridged by the evaluative research which could provide a rational basis for practice (Richards 1975).

Obstetricians (and their paediatric colleagues) have generally worked against a background of falling maternal and perinatal mortality rates. Sometimes they have been too ready to attribute these improvements to their own activities and to use them to justify more intervention without seeking evidence to support causal associations. In the heat of the debate on the maternity services in Britain, some professionals turned to vital statistics to defend their position. An editorial in The Lancet (1975) reviewed the most recent report on confidential enquiries into maternal deaths (Department of Health and Social Security 1975) and suggested that it was a reminder 'that those who advocate any move away from organised obstetric teams should be careful not to lead less well-informed women into danger'. The writer went on to attribute a striking fall in the number of maternal deaths to 'advances in scientific obstetrics, the findings of previous enquiries, improved health in the population, limitations in family size, and the habit of having babies in hospital'. Subsequent correspondence (Newcombe, Campbell, and Chalmers 1975) pointed out that at least one third of the decline in the maternal mortality rate over the 9 years between 1964 and 1972 could be accounted for by changes in the age and parity of the parturient population and that effects of similar magnitude might be attributed to changes in socio-economic status and the gestational age at which abortions occur. Only after such standardization had been undertaken would it be possible to assess the relative importance of social and medical changes in contributing to the fall. More recently, an editorial in the *British Medical Journal* (1976) claimed that technological innovation in obstetrics had been proved to be effective and that 'every drop of even 0·1% in perinatal mortality should mean a drop in the numbers of babies surviving with physical or mental defects'. These claims prompted correspondence (Campbell, Lowe, and Cochrane 1976; Costello 1976; Kirke 1976) suggesting that such unsubstantiated statements did great discredit to a profession which thought of itself as scientific.

Other studies have indicated that caution is necessary in using observational data as evidence of the effectiveness of interventions. An analysis of trends in the management and outcome of pregnancy in nearly 40 000 deliveries to women resident in Cardiff between 1965 and 1973 revealed no striking change in either the total perinatal death rate or the timing and cause of perinatal deaths (Chalmers, Zlosnik, Johns, and Campbell 1976). A comparison of the work and results of two obstetric teams in the same city over a five-year period failed to demonstrate any advantage of a policy characterized by a wider use of induction of labour and ante-partum monitoring with urinary oestrogen assay and serial ultrasound cephalometry (Chalmers, Lawson, and Turnbull 1976).

The establishment of causal relationships using such observational data is fraught with difficulty. These difficulties have been well reviewed by Susser (1973) who lists five separate criteria for judging observed relationships to be causal. The *time sequence* in the relationship must be correct; there must be *consistency* of association on replication; the *strength* and *specificity* of the association should be consistent with a causal hypothesis; and there should be a *coherent explanation* of the presumed causal nature of the association in the light of current knowledge. The difficulties in handling observational data should not (and do not) daunt those who must in the end make judgements of causality to guide clinical action. However, there is a need for a more general acknowledgement of the limitations of such data in permitting these inferences.

In contrast, experimentally derived data are far more robust in attempts to establish causal relationships. Because of the considerable biological variability in the circumstances of medical practice, the preferred means of conducting valid experiments is to assign different treatments (one of which should be standard, current practice) at random, to comparable groups of patients. The introduction of this technique led to a leap forward in medical research which has been compared to the progress made following the invention of the microscope (Susser 1973). In spite of this, the vast majority of medical interventions remain unevaluated by randomized controlled trials (Cochrane 1972).

In part this is due to the undoubted difficulties in setting up and conducting such trials, and there is certainly an urgent need for other forms of experiment to be designed and introduced into clinical medicine. Furthermore, such randomized controlled trials can usually only answer one specific question at a time, whereas the pace of medical innovation is such that it seems necessary to answer many questions simultaneously. Nevertheless, much of the failure to employ this technique seems to have arisen from a basically unscientific approach to clinical research, combined with an unwillingness among individualistic, ambitious research workers to engage in the kind of large-scale, collaborative studies which are needed to test many relevant hypotheses.

Another hurdle to be negotiated by those proposing experimental studies in clinical practice is the question of ethics. The boundary between ethical and unethical clinical research has the potential for considerable mobility— but how has it affected decisions to conduct the kind of experimental research outlined above? First, ethical judgements may be influenced by the danger of malpractice suits, either for not preserving conservative ('established') practice or, alternatively, for not being in the forefront of innovation. Secondly, because high status within the medical profession is accorded to innovators, suggestions that a new treatment should be evaluated by randomized controlled trial is countered with suggestions that it would be unethical to deny a group of patients the 'benefit' claimed for the technique. In these circumstances, the ethical starting-point of the innovator is that doctors do more good than harm. The unwillingness to conceptualize iatrogenic morbidity is well illustrated by the reaction of hospital physicians to the presentation of preliminary results of a clinical trial comparing home and hospital management of acute myocardial infarction (Mather *et al.* 1976). When results were presented suggesting an improved outcome for hospital cases, but failing to reach statistical significance, a hospital physician suggested that to proceed with the trial would be unethical. When it was revealed that the slide illustrating the data had been incorrectly labelled and that the home treatment group was in fact doing slightly better than the hospital treatment group, there was no amended suggestion that it would be unethical to continue admitting cases to the hospital! (Cochrane 1972). In the final analysis, ethical considerations suggest that randomized trials are more suitable than uncontrolled innovation and experimentation in protecting the interests of patients (Byar, Simon, Friedewald *et al.* 1976, Shaw and Chalmers 1970).

Perinatal medicine, like medicine as a whole, suffers from a dearth of experimentally derived knowledge upon which rational practice can be based. The current public and professional debate on modern obstetrics in Britain has highlighted the reality of this situation. It is true that some randomized controlled trials have been performed in obstetrics and neonatal paediatrics (see special references at the end of this chapter) and there is some evidence that such experimental research is now being conducted more frequently. However, it still constitutes a pitifully small proportion of the total research effort in perinatal medicine.

Part of the difficulty lies in the selection of suitable measures of outcome. Even if one leaves aside the important question of how to measure satisfaction among women using the perinatal health services, problems in choosing physical outcome variables remain. Both perinatal and maternal deaths are now comparatively rare events, and the validity and long-term significance of current measures of neonatal morbidity is the subject of considerable difference of opinion. But these difficulties are not insuperable. Mortality rates can still be useful outcome measures in the context of multicentre trials, and adequate follow-up studies of infants and children will indicate which neonatal variables are the most appropriate indicators of significant morbidity.

Some questions are probably not amenable to resolution by experimental research. For example, it is highly unlikely that it will ever be possible to conduct a satisfactory randomized controlled trial to compare home with hospital confinement. Even if such a trial was mounted, the extrapolation of the findings to communities with different population densities and transport facilities would prove a hazardous exercise. Judgements concerning the relative safety of home and hospital confinement must continue to rely on the observational approach adopted by Ashford (see Chapter 2 of this book) and Tew (see Chapter 4 of this book), although it is possible that the implications of their findings will be modified by developments in intensive intra-partum foetal monitoring in low-risk pregnancies (Parsons, 1977, unpublished). But even if the issue to which this book addresses itself cannot be resolved by experimental research, many other unanswered questions can. It is certain that doctors and nurses working with pregnant women and neonates must sometimes question the value of certain widely accepted and routinely performed procedures.

For example, what are the advantages of the various elements of antenatal care? Under what circumstances are the interventions which characterize modern management of labour, for example, perineal shaving and episiotomy, beneficial? In what circumstances do the risks of Caesarean section outweigh the benefits? What kind of support does a mother need to establish lactation successfully? Which infants derive net benefit from admission to a special-care unit? Only when these and other similar questions are answered will we begin to have health services which are based on a rational use of our limited resources.

If one lesson that emerges from the British debate on obstetric practice is that there is a need to establish the effects of interventions in perinatal medicine, then the other is that a maternity service which loses touch with the feelings and expectations of its clients will not meet their needs. The two main concerns of all those involved in the provision of perinatal care should be to use effective therapy appropriately and ensure that such therapy, together with the 'caring' element of the service, is acceptable to both health service users and personnel.

In the final analysis, the doctors, midwives, and nurses working in the clinical setting hold the key to progress. It is they who have contact with clients and can seek their views. Only they are in a position to conduct the experimental studies which are so urgently required. They are more likely than outsiders to develop the lines of thought upon which further advance depends. It is also they who need the courage and humility to challenge elements of their current practice which are of doubtful value.

References

General references
Bardon, D. (1973). 'Psychological implications of provision for childbirth'. *Lancet* ii, 555.

Beard, R., Brudenell, M., Dunn, P., and Fairweather, D. (1976). *The management of labour*. Royal College of Obstetricians and Gynaecologists, London.

British Medical Journal (1975). Editorial: 'Medicine on television' i, 539.

—— (1976). Editorial: 'A policy of despair' i, 787.

Byar, D. P., Simon, R. M., Friedewald, W. T. *et al.* (1976). 'Randomized clinical trials'. *New England Journal of Medicine* **295**, 74.

Campbell, H., Lowe, C. R., and Cochrane, A. L. (1976). 'Priorities for health and social services'. *British Medical Journal* i, 1013.

Chalmers, I., Lawson, J. G., and Turnbull, A. C. (1976). 'An evaluation of different approaches to obstetric care'. *British Journal of Obstetrics and Gynaecology* **83**, 921.

——, Zlosnik, J. E., Johns, K. A., and Campbell, H. (1976). 'Obstetric practice and outcome of pregnancy in Cardiff residents, 1965–1973'. *British Medical Journal* i, 735.

Cochrane, A. L. (1972). *Effectiveness and efficiency*. Oxford University Press for the Nuffield Provincial Hospitals Trust.

Costello, A. (1976). 'Priorities for health and social services'. *British Medical Journal* i, 1013.

Department of Health and Social Security (1975). *Report on confidential enquiries into maternal deaths in England and Wales 1970–1972*. Report on Health and Social Subjects, No. 11. H.M.S.O. London.

The Guardian (1974). Statement of the President of the National Childbirth Trust 9 December.

Illich, I. (1974). *Medical Nemesis*. Calder & Boyars, London.

Kirke, P. (1976). 'Priorities for health and social services'. *British Medical Journal* i, 1014.

Kitzinger, S. (1971). 'Crystal womb'. *New Society* 25 November.

The Lancet (1974). Editorial: 'A time to be born' ii, 1183.

—— (1975). Editorial: 'The cold facts of childbirth' ii, 963.

Maclean, U. (1975). 'Patient delay: some observations on medical claims to certainty'. *Lancet* ii, 23.

Massey, G. and Bates, R. (1975). 'Medicine on television'. *British Medical Journal* i, 732.

Mather, H. G., Morgan, D. C., Pearson, N. G., *et al.* (1976). 'Myocardial infarction: a comparison between home and hospital care for patients'. *British Medical Journal* i, 925.

Ministry of Health (1961). *Human relations in obstetrics*. H.M.S.O., London.

Morris, N. (1960). 'Human relations in obstetric practice'. *Lancet* i, 913.

Newcombe, R. G., Campbell, H., and Chalmers, I. (1975). 'Maternal deaths'. *Lancet* ii, 1099.

Reid, R. (1975). 'Medicine on television'. *British Medical Journal* i, 732.

Richards, M. P. M. (1975). 'Innovation in medical practice: obstetricians and the induction of labour in Britain'. *Social Science and Medicine* 9, 595.

Robinson, J. (1974). 'Consumer attitudes to maternity care'. *Oxford Consumer* May 1974.

—— (1975). 'Elective induction of labour'. *Lancet* i, 1088 and 1242.

Shaw, L. W. and Chalmers, T. C. (1970). 'Ethics in co-operative clinical trials'. *Annals of the New York Academy of Science* 169, 487.

Stacey, M. (1972). 'Beliefs and practices about illness and treatment as they affect the hospital care of children and women'. Read before the Third International Conference, Social Science and Medicine, Elsinore, Denmark, August 1972.

Susser, M. W. (1973). *Causal thinking in the health sciences*. Oxford University Press.

Swansea Women and Health Group (1974). 'Having a baby'.

Walker, J. (1972). 'The modern midwife: ideology and interaction in hospital'. Read before the Third International Conference, Social Science and Medicine, Elsinore, Denmark, August 1972.

Examples of experimental research in perinatal medicine

Blackwell, R. Q., Chow, B. F., Chinn, K. S. K., Blackwell, B-N., and Hsu, S. C. (1973). 'Prospective maternal nutrition study in Taiwan: rationale, study design, feasibility, and preliminary findings'. *Nutrition Reports International* 7, 517–32.

Bland, R. D., Clarke, T. L., and Harden, L. B. (1976). 'Rapid infusion of sodium bicarbonate and albumin into high-risk premature infants soon after birth: a controlled, prospective trial'. *American Journal of Obstetrics and Gynaecology* 124, 263–7.

Caldeyro-Barcia, R., Schwarcz, R., Belizan, J. M., Martell, M., Nieto, F., Sabatino, H., and Tenzer, S. M. (1974). 'Adverse Perinatal Effects of Early Amniotomy during Labour'. In *Modern perinatal medicine* (ed. L. Gluck), p. 431. Chicago University Press.

Cole, R. A., Howie, P. W., and Macnaughton, M. C. (1975). 'Elective induction of labour: a randomised prospective trial'. *Lancet* i, 767–70.

Coxon, A., Fairweather, D. V. I., Smyth, C. N., Frankenberg, J., and Vessey, M. (1973). 'A randomized double blind clinical trial of abdominal decompression for the prevention of pre-eclampsia'. *Journal of Obstetrics and Gynaecology of the British Commonwealth* 80, 1081–5.

Durbin, G. M. Hunter, N. J., McIntosh, N., Reynolds, E. O. R., and Wimberley,

P. D. (1976). 'Controlled trial of continuous inflating pressure for hyaline membrane disease'. *Archives of Disease in Childhood* **51**, 163.

Ferguson, J. H. (1953). 'The effect of stiboestrol on pregnancy compared to the effect of a placebo. *American Journal of Obstetrics and Gynaecology* **65**, 592–601.

Fletcher, J., Curr, A., Fellingham, F. R., Prankerd, T. A. J., Brant, H. A., and Menzies, D. N. (1976). 'The value of folic acid supplements in pregnancy'. *Journal of Obstetrics and Gynaecology of the British Commonwealth* **78**, 781–5.

Johnston, R. A. and Sidall, R. S. (1922). 'Is the usual method of preparing patients for delivery beneficial or necessary?' *American Journal of Obstetrics and Gynaecology* **4**, 645–50.

Leather, H. M., Humphreys, D. M., Baker, P., and Chadd, M. A. (1968). 'A Controlled trial of hypotensive agents in hypertension in pregnancy'. *Lancet* ii, 488–90.

Liggins, G. C. and Howie, R. N. (1974). 'The prevention of RDS by maternal steroid therapy'. In *Modern perinatal medicine* (ed. L. Gluck), p. 415. Chicago University Press.

Parsons, R. J. (1977). 'Continuous fetal monitoring: what is its value?' Paper read before 21st British Congress of Obstetrics and Gynaecology, Sheffield.

Patterson, W. M. (1971). 'Amniotomy, with or without simultaneous oxytocin infusion'. *Journal of Obstetrics and Gynaecology of the British Commonwealth* **78**, 310–16.

Redman, C. W. G., Beilin, L. J., Bonnar, J., and Ounsted, M. K. (1976). 'Fetal outcome in trial of antihypertensive treatment in pregnancy'. *Lancet* ii, 753–6.

Renou, P., Chang, A., Anderson, I., and Wood, C. (1976). Controlled trial of fetal intensive care. American Journal of Obstetrics and Gynaecology, **126**, 470–6.

Shepherd, J., Sims, C., and Craft, I. (1976). 'Extra-amniotic prastaglandin E_2 and the unfavourable cervix'. *Lancet* ii, 709–10.

Sood, S. K., Ramachandran, K., Mathur, M., Gupta, K., Ramalingaswamy, V., Swarnbai, C., Ponniah, J., Mathan, V. I., and Baker, S. J. (1975). 'The effects of supplemental oral iron administration to pregnant women'. *Quarterly Journal of Medicine*, New Series **44**, 241–58.

Spellacy, W. N., Buhi, W. C., and Birk, S. A. (1975). 'The effectiveness of human placental lactogen measurements as an adjunct in decreasing perinatal deaths. Results of a retrospective and a randomised controlled prospective study'. *American Journal of Obstetrics and Gynaecology* **121**, 835–44.

Tabb, P. A., Inglis, J., Savage, D. C. L., and Walker, C. H. M. (1972). 'Controlled trial of phototherapy of limited duration in the treatment of physiological hyperbilirubinaemia in low-birthweight infants'. *Lancet* ii, 1211–12.

Thalme, B., Belfrage, P., and Raabe, N. (1974). 'Lumbar epidural anaesthesia in Labour: 1, acid–base balance and clinical condition of mother fetus and newborn child'. *Acta Obstetrica et Gynecologia Scandanavica* **53**, 27–35.

Wu, P. Y. K., Teilmann, P., Gabler, M., Vaughan, M., and Metcoff, J. (1967). '"Early" versus "Late" feeding of low birth weight neonates: effect on serum bilirubin, blood sugar, and responses to glucagon and epinephrine tolerance tests'. *Pediatrics* **39**, 733–9.

4

The case against hospital deliveries: the statistical evidence

The 1970 Peel Report recommended that the goal should be 100 per cent hospital confinements, but did not publish any figures on which it based these conclusions. Since that date official policy has been based on these recommendations. In this chapter Marjorie Tew analyses the Registrar General's statistics on perinatal mortality to find the statistical basis for the Peel Committee recommendation. She was surprised to find no evidence for the desirability of a 100 per cent hospital confinements. In this chapter she explains what she discovered.

Introduction

In the nineteenth century, hospitals offered a much less safe environment for childbirth than did the home, where most deliveries took place. During the twentieth century conditions in both places improved greatly. The proportion of institutional confinements increased until by 1950 about half of all births were taking place in National Health Service (NHS) hospitals, and this proportion rose steadily to 94 per cent in 1975.

Many mothers who have their babies in hospital would prefer to have them at home, if they were not pressed to do otherwise by medical advice and the lack of domiciliary midwifery services (see Kitzinger, Chapter 10 of this book). Moreover, the immediate cost to the taxpayer of hospital confinements is much greater than that of home confinements (see Ashford, Chapter 2 of this book; Goldthorp and Richman 1974). There are, therefore, powerful arguments, personal and financial, against hospital confinements. To justify the great change that has come about during this century, there must be an even more powerful argument in their favour. The argument which became the basis for official policy and through much repetition widely accepted as true was stated in unequivocal terms in 1970, in the Report of the Peel Committee (Standing Maternity and Midwifery Advisory Committee 1970):

Para. 248. We consider that the greater safety of hospital confinement for mother and child justifies the objective of providing sufficient hospital facilities for every woman who desires or needs to have a hospital confinement. Even without specific policy direction the institutional confinement rate has risen from 64·6 per cent in 1957 to 80·7 per cent in 1968, and shows every sign of continuing to rise, so that discussion of the advantages and disadvantages of home or hospital confinement is in one sense academic.

and

Para. 277. We consider that the resources of modern medicine should be available to all mothers and babies, and we think that sufficient facilities should be provided to allow for 100% hospital delivery. The greater safety of hospital confinement for mother and child justifies this objective.

The Committee did not actually substantiate its assertions with statistical evidence, but it drew attention in para. 29 to the rising trend in institutional confinements on the one hand and the falling trends of perinatal and maternal mortality on the other.

Examination of statistics

It is well known, however, that correlations between time series, in which there is a trend in each of the related variables, are likely to be spurious (Granger and Newbold 1974): the secular decline in the mortality rates could as readily be shown to correlate with the secular increase in motorway mileage or television licences. If one variable is dependent on another, any change in the independent variable will be associated with an appropriate change, in direction and quantity, in the dependent variable. If no significant correlation can be established between the change from one year to the next in each of the variables, a dependent relationship is very unlikely to exist between them.

In particular, to support the hypothesis put forward by the Peel Committee—that an increase in the rate of births in hospital will bring about a reduction in the perinatal or maternal mortality rate—there must be a significant negative correlation between the annual change in the proportion of births taking place in hospital on the one hand and the annual change in these mortality rates on the other. The rates under consideration are set out in Table 4.1, together with the annual changes in the value of each (first differences). It is clear that the annual changes in the hospitalization rate bear little relation to the annual changes in either of the mortality rates and statistically the correlation coefficients, in both cases -0.26, are not significant ($P < 0.05$). When the same statistical procedure is applied in turn to the data over the same period for the two pairs of variables in each of the 15 hospital Regions, in no case is a significant negative correlation established and, indeed, in more than half of the 30 cases the correlation is positive.

Correlations are the more reliable the greater the number of observations included. If, to secure larger numbers from limited data, all the annual pairs of observations in all the Regions are aggregated into one single correlation between hospitalization rates and perinatal and maternal mortality rates respectively, both the resulting coefficients are found to be small but positive.

Although such an analysis of their trends cannot by itself prove beyond doubt that a dependent relationship between the variables does not exist, it affords no support for the alternative hypothesis, that a dependent

Table 4.1 Percentage of births in hospital and rates of perinatal and maternal mortality, showing annual changes, England and Wales

| | Births in hospital | | Mortality per 1000 births | | | |
| | | | Perinatal | | Maternal | |
	Per-centage	Annual change	Rate	Annual change	Rate	Annual change
1962	63·3		30·8		0·350	
		+2·6		−1·8		−0·070
1963	65·9		29·3		0·280	
		+3·0		−1·1		−0·025
1964	68·9		28·2		0·255	
		+1·4		−1·3		−0·003
1965	70·3		26·9		0·252	
		+3·4		−0·6		+0·006
1966	73·7		26·3		0·258	
		+2·0		−0·9		−0·054
1967	75·7		25·4		0·204	
		+2·3		−0·7		+0·037
1968	78·0		24·7		0·241	
		+5·2		−1·3		−0·049
1969	83·2		23·4		0·192	
		+2·0		0·0		−0·008
1970	85·2		23·4		0·184	
		+3·5		−1·1		−0·019
1971	88·7		22·3		0·165	

Sources of Tables 4.1 and 4.2: Department of Health and Social Security and Office of Population Censuses and Surveys, Report on Hospital In-patient Enquiry, 1971, Table M2; Registrar General's Statistical Reviews 1962–71, Table 13 and Appendix F1.

relationship between the variables does exist and that the degree of dependence is strong.

Another approach is to analyse the data in cross-section: i.e., in each year the percentage of hospital births and the two mortality rates in each of the 15 hospital Regions can be correlated. The results are shown in Table 4.2 and confirm the previous findings—not only that there is an absence of significant negative correlation, but also that high mortality rates are most often associated with high rates of births in hospital.

Perinatal mortality is made up of still births plus deaths in the first week of life. Of the causes of early neonatal death one might expect those in-

Table 4.2 Correlation coefficients (*r*) between percentage of births in hospital and mortality rates in 15 Hospital Regions†

	Percentage of births in hospital correlated with	
	perinatal mortality rate	maternal mortality rate
1963	+0·28	+0·18
1964	+0·19	+0·13
1965	+0·34	−0·01
1966	+0·23	+0·07
1967	+0·11	+0·14
1968	+0·39	+0·06
1969	+0·33	−0·25
1970	+0·19	−0·01
1971	+0·23	+0·26

† Wessex excluded from 1966.

cluded in the group, birth injury, difficult labour, and other anoxic and hypoxic conditions, to be especially sensitive to conditions at delivery.† If hospital births are indeed safer, one might expect increases in the rate of hospital births to be associated to a significant degree with decreases in the death-rate from these causes. But when all the same statistical procedures as before are applied in turn to these death-rates and to the still-birth rates, again in not one single instance is a significant negative correlation established between hospitalization rates and mortality rates; indeed, the correlation coefficients, though not significant, are more often than not positive.

Is there other evidence to support the contention that hospital deliveries are safer? The British perinatal mortality survey (Butler and Bonham 1963) gathered a great deal of information about every singleton birth (= mothers delivered) in Great Britain in 1 week in March 1958 and about every neonatal death in the ensuing 3 months. Of the births, 41 per cent were booked for delivery in consultant hospitals, and 40 per cent for delivery at home, though 16 per cent of the home bookings were transferred late in pregnancy or in labour to hospital.‡ Mortality in each group, as throughout the survey, was measured in terms of survey mortality ratios—a series of index values expressing mortality rates in each sub-class as a percentage of the overall mortality rate (= 100).

† *International Classification of Diseases*, 8th revision, B43; before 1968, 7th revision, B42, birth injury, post-natal asphyxia, and atelectasis.
‡ For reasons of space and simplicity, the general practitioner hospitals have been omitted from this analysis.

The mortality ratio for cases booked for and delivered in hospital (103) was slightly above the overall average, for cases booked for and delivered at home (49) was much below it, but for the late transfers to hospital (336) very much above it. However, even if it is accepted that death following transfer should properly be attributed to the place of booking (and the

Table 4.3 Perinatal survey mortality ratios (1958) by risk factor and place of booking/delivery

	Parity†				Standardized ratios
	0	1,2	3+	All	
Hospital	98	90	164	103	106
Home (including transfer)	105	72	113	88	91

	Social class				
	1,2	3	4, 5, and illeg.	All	
Hospital	83	99	119	103	102
Home (including transfer)	68	86	102	88	89

	Toxaemia				
	None	Mild	Other	All	
Hospital	84	85	183	103	102
Home (including transfer)	68	85	161	88	94

† Parity denotes the number of previous births, live or still
Source: Butler and Bonham (1963)

propriety of this attribution can be contested), the combined mortality ratio for home (88) remained well below the hospital value (which also excluded unbooked cases). It is contended that the discrepancy between these crude ratios is to be explained by the greater proportion of high-risk cases among hospital births.

The survey quantified many of the risk factors in childbirth, but of those known early enough in pregnancy to influence booking only three, maternal parity, social class, and toxaemia, were so cross-classified. Table 4.3 shows how perinatal risk varies with each of these factors and how, in the sub-classes at high risk as well as at low, the ratios for home bookings are in most cases lower than for hospital. To allow for differences in the pro-portion of births in each sub-class in hospital and at home, standardized ratios can be calculated, assuming that both places had the same proportion in each sub-class as the overall average. These 'risk-standardized' ratios given in the final column show that only a very small part of the difference between the home and hospital crude ratios is explained by the greater proportion in hospital of cases at high risk on account of these specific factors.

If the hospital bookings included a preponderance of cases at high pre-delivery risk, it must have been on account of maternal characteristics for which analysis by place of delivery was not published. Some of these, notably adverse obstetric history and certain diseases of the mother, are strongly associated with perinatal loss and such cases may well have been concentrated in hospital. Without data, there is no means of knowing what effect standardizing for such risk factors might have had.

Current investigation of the original, unpublished, 1958 material (Fedrick 1977, personal communication) reveals that the mothers, who were at the lowest risk in every one of the significant factors measured, made up a con-siderably greater proportion of the home than of the hospital bookings, and for this group at minimal risk it was the hospitals which had the lower mortality rate. In contrast, the published analysis shows that for the out-come measures, length of gestation and birthweight, it was in the groups at highest risk that mortality in hospital greatly exceeded that at home. At gestations under 38 weeks the hospital ratio was 515, compared with 441 at home; for known birthweights under 2·001 kg the hospital ratio was 1976, compared with 1866 at home.

Clearly what we as yet know from the 1958 survey is not enough to decide the issue. But in any case its evidence may no longer be relevant: the expansion of the hospital service and the contraction of the domiciliary maternity service mean that births in hospital have come to include many at low risk, because there is no alternative, while techniques of treatment have changed radically, and much more so in hospital than in the home.

Since 1958 there has been a dearth of studies yielding data which enable mortality rates of hospital and home born infants to be compared, allowance being made for differences in risk in the two populations. In the survey of British births in 1970 (Chamberlain and Chamberlain 1975) there were too few deaths in the sample to permit mortality analyses by place of delivery and risk factors, though the wide disparity between the perinatal mortality rate per 1000 total births for infants born at home (4·3) and in NHS consultant units (27·8) could be explained only by an overwhelming weight of risk factors among the hospital deliveries and, unless the home population was an unrepresentative sample, it must have included some mothers at high risk, for of all births at home in 1970 5·3 per cent were to mothers aged 35 and over, 13·8 per cent to mothers of parity 3+, and 4·1 per cent were illegitimate (Registrar General 1962–73).

Table 4.4 Maternal mortality rates per 100 000 maternities by age and place of booking/delivery 1967–9

	Ages (years)							Standardized rates
	All	<19	20–24	25–29	30–34	35–39	40+	
Hospital	21	7	12	19	29	47	89	21
Home†	14	5	10	14	21	27	52	15

† Includes transfers
Source of Table 4.4 and 4.5: Department of Health and Social Security, Report on Confidential Enquiries into Maternal Deaths, 1967–9

Table 4.5 Maternal mortality rates per 100 000 maternities by parity† and place of booking/delivery 1967–9

	Parity						Standardized rate
	All	0	1	2	3	4+	
Hospital	21	17	16	24	25	54	21
Home‡	14	37	7	10	21	38	15

† For definition see Table 4.3
‡ Includes transfers

Triennial reports on confidential enquiries into maternal deaths have analysed mortality by place of booking and delivery, but only in the 1967–1969 report do the statistics as presented permit the comparison to be made between deliveries at home and in consultant hospitals, attributing death to the place of booking even if delivery took place in hospital. Maternal mortality by place of booking/delivery was cross-classified with age and parity groups. Tables 4.4 and 4.5 show that the crude rate and the rate in nearly all sub-classes, including those where the risk was highest, were lower for home than for hospital bookings. The standardized rates (calculated as above but expressed as a rate) show that only a very small part of the disparity between the crude rates can be explained by differences in the proportional distribution of age or parity groups in the respective populations. Similarly the statistics, published annually by the Registrar General, show that over the 5 years 1969–73 births in hospital, which by then made up 76 per cent of the total, included a slightly greater proportion to mothers of high-risk age and (because of the heavy preponderance of first births there) a much greater proportion to mothers of high-risk parity. But more importantly they show that, for age and parity alike, in both the high-risk group (with above-average rates) and the low-risk group (with below-average rates), the still-birth rate in hospital was much higher than at home (Table 4.6).

Table 4.6 Distribution of births and stillbirth rates at home and in consultant hospitals by maternal age and parity† (legitimate births, England and Wales, 1969–73)

Risk group	Percentage of total births		Still births per 1000 total births	
	Home	Hospital	Home	Hospital
Age (years)				
30 and over (high)	22	24	6·7	19·2
under 30 (low)	78	76	3·8	13·5
all ages	100	100	4·5	14·8
Parity†				
0, 3, and over (high)	23	56	8·4	16·1
1, 2 (low)	77	44	3·3	13·3
all parities	100	100	4·5	14·8

† The Registrar General uses parity to mean the number of previous live-born infants only. Source of Tables 4.6–4.8: Registrar General's Statistical Reviews (1969–73), Part 11, Appendices B2 and B3.

Since the evidence of single risk characteristics does not support their case, the second line of defence of the advocates of hospitalization is that hospital rates are higher because a relatively greater proportion of births there have more than one high-risk characteristic. The data considered earlier permit standardization for only one risk factor at a time. But for still births the Registrar General makes it possible for the analysis to be carried further and deal with two factors at a time. His cross-classification of age and parity groups again confirms that the proportion of births which fell into the high-risk group for both characteristics was greater in hospital. But again, the rates for both high-risk and low-risk groups were much higher in hospital than at home (Table 4.7). From Tables 4.6 and 4.7 it is clear that in both places the proportion of births was much lower and the still-birth rate somewhat higher in the double high-risk group than in either of the single high-risk groups. This is as far as the Registrar General's analysis of English data goes. But the Registrar General for Scotland analyses overall perinatal mortality according to three maternal characteristics, age, parity, and social class. The proportion of births at high risk in all three categories is much less than the proportion at high risk in any two and amounted in the 5 years 1970–4 to 4·5 per cent of all births. For those at triple high risk the death-rate was higher than for those at double high risk, but the margin between them was considerably smaller than the margin between the rates of the double- and single-high-risk groups. For those in more than three high-risk categories one can infer that the proportion of births affected would be extremely small and, though their death-rate would be higher than for the triple-risk group, it would probably not be much higher.

Table 4.7 Distribution of births and still-birth rates at home and in consultant hospitals by combined maternal age and parity (legitimate births, England and Wales, 1969–73)

	Percentage of total births		Still births per 1000 total births	
Risk group	Home	Hospital	Home	Hospital
Age 30+ Parity (high) 0, 3+	8	12	10·2	21·8
Remainder (low)	92	88	4·0	13·9
All ages/parities	100	100	4·5	14·8

Age, parity, and social class are not the only characteristics associated with variations in the still-birth rate; others include the general health status and physique of the mother; diseases such as toxaemia arising out of pregnancy; previous obstetric history; birthweight of the infant. All these characteristics, however, are to a greater or lesser degree interdependent: multiparous mothers tend to be the older ones who have had more time to accumulate an adverse obstetric history or to develop diseases such as hypertension; a relatively great proportion of social class 4 and 5 mothers are in high-parity groups and the general health status and physique of these mothers is relatively poor; toxaemia occurs most often in first, fourth, and subsequent pregnancies; low birthweight babies are born most often to mothers of poor physique and least often to those aged 20–29. Taking account of the risks associated with age or parity takes account of most of the risk associated with one or more additional characteristics; as the multiplicity of high-risk factors suffered increases, the still-birth rate is likely to increase, but by diminishing margins. At the same time the proportion of births affected decreases, so that the net effect on overall averages is small. This general principle is as applicable to early neonatal and maternal mortality as to still births.

Table 4.8 Hypothetical still-birth rates in consultant hospitals and at home (Legitimate births, England and Wales, 1969–73)

	Hospital			Home
	Total births	Still births	Rate	Rate
Actual	2 612 492	38 659	14·8	4·5
20 per cent at multi-high risk	522 498	26 125	50·0	—
Remainder	2 089 994	12 534	6·0	4·5

Unfortunately no data have yet been analysed which would enable us to quantify and compare the weighted average pre-delivery risk of births in hospital and at home, but the following hypothetical calculation indicates how great the excess of births in hospital at multi-high risk would have to be to explain the excess in their overall mortality rate. Let us suppose that between 1969 and 1973 as many as 20 per cent of hospital births had three or more high-risk characteristics and that the average still-birth rate for this multi-high-risk group was 50 per 1000; i.e., not just a little higher than the rate for the double-high-risk group, but more than twice the rate in hospital and nearly five times the rate at home; at the same time let us suppose that of the home births none had more than two high-risk characteristics. Table 4.8 shows that the remaining 80 per cent of hospital births with less than three high-risk characteristics would still have had a still-birth rate one-third higher than the home still-birth rate. It therefore seems unlikely that any combination of high-risk factors in the hospital births could explain the wide disparity between the hospital and home still-birth rates. Moreover, such evidence as exists suggests that what obtains for still births obtains equally for neonatal and maternal deaths.

However, probably 20 per cent of births are to mothers with no high-risk factor identifiable before delivery, yet about 10 per cent of perinatal deaths are to such mothers. To ensure that these unpredictable dangerous births take place in consultant hospitals, obstetricians recommend that all births should take place there, for they claim that the chances of a successful outcome are then improved. However valid the claim may be in individual cases, the available statistical evidence does not support it in general. It does not show that an increased rate of hospitalization promotes the objective of reducing overall mortality.

Conclusion

The Peel Committee considered that '... discussion of the advantages and disadvantages of home and hospital confinement is in one sense academic.' Far from this being so, there is strong reason to question whether the official policy is soundly based of providing for 100 per cent hospital confinement; the published statistics, so far as they go, show that the risks for infant and mother are in many categories lower when the birth takes place at home. There is urgent need for critical and impartial investigation into unpublished as well as published data, to find a valid explanation of the much higher mortality in consultant hospitals and to identify the circumstances where it is lower, so that future policy for maternity care may be directed towards providing a balance between home and hospital confinement that is based on demonstrable fact.

References

Butler, N. R. and Bonham, D. G. (1963). *Perinatal mortality*. Livingstone, Edinburgh.

Chamberlain, R. and Chamberlain, G. (1975). *British births 1970*. Heinemann, London.

Department of Health and Social Security (1967–9). *Reports on confidential enquiries into maternal deaths in England and Wales, 1967–1969*. H.M.S.O., London.

Department of Health and Social Security and Office of Population Censuses and Surveys (1971). *Report on hospital in-patient enquiry 1971*, Table M2. H.M.S.O., London.

Goldthorp, W. O. and Richman, J. (1974). 'Maternal attitudes to unintended home confinement'. *Practitioner* **212**, 845.

Granger, C. W. J. and Newbold, P. (1974). 'Spurious correlations in econometrics'. *Journal of Econometrics* **2**, 111–20.

Registrar General (1962–73). *Registrar General's Statistical Reviews of England and Wales:* Part I, Tables 13, 19, Appendix F1, 1962–71; and Part II, Tables Appendix B2, B3, B5, 1969–73. H.M.S.O., London.

Registrar General of Scotland (1970–4). *Annual Reports 1970–74*, Table H2.2.

Standing Maternity and Midwifery Advisory Committee (1970). *Report on domiciliary midwifery and maternity bed needs* (The Peel Report). H.M.S.O., London.

A place of safety?
An examination of the risks of
hospital delivery

A proportion of mothers need the care that can be provided by a fully
equipped hospital and the skills of those trained and experienced in obstetrics
in which there are deviations from the normal.

Yet not all hospitals are equipped or staffed in this way. The public image of
the hospital is a place of safety. In the following chapter Martin Richards
questions whether in some cases this is really so.

Introduction

Almost all the arguments that have been used to justify the increasing proportion of hospital deliveries are based on the unexamined assumption that
any hospital is always safer than any domiciliary confinement. In this
chapter I want to examine this assumption and hope to show that the evidence is far from convincing. I shall first consider the question of perinatal and maternal mortality and then proceed to issues related to morbidity.

At first sight, the answer to the question that I am raising, about the safety
of hospital delivery might seem to be self-evident—and, indeed, would seem
to be the majority view. Hospitals can provide many facilities that are not
available for a home confinement, as well as skilled doctors and nurses, so
is it not reasonable to suppose that any mother is likely to be better off
where help is close at hand? I am not doubting that risk cases should be
delivered in hospital (say about 60 per cent of mothers in Britain, extra-
polating from Dutch experience (see Chapter 6 of this book) and allowing
for our higher incidence of pre-term and low-birthweight babies). But what
about the 40 per cent of uncomplicated cases: are we justified on the
grounds of safety in suggesting that they all should go to hospital as well?
Ideally the matter could be settled by a randomized controlled trial in which
comparable groups of women would be delivered at home or in a hospital
and data collected to compare the outcomes. Unfortunately, as is so often
the case in obstetrics, nobody has done such a trial, so we must look to
less direct indications. However, it is worth noting that when such trials have
been carried out elsewhere in medicine to establish the effectiveness of
hospital treatment, some rather counter-intuitive results have been obtained.
Most of the same assumptions that have been made about childbirth apply

to the treatment of heart attacks. Hospital coronary care units offer monitoring equipment, expert medical and nursing aid, and other advantages over home care—or so it was believed. But when the situation was assessed in a trial, it was found that heart attack patients who remained at home looked after by their families and general practitioners (GPs) had a slightly better prognosis than those admitted to a specialized hospital unit (Mather *et al.* 1971). If nothing more, this study should make us rather sceptical of theoretical claims about the advantages of hospitals which are not supported by concrete evidence.

Perinatal mortality

Arguments about perinatal mortality† dominate the hospital versus home debate. Evidence from international comparisons between industrialized countries does not provide any *prima facie* case that the proportion of hospital delivery has much bearing on the matter.

Table 5.1 shows that there is quite wide variation in the perinatal mortality figures but attempts to explain this variation by the proportion of hospital

Table 5.1 Perinatal and maternal mortality in various countries

	Perinatal mortality		Maternal mortality per 1 000 000 births
	1969	1973	
United States	27·1		24·5
England and Wales	23·7	21·3	19·4
Scotland	25·6	22·7	14·4
Northern Ireland	29·2	25·9	15·4
Republic of Ireland	27·0		31·8
Sweden	16·3	12·9 (1974)	10·2
Norway	20·7	16·8	14·8
Finland	18·9		14·8
Netherlands	19·6	16·4	19·4
Belgium	25·1		20·5
France	25·4		24·9
Italy	32·4		60·6
West Germany	25·2	23·2	53·1
Switzerland	19·5	15·5	29·3

Source: Maxwell (1974)

† Perinatal mortality is the rate per 1000 births of still births of more than 28 weeks of gestation, together with liveborn infants that die within the first week of life.

confinements, or by a number of other indices of the medical services provided, have been unsuccessful. Sweden has virtually 100 per cent hospital confinements and excellent perinatal figures while the United States with a similar hospital emphasis does very poorly. The Netherlands, which has one of the lowest perinatal mortality rates, has about half of all births at home. Italy is an interesting case because it has the highest perinatal and maternal mortality of the countries listed but it also has the largest numbers of doctors per head of population. Of course, many factors beyond the provision of medical services determine perinatal mortality rates. What international comparisons do show is that the 'extra-medical' factors are dominant. The figures given in the table do correlate with the standard of living in the various countries and, more particularly, with the equality of distribution of income. It is countries with high standards of living and relatively equal distribution that come out best. Though the pattern is somewhat different, much the same argument applies to maternal mortality.

The most important factor in determining the perinatal mortality rate is the proportion of low-birthweight deliveries. In Britain (Table 5.2) about 60 per cent of neonatal mortality arises from the 6 per cent of births of infants weighing less than 2·500 kg.

Table 5.2 Birthweight and perinatal mortality

Birthweight (kg)	Percentage of births	Perinatal mortality rates
1·000 and under	0·3	931·0
1·001–1·500	0·6	613·2
1·501–2·000	1·2	260·9
2·001–2·500	4·7	69·1
2·501–3·000	18·9	18·0
3·001–3·500	39·1	6·7
3·501–4·000	26·8	4·2
4·000 +	8·3	6·5

Source: Chamberlain *et al.* 1975

A further 20 per cent of all deaths are related to congenital malformations (Chamberlain *et al.* 1975). Thus the perinatal mortality rate is largely determined by the *incidence* of low birthweight and congenital malformations. The place of delivery will have no influence on the latter and only a marginal effect on the former, so the relationship between perinatal mortality and place of confinement is indirect. Of course, though the place of delivery will have very little influence on the incidence of low birthweight, it may well affect the survival of these babies. Again we lack direct evidence but it seems reasonable to suppose that very small babies (under 2000 kg) are better off in a hospital with a special-care baby unit. However, many of the 'large prems' (i.e. 2·000–2·500 kg) can be and are successfully nursed at home. The British births survey of 1970 (Chamberlain *et al.* 1975) shows that only 16 per cent of the babies in this weight range born at home were admitted to a special-care baby unit.

Another way of looking at mortality is to seek evidence of improvements with the increasing proportion of hospital deliveries. As hospital confinements have increased, perinatal mortality has fallen (Table 5.3).

Table 5.3 Place of delivery and perinatal mortality

Place of delivery	1946	1958	1970
	(per cent)	(per cent)	(per cent)
Home	42·4	36·1	12·4
NHS consultant hospital:			
„ consultant bed	40·6	48·5	66·3
„ GP bed	—	—	3·1
GP unit	—	12·4	15·4
Private	13·1	2·9	1·2
Perinatal mortality	38	33	23

Source: Chamberlain *et al.* 1975

Clearly overall there is a statistical relationship (see Ashford, Chapter 2 of this book) but we cannot conclude that there is any direct causal link. If one looks at the breakdown of the causes of death in newborns, 70 per cent are accounted for by intrauterine asphyxia, respiratory distress syndrome, and malformations. In spite of the fact that high rates of hospital delivery have been justified because they are said to reduce the mortality from the first two causes, the figures have remained unchanged from 1958 to 1970 despite a reduction in home confinements from 36 per cent to 12 per cent. Evidence from the Cardiff births survey (Chalmers 1975) confirms this pattern and indicates that a virtually 100 per cent hospital delivery rate may produce no reduction in these infant deaths.

What, I think, any discussion of perinatal mortality makes clear, is that, assuming there is an adequate selection of high-risk cases, there is no strong evidence to suggest that hospital confinement rates of more than about 60 per cent are likely to make a significant difference—at least on the basis of standards of care available in Britain today. The selection of risk cases in Britain has not been good (e.g. Butler and Bonham 1963; Arthure, Tomkinson, Organa, Lewis, Adelstein, and Weatherall 1975; Cox, Fox, Zinkin, and Mathews 1976) but, following the example of the Dutch, there is no reason to think it could not be improved given the motivation to do so.

For the remainder of this chapter I want to confine the discussion to the 40 per cent or so of low-risk mothers. My remarks are based on the assumptions of an adequate selection process for risk cases and the provision of 'flying squads' to cover emergencies in domiciliary births. Though neither of these obtain at present† there are neither theoretical nor over-riding practical difficulties that might prevent these assumptions being met.

Delivery at home and in hospital

As other chapters in this book describe, there are major differences from the mother's point of view between a home and hospital confinement.‡ At home a mother is in a familiar place, surrounded by familiar people. Even if those attending her wished to do so, they could not reproduce the insti-tutional atmosphere of a hospital.

The mother's attendants are visitors in her home; she is not staying tem-porarily in the institution *they* run. This means that many of the pro-cedures and routines that a mother is forced to accept by social pressures in hospital are avoided in the home. At home social relationships are not influenced by the demands of large bureaucratic structures dominated by an ethos of technical efficiency; instead they result from the needs and wishes of the individuals concerned. This is a point of overwhelming importance and it is hardly surprising that where women have experience of both, and some genuine choice, a majority opt for home confinement (Riley 1975).

Even where determined efforts are made, it is impossible to reproduce the conditions of a home in a hospital labour ward. The provision of bright furnishings, for example, may make things look more cheerful, but is unlikely to change the social relationships found in hospitals. Hospitals are complex social structures with hierarchical organizations. This has at least two implications from the patients' point of view. First, there are clearly recognized routines for the division of time and space. So on each ward patients are usually required to do the same things at the same time. Patients wake, sleep, and are fed at times determined by the hospital routine. A recent survey showed that three-quarters of all mothers in hos-pital were required to feed their babies at set times. Visitors to hospitals are usually restricted to set times regardless of the individual needs of

† At present flying squad provision does not meet the required standards. The Confidential Enquiries into Maternal Deaths have revealed that at least one death has been associated with the avoidable factor of a consultant who failed to provide a flying squad in his area (Arthure *et al.* 1975).

‡ Here I am not going to consider general practitioner units. Much of what I have to say will apply to these but other factors are also involved and these units deserve a separate dis-cussion.

mothers and/or of visitors. One can find similar patterns in the use of space so that, for example, patients are encouraged to move to day-rooms at certain times of day. It might be thought that this degree of organization was a consequence of the fact that many hospitals still have large wards where some degree of routine is probably essential. However, there appears to be very little difference between such hospitals and those that have single rooms for mothers, suggesting that routines stem from features of the social organization of the whole hospital. The second feature of hospitals is that patients tend to lose their individual identity and are treated as uniform members of larger category groups: 'mothers', 'grand multips', 'elderly primips', and so on. Of course, a mother's individual needs, especially at an emotional level, may not be those that are thought typical of her group. Given that so much of our personal identity depends on our idiosyncratic relationships with others, it is not surprising that many patients become quite disturbed by their experiences in hospital as their identities are reduced to 'the caesar in the end bed'.

In hospital a mother is on the doctors' and, more importantly, the nurses' territory and so is under strong pressures, direct and indirect, to follow their ways of doing things. At best, she is likely to find that hospital routines can be bent only to a small degree to accommodate her individuality. For those who do not toe the line, there is the constant threat of being branded as a 'difficult' patient. This pressure tends to mute and modify the comments of patients to hospital staff about the care they have received. So staff are often misled about the acceptability of hospital routines.

For many years, there has been concern about the treatment of maternity patients (e.g. Department of Health and Social Security 1961). Charges of insensitive or inhumane treatment have often been answered by the suggestion that they result from staff shortages. However, recent events have shown that this cannot be the root cause, as the maternity services now have a more generous provision of staff than almost any other part of the health service. Staffing levels in maternity hospitals have not been reduced in parallel with the declining birth-rate and most units are now working with a bed occupancy rate of about 60 per cent. At the same time maternity services are among the highest spenders on the 'hotel' side of hospital costs. Also there is evidence to suggest that when nursing work-loads are reduced, contact with patients does not improve unless special efforts are made.

Given the generous provision of resources for maternity hospitals, these are ideally placed to move towards systems of management that are as acceptable to patients as possible. The Department of Health and Social Security is now planning to cut spending in maternity services but this should not be any threat to improved staff–patient relations, as very considerable savings could be effected by reducing lengths of stay and the bed provision. After a long period of decline, lengths of stay are now increasing again and are, on average, about a week. American experience has shown that stays can be reduced to less than half this average without affecting the health of mothers or babies. Costs are related to lengths of stay so that by shortening these one could save money without reducing staff–patient ratio. Modification in lengths of stay can also be used as a buffer against long- and short-term fluctuations in the number of births.

None of what I have said is intended to suggest that we should not do our utmost to make hospitals as comfortable and welcoming as possible. However, we should not pretend that a hospital can ever be the same as one's own home and we must recognize the limitations imposed by the nature of hospitals as complex social institutions and by the divergent interests of patients and staff.

The other major disadvantage of hospital care is that the mother is much more likely to be exposed to unnecessary intervention than at home. Here we are not dealing with something like the comparative comfort of home and hospital which might be given a relatively low priority from a narrow medical point of view, but a potential source of differential morbidity and mortality. It is unnecessary intervention that must arouse serious doubts about the claims of the greater safety of hospital for 'low-risk' mothers.

The active management of labour

A very general feature of modern medicine is that techniques that do pro-vide benefits for particular groups of patients tend to get used for wider and wider indications so one may eventually reach a point where people who do not require treatment at all are being given it. As this latter group will have nothing to gain from the technique they will be worse off than if left alone if the technique carries any risk. This feature of modern medical practice can be demonstrated in several aspects of maternity care (Richards 1975b, 1977a, b).

A paradigm case of the over-use of a potentially valuable technique is the induction and acceleration of labour. Induction (the initiation of labour before it begins spontaneously) can be life-saving in a few specific situations as when a mother has toxaemia or the baby is very overdue, but as the technique carries risks, it will benefit neither mother nor child when it is used in the absence of medical or pressing social indications. Though inductions involving artificial rupture of the membranes are sometimes carried out at home deliveries, induction and acceleration (the speeding up of labour, generally with oxytocic drugs) are very seldom, if at all, carried out at home, so the hazard of unnecessary induction is more or less confined to hospital practice. We do not know how prevalent active management of labour (induction plus acceleration) may be, as national statistics are not collected. However, induction is recorded and this has risen from 13·75 per cent in 1963 to 37·2 per cent in 1973 (provisional Department of Health and Social Security figures for 1974 suggest a rate of 40·7 per cent). Fourteen per cent of induced births is about the level that might be expected on the basis of the incidence of complications† that could be alleviated by induction so the increase beyond that figure represents the use of the technique where no clear medical reasons exist.‡ On top of this figure one must add an unknown number of cases where labour begins spontaneously but is then accelerated. Judging by practice in a few hospitals that have published figures, where around 30 per cent of births are induced, a further 20–30 per cent of labours will be accelerated.

Table 5.4 Queen Charlotte's Maternity Hospital Statistics
(1972 records incompletely coded)

	1969	1970	1971	1973	1974
Induction (per cent)	17·0	15·1	31·4	27·0	26·0
Caesarean sections (per cent)	5·5	5·8	6·3	7·2	9·2
Forceps (per cent)	13·7	13·7	14·8	25·5	29·1
Epidurals (per cent)	Not recorded	3·7	16·1	46·9	58·5
Perinatal mortality rate (per 1000)	24·2	23·2	19·1	15·4	15·5
Deliveries	3430	3341	3201	3209	3049

Source: Craft (1976)

A fairly typical pattern of changing obstetric practice is shown in Table 5.4 which gives statistics from Queen Charlotte's Maternity Hospital in London. This hospital might be described as having a relatively selective induction policy but has an unusually high rate for the use of epidural anaesthesia.

As no randomized trial of active management has been carried out in Britain, one cannot state with certainty the prevalence of the complications of the techniques. However, available evidence suggests that they may be

† A recent report of a series from Ireland suggests that even this figure may be too high (O'Driscoll, Carroll, and Coughlan 1975).

‡ Post-maturity of the foetus is the most common indication given for induction. One would expect that as the technique has become more widespread the number of post-mature babies would fall. However, a comparison of the 1958 and 1970 perinatal mortality surveys shows only a very slight change. In 1958 11·5 per cent of babies were estimated to be of more than 42 weeks gestation and 9·3 per cent weighed more than 4000 g, the respective figures in 1970, with more than double the number of inductions, were 11·0 per cent and 8·2 per cent. This suggests that the technique is used very non-selectively and that cases where it might be used with benefit are being missed and is confirmed by other evidence (figures from Butler and Bonham (1965) and Chamberlain *et al.* (1975)).

associated with a raised incidence of Caesarean sections, forceps deliveries, and maternal infections, greater use of narcotic analgesics and epidural anaesthesia, more immaturity, respiratory depression, and jaundice in the babies, and higher rates of admission to special-care nurseries.

Against these 'costs' one may set the advantages of the induction for those cases where there is a medical reason for it. In addition, there is the question of convenience. As far as mothers are concerned there are undoubtedly some women who would like to have their baby on a certain day. However, on the evidence of mothers' complaints about induction, this group is clearly smaller than the number who are actually induced for non-medical reasons. The group might be smaller still if all mothers were told of the risks of the technique to themselves and their babies (see Kitzinger 1975). The same point can be made about the use of acceleration techniques in spontaneous labours. It is obviously a great boon that very long labours can be avoided but the use of acceleration is now far more general than can be accounted for by selective application to cases of potentially long labour. There is also the question of the possibility of greater convenience for maternity hospital staff. In spite of a falling birth-rate, the wider use of active management has not apparently resulted in any reduction in staffing maternity hospitals (though hours of work may have been reduced). Although accelerated labours are shorter, a greater degree of supervision is required. At least one study (Cole, Howie, and Macnaughton 1975) suggests that the proportion of night-time deliveries is not significantly reduced. If one takes into account the probable greater need for specialized paediatric care after induction (see below) the overall effect for maternity hospitals may well be a greater work-load for staff.†

The increase in Caesarean sections during labour after induction (Bonnar 1975) which presumably follows foetal distress with the stronger contractions of an accelerated labour is a potentially serious hazard for the mother.† The proportion of Caesarean sections has risen from 3·4 per cent of all deliveries in 1964 to 4·9 per cent in 1972 while the fatality rate has fallen from 1·3 per 1000 sections to 1·0 over the same period (Arthure et al. 1975). Once a mother has had a section she is much more likely to require one in future deliveries so the risk for her and her children is cumulative. As well as the

---

† One could argue that the use of intervention techniques that increase staff work may be encouraged by the falling work-load resulting from the decline in the birth-rate. Their use may represent an attempt to stretch work to fill the available time. By analogy, one might note that the use of labour-saving devices in the home has not reduced the time spent doing housework.

† The Cardiff birth survey (Chalmers 1975) suggests a rapid rise in the incidence of foetal distress in labour (from about 8 per cent in the late 1960s to more than 20 per cent in 1972). Not all the increase can be explained by the rise in inductions and accelerated labour. (See also Richards (1977b).)

‡ Surgical induction itself is found to be painful by a substantial minority of women (Caseby 1974).

very small risk of death from this operation, one has also to consider the considerable discomfort of the recovery period and the difficulties in mobility and in nursing the baby.

The rise in forceps deliveries (which carried hazards for the baby; see e.g. O'Driscoll (1975)) may not be a direct consequence of active management but may follow the use of epidural anaesthesia which is often associated with this style of obstetrics. The increasing use of forceps may account for the rising incidence of lacerations in mothers (from 4·3 per 1000 deliveries in 1970 to 8·1 in 1973) which has occurred in spite of increasing use of episiotomy. These have increased from 24·3 per cent of deliveries in 1970 to 37·0 per cent in 1973.

Active management produces stronger and more painful contractions of the uterus so higher levels of pain-killing drugs tend to be used (e.g. Chalmers 1975). All the usual drugs given to relieve pain in labour pass, via the placenta, to the baby. Most of them have the effect of depressing the baby's breathing at birth and inhibiting sucking during the first week or more of life (Bowes, Brackbill, Conway, and Steinschneider 1970; Aleksandrowiz 1974; Scanlon 1974; Richards 1977c). Some much longer-lasting psychological effects on the baby have been reported but too little research has yet been done to assess the prevalence or significance of these. Because of the depressive effect on infant sucking, lactation may be harder to establish (Dunn and Richards 1975) and the initial relationship of mother and baby may be made more difficult. Of course, drugs are also used at home deliveries but because active management is not used and more psychological support is usually given there is less need for them. Epidural anaesthesia, which seems to be particularly bad for the baby's sucking abilities, is never given outside a hospital. As hospital deliveries have risen, the use of drugs has gone up. In 1958, 56 per cent of mothers received Pethidine in some form, whereas 68 per cent did so in 1970 (Butler and Bonham 1965; Chamberlain et al. 1975). This increase in the use of Pethidine has occurred despite a much wider employment of epidurals which one might have expected to act as a substitute.

Much confusion surrounds the use of analgesics in labour. For example, Pethilorfan (a combination of Pethidine and a narcotic antagonist, levallorphan) was used in 23 per cent of deliveries in 1970, despite the publication of a number of studies showing that it has a much more depressive effect on babies than Pethidine (e.g. Campbell, Masson, and Norris 1965) and is a less effective analgesic (e.g. Schott and Herz 1970). An even more disturbing picture is revealed for the narcotic antagonist, Lethidrone (Nalorphine). This drug, when given to a baby at birth, can counteract some of the effects of narcotics like Pethidine. However, when it is given to a baby with respiratory depression that does not arise from narcotic use, it makes matters worse. The British births survey of 1970 (Chamberlain et al. 1975) showed that 136 of the mothers whose infants were given this drug (of the total of 409) had not been given Pethidine. Again, we do not know whether these potentially dangerous mistakes were made at home deliveries or in hospital, but the latter seems most likely.

The greater respiratory depression of induced babies is documented in the British births survey of 1970 (Table 5.5).

Table 5.5 Induction and respiratory depression in infants

Method of induction	Respiratory depression ratio†
Artificial rupture of the membranes: alone	5·3
: with other methods	9·0
Intravenous oxytocin: alone	7·7
: with other methods	9·1
Oxytocin by mouth: alone	7·7
: with other methods	9·1
No induction	3·6

Source: Chamberlain *et al.* 1975
†The number of babies taking more than 3 minutes to the onset of respiration experienced as a percentage of the total number of babies in that group.

The table indicates that the commonest technique of active management, artifical rupture of the membranes and intravenous oxytocin, produced three times the rate of depressed babies found in the non-induced group. Of course, some allowance must be made for cases where the induction was carried out for genuine medical reasons where the baby may have already been at risk. However, there is little doubt that the combination of greater use of analgesic drugs and the more violent contractions of the accelerated labour can produce more depressed babies (see also Liston and Campbell (1974)).

Some of the increase in respiratory depression may result from the relative immaturity of the induced babies. By definition an induced birth takes place earlier than it would have done without interference and in rare cases where the gestational age is incorrectly assessed, a seriously pre-term infant may be produced. However, it is possible that even a slight degree of immaturity may be significant for the infant's respiration at birth. Though the process is far from understood, it seems that the infant plays some part in initiating his own birth (when spontaneous). The adrenal hormones that appear to be involved in this process also play a part in the mechanism that ensures the lungs are mature at birth. We do not know how far the reduction in the length of gestation produced by induction is important, but it is possible that it may be related to respiratory depression in induced infants. What is established is that a few full-term babies develop serious respiratory distress syndrome after induction.

Because of the potential hazards to the foetus of induction and acceleration techniques, some obstetricians consider that active management should not be undertaken unless foetal monitoring is also used (though, at present, many actively managed labours are not monitored). There are disadvantages associated with its use. Attachment to monitoring devices means that the mother must be relatively immobile and the electrodes attached to the baby's head can give rise to complications (Atlas and Serr 1976).

Another reason why babies born after induction may be in less good condition than after a spontaneous delivery is that intact membranes may afford some protection to the foetus during labour. In labour with intact membranes placental circulation appears to be better than after rupture and the forewaters reduce pressures on the baby's head (Calder 1976).

Jaundiced infants have become much more common in recent years. At Queen Charlotte's Maternity Hospital, for example, the rate of 'significant' jaundice has risen from 8 per cent in 1971 to 15 per cent in 1973 (Campbell, Harvey, and Norman 1975). The reasons for this are uncertain but it does seem to be associated with the use of oxytocin for induction and acceleration (Chalmers, Campbell, and Turnbull 1975), epidurals and forceps delivery (Campbell *et al.* (1975); but see also Gould, Mountrose, Brown, and Whitehouse 1974). One possible connecting factor may be bruising of the infant (Friedman and Sachtelben 1976). Though jaundice is treatable it can require intensive intervention, including exchange blood transfusion for serious cases, and it is a frequent cause for the admission of a baby to a special-care unit.

Many of the hazards of induction and acceleration for the baby create problems that require specialized paediatric care so it is not surprising that rates of admission to special-care baby units are rapidly rising. In 1970 12 per cent of babies born in England and Wales were admitted to such a unit compared with 18·4 per cent in 1975 (Department of Health and Social Security statistics). Not all this rise can be explained by problems associated with induction, but some probably can.

Liston and Campbell (1974) showed that babies from mothers who had received oxytocin were more often distressed during labour, depressed at birth, and were more likely to be admitted to a special-care unit (Table 5.6).

In this study, some of the babies' problems may have arisen from conditions that led to the induction being undertaken rather than from the induction itself. But as so many of the complications of induction and acceleration give rise to problems in the neonatal period (see Richards 1977b), a direct link between active management techniques and admission to a special-care unit would not be unexpected.

One factor that may have contributed to the rapid increase in the use of

Table 5.6 Special-care nursing admissions

	Proportion of cases admitted (per cent)
Normal spontaneous labour	3·7
Artificial rupture of the membranes but no oxytocin	8·8
Low dose of oxytocin	12·6
High dose of oxytocin	23·8

Source: Liston and Campbell (1974)

induction and acceleration techniques is that these are readily available in most hospitals. If a technique is available the general tendency in medicine seems to be to use it even though the benefits may be marginal or non-existent. This phenomenon can be illustrated by the pattern of use of X-rays in pregnancy. In the late 1950s evidence was produced which linked exposure to X-rays during pregnancy to later cancers in the children, and this led to a big decrease in the use of X-rays for diagnosis. More recently ultrasound techniques have come into wide use and it was hoped that these, in part, might serve as a substitute for X-rays. However, in many hospitals X-rays are now being used as widely as in the early 1950s (though the doses of X-rays employed may be lower) and in some areas as many as 35 per cent of all pregnant women are exposed (Carmichael and Berry 1976). There is very little reason to think that rates of exposure as high as this can be justified in terms of medical benefits. As Carmichael and Berry comment,

'It seems that where a patient attends a hospital with readily accessible X-ray facilities, these facilities will be used. At [one] hospital, the X-ray set was withdrawn, and the patients had to be sent to a nearby hospital. This small barrier to the use of X-rays may partly explain why only 8·6% of pregnancies delivered in [this] hospital were examined by X-ray.' Another reason why X-ray use is so high may be the increasing use of induction because this technique is often employed to assess the maturity of the foetus in an attempt to avoid the possibility of an unnecessarily pre-term birth.

With rising rates of hospital confinements and the tendency for antenatal care to be increasingly based in hospitals, wider use is being made of a whole range of diagnostic techniques during pregnancy. There is little reason to believe that the more general use of such techniques offers substantial benefits to mothers or children (see Chalmers 1975). Apart from possible hazards associated with their use, these diagnostic facilities are very expensive to provide and may partly account for the rapidly rising costs of maternity services at a time when the birth-rate is dropping dramatically. In addition pregnant women are being required to make more visits to hospital clinics and to spend many hours in waiting rooms. A thorough investigation of the costs and benefits of all aspects of antenatal care has now become an urgent matter.

This brief discussion of induction suggests that the technique carries significant morbidity for both mother and infant. We know that for many mothers the induction is not performed for medical reasons.† If the mother had had a home confinement the active management would have been avoided and she would not have been unnecessarily exposed to the dangers of the technique. A feature of the induction situation which is found elsewhere in medicine is that the iatrogenic (doctor-created) problem following one intervention requires further intervention for its treatment. So the use of medical facilities increases at a compound rate. But to make matters worse, admission of a baby to a special-care unit is not the end of the induction story because this treatment itself seems to carry significant iatrogenic risks. It is now reasonably well established that the separation of mother and baby that follows admission to a special-care unit may have deleterious consequences for the mother's relationship with her child for many months after delivery (Kennell, Jerauld, Wolfe, Chester, Kreger, McAlpine, Stelfa, and Klaus 1974; Ringler, Kennell, Jarvella, Navojosky, and Klaus 1975; Whiten 1977; Richards 1975a; Brimblecombe, Richards, and Roberton 1977). Thus, the repercussions of foetal distress and other complications of active management could be very long lasting.

We should also note in passing that special-care nurseries are very expensive facilities. Increasing use of active management of labour and relaxation of criteria of admission to special-care units undoubtedly cause extra expense for the Health Service. The net effect is that less money is available for other desirable facilities.

Admission to a special-care unit, like induction, is used more widely than it should be for the maximally beneficial effects. As induction has increased so have admissions to these units but on top of this the criteria for admission seem to have been relaxed so that a considerable number of full-term well babies are being admitted to some units. Presumably, these units' function has been modified from a place where highly specialized treatment can be given to that of an observation ward. Given the potential hazards of early separation of mother and infant, this is a very undesirable practice. As one might expect, this 'excess' of admissions comes almost exclusively from babies born in hospitals where there are special-care units—it is all too easy to wheel a cot down a corridor but much more substantial reasons

† Here it is worth emphasizing the distinction drawn earlier between essential and non-essential inductions. There are cases where induction is medically desirable for the mother, her baby, or both. However, the number of such cases is far less than the number of inductions currently performed. An induction is medically desirable when the risks of the procedure are less than those expected if the pregnancy was allowed to continue.

are required before an ambulance is called and a newborn baby is carried on a long journey (Chamberlain *et al* 1975). A reason that may have encouraged the ever-increasing number of babies to these units is the falling birth-rate. Nature, it is said, abhors a vacuum, and clinicians appear to abhor empty beds. If one looks at admission figures for these units one typically finds that the number of babies coming in is more or less constant from year to year. But, as the birth-rate is falling rapidly, this will mean that the criteria for admission are being relaxed and more fit babies are admitted (Brimblecombe, Richards, and Roberton 1977).

Again, like induction, special-care units can be literally life-saving for some babies but the admission of fit babies can only be potentially harmful. As almost all the fit babies come from maternity hospitals to which these units are attached, unnecessary admission is a hazard of hospital, not home, deliveries.

Other separation of mother and baby may stem from hospital routines. Of course, not all mothers want to be with their babies day and night during the first few days after delivery but the significant point about a hospital is that only very seldom will the routine be one that a mother has chosen for herself. If a mother in hospital has a sudden wish to see or hold her baby, she is only able to do this in so far as her wish conforms with the hospital routine. At home, of course, there are no such requirements for conformity.

An important consequence of hospital routines is that a mother is seldom able to take real responsibility for her own child—she cannot always feel it is really hers. Research in Sweden has demonstrated that where there are routines that regulate a mother's contact with her child and the choice of feeding times, mother's confidence to cope with her child when she goes home is reduced (Greenberg, Rosenberg, and Lind 1973).

Conclusion

The wider use of induction and acceleration and changes in admission policies of special-care units means that mothers who could have had normal uncomplicated deliveries at home are being exposed to unnecessary risks in hospital. As these dangers can be avoided by a domiciliary confinement, this situation casts considerable doubt on the supposed superior safety of hospital delivery for uncomplicated cases. As I said earlier, controlled studies have not been carried out either comparing home and hospital delivery or to assess the overall advantages and disadvantages of induction and acceleration, so we cannot state with certainty what the risks of hospital delivery are, and, of course, the situation will vary from place to place depending on the policies of the local hospital. It might be argued that contemporary risks in hospitals represent a temporary situation and that when the complications of induction and unnecessary admission to a special-care baby unit are more widely known, these techniques will be used more selectively, so that mothers and babies will not be exposed to unnecessary hazards. Practice does seem to be changing and induction rates may be falling in the face of widespread adverse comment in the press and on radio and television. Significantly, some of the obstetricians who were most closely involved in pioneering the techniques are now urging caution to their colleagues. However, this does not detract from a more general point that can be made about modern medicine. The pattern we see for the introduction of induction for clearly defined reasons, and then a general increase beyond a point where beneficial returns can be expected, is all too typical of much of present-day medical practice. Feedback mechanisms seem to operate very slowly to curb the over-enthusiastic use of potentially valuable techniques. Usually considerable excesses occur before the situation settles down to a more rational policy.

In obstetrics this feature has been present from the earliest days. Two centuries ago William Hunter, the best-known of the 'man midwives', used to show his student a pair of obstetrical forceps, rusty from disuse: 'where they save one, they murder twenty'. Today the situation has got worse because the rate of introduction of new techniques leaves little time for effective assessment, and few seem to have the time or facilities for such work. The temptations of over-enthusiasm are greater in obstetrics because of the mixture of complicated and uncomplicated cases that are treated side by side in the hospital. As the whole ethos of hospital treatment involves intervention it may be very difficult to avoid unnecessary intervention in normal cases. So even though the current over-use of induction and special-care nurseries may be curbed, unless there is a basic change in the traditional attitudes of doctors, the future is likely to bring further epidemics of iatrogenic illness in hospitals. Obviously, we must try to prevent this happening by all possible means. One strategy is not to expose women and babies to the risks, by delivering uncomplicated cases at home. Given the technical limitations and general philosophy of midwife and GP care, unnecessary intervention is a much less serious problem. A movement towards a 60:40 per cent hospital/home system has many other advantages. Not only does it offer the degree of choice women want and might reasonably be given, but it minimizes the 'institutional' influences on mother and baby. Though, as I have pointed out above, we must do all we can to minimize these, we can never pretend that a hospital is like a home. The existence of a home delivery service for a significant minority of mothers might continue to have beneficial effects on hospitals by providing a standard against which the acceptability of hospital practices to patients can be assessed. It is unlikely to be coincidental that countries like the United States which have had no tradition of home delivery for many decades also seem to display the most excessive features of institutionalized delivery with extensive intervention and reliance on routines.

A final comment about costs: as Ashford (Chapter 2 of this book) has demonstrated, hospital confinement is much more expensive than home delivery. The development of medical facilities is limited by cost and at present we are wasting resources by providing hospital facilities for delivery for women who neither want them nor require them on medical grounds. The money could be much better used elsewhere in the health service. In effect, the provision of unnecessary maternity facilities is depriving other kinds of patients of valuable and much-needed treatment. This has to be added to the list of disadvantages of a policy of 100 per cent hospital delivery.

Patients have never played an important part (indeed very little part at all) in making policy for maternity care. A great weakness of our new reorganized Health Service is that they are still denied any significant degree of democracy in its government. However, pressure groups can exert some influence on policy and this is the only means available to try to create a more rational system of maternity care. Consumers must attempt to influence policy at every level from Parliament and the Department of Health and Social Security through the Community Health Councils to individual doctors and nurses. For too long they have been passive in the face of changes foisted on them by the medical profession.

References

Aleksandrowicz, M. K. (1974). 'The effects of pain relieving drugs administered during labor and delivery on the behavior of the newborn: a review'. *Merrill-Palmer Quarterly* **20**, 121–41.

Arthure, H., Tomkinson, J., Organe, G., Lewis, E. M., Adelstein, A. M., and Weatherall, J. A. C. (1975). 'Report on confidential enquiries into maternal deaths in England and Wales 1970–72'. Department of Health and Social Security Report on Health and Social Subjects No. 11. H.M.S.O., London.

Atlas, M. and Serr, D. M. (1976). 'Hazards of fetal scalp electrodes'. *The Lancet* i, 648.

Bonnar J. (1975). 'Induction and acceleration of labour in modern obstetric practice'. Paper presented at a Study Group on Problems in Obstetrics organized by the Medical Information Unit of the Spastics Society. Tunbridge Wells, April 1975.

Bowes, W. A., Brackbill, Y., Conway, E., and Steinschneider, A. (1970) (eds). 'The effects of obstetrical medication on foetus and infant'. *Monographs of the Society for Research in Child Development* **137**, No. 4.

Brimblecombe, F. S. W., Richards, M. P. M., and Roberton, N. R. C. (1977) (eds). *Early separation and special care nurseries. Clinics in developmental medicine.* Spastics Publications/Heinemann Medical Books, London. (In press.)

Butler, N. R. and Bonham, D. G. (1963). *Perinatal mortality.* Churchill Livingstone, Edinburgh.

Calder, A. A. (1976). 'Augmentation of uterine action in spontaneous labour'. In *The management of labour* (ed. R. Beard, M. Brudenell, P. Dunn, and D. Fairweather). Royal College of Obstetricians and Gynaecologists, London.

Campbell, N., Harvey, D., and Norman, A. P. (1975). 'Increased frequency of neonatal jaundice in a maternity hospital'. *British Medical Journal* iii, 548–52.

Campbell, D., Masson, A. H. B., and Norris, W. (1965). 'The clinical evaluation of narcotic and sedative drugs. II. A re-evaluation of pethidine and pethilorphan'. *British Journal of Anaesthesia* **37**, 199.

Carmichael, J. H. E. and Berry, R. J. (1976). 'Diagnostic X-rays in late pregnancy and in the neonate'. *Lancet* i, 351.

Caseby, N. (1974). 'Epidural analgesia for the surgical induction of labour'. *British Journal of Anaesthesia* **46**, 747–51.

Chalmers, I. (1975). 'Evaluation of different approaches to obstetric care'. Paper presented to a seminar on Human Relations and Obstetric Practice, University of Warwick, October 1975.

——, Campbell, H., and Turnbull, A. C. (1975). Use of oxytocin and incidence of neonatal jaundice. *British Medical Journal* ii, 116–18.

Chamberlain, R., Chamberlain, G., Howlett, B., and Clamaux, A. (1975). *British Births 1970*. Heinemann Medical Books, London.

Cole, R. A., Howie, P. W., and Macnaughton, M. C. (1975). 'Elective induction of labour. A randomised, prospective study'. *The Lancet* i, 767–70.

Cox, C. A., Fox, J. S., Zinkin, P. M., and Mathews, A. E. B. (1976). 'Clinical appraisal of domiciliary obstetric and neonatal practice'. *British Medical Journal* i, 84–6.

Craft, I. (1976). 'Induction of labour'. *Midwife, Health Visitor and Community Nurse* **12**, 42–4.

Department of Health and Social Security (1961). *Human relations in obstetrics*. H.M.S.O., London.

Dunn, J. and Richards, M. P. M. (1977). 'Observations on the developing relationship between mother and baby in the neonatal period'. In *Studies in mother-infant interaction* (ed. H. R. Schaffer). Academic Press, London. (In press.)

Friedman and Sachtelben, M. R. (1976). 'Neonatal jaundice in association with oxytocin stimulation of labour and operative delivery'. *British Medical Journal* i, 198–9.

Gould, S. R., Mountrose, U., Brown, D. J., Whitehouse, W. L., and Barnardo, D. E. (1974). 'Influence of previous oral contraception and maternal oxytocin infusion on neonatal jaundice'. *British Medical Journal* iii, 228–30.

Greenberg, M., Rosenberg, I., and Lind, J. (1973). 'First mothers rooming-in with their newborns'. *American Journal of Orthopsychiatry* **43**, 783–8.

Kennell, J. K., Jerauld, R., Wolfe, H., Chester, D., Kreger, N. G., McAlpine, W., Steffa, M., and Klaus, M. H. (1974). 'Maternal behavior one year after early and extended post-partum contact'. *Developmental Medicine and Child Neurology* **16**, 172–9.

Kitzinger, S. (1975). *Some mothers' experience of induced labour*. National Childbirth Trust, London.

Liston, W. A. and Campbell, A. J. (1974). 'Dangers of oxytocin-induced labour to foetuses'. *British Medical Journal* iii, 606–7.

Mather, H. G., Pearson, W. G., Read, K. L. Q., Shaw, D. B., Steed, G. R., Thorne, M. G., Jones, S., Guerrier, C. J., Erant, C. D., McHugh, P. M., Chowdhury, N. R., Jafory, M. H., and Wallace, T. J. (1971). 'Acute myocardial infarction: home and hospital treatment'. *British Medical Journal* ii, 334.

Maxwell, R. (1974). *Health care. The growing dilemma*. McKinsey, New York.

O'Driscoll, K., Carroll, C. J., and Coughlan, H. (1975). 'Selective induction of labour'. *British Medical Journal* iv, 727–9.

—— (1975). 'An obstetrician's view of pain'. *British Journal of Anaesthesia* **47**, 1053–9.

Richards, M. P. M. (1975a). 'The one-day old deprived child'. In *Child alive* (ed. R. Lewin). Temple-Smith, London.

—— (1975b). 'Obstetricians and the induction of labour in Britain'. *Social Science and Medicine* **9**, 595–602.

—— (1977a). Towards a national illness service. (Book in preparation.)

—— (1977b). 'The induction and acceleration of labour. Some benefits and complications'. *Early Human Development* **1**, 3–17.

—— (1977c). 'Effects on infant behaviour of analgesics and anaesthetics used in obstetrics'. Paper presented at the 5th Conference of the European Teratology Society, Italy. (In press.)

Riley, D. (1977). 'What do women want? The question of choice in the conduct of labour'. *In Benefits and hazards of the new obstetrics* (ed. T. Church and M. P. M. Richards). *Clinics in Developmental Medicine*, Heinemann Medical Books, London. (In press.)

Ringler, N. M., Kennell, J. H., Jarvella, R., Navojosky, B. J., and Klaus, M. H. (1975). 'Mother-to-child speech at 2 years—effects of early postnatal contact'. *Journal of Paediatrics* **86**, 141–4.

Scanlon, W. W. (1974). 'Obstetric anaesthesia as a neonatal risk factor in normal labor and delivery'. *Clinics in Perinatology* **1**, 465–82.

Schott, K. A. M. and Herz, A. (1970). 'Interaction between morphine and morphine antagonists after systemic and intraventricular application'. *European Journal of Pharmacology* **12**, 53–64.

Whiten, A. (1977). 'Assessing the effects of perinatal events on the success of the mother–infant relationship'. In *Studies in mother–infant interaction* (ed. H. R. Schaffer). Academic Press, London. (In press.)

G. J. KLOOSTERMAN

6

The Dutch system of home births

Do you think you can take over the universe and improve it?
I do not believe it can be done.
The universe is sacred.
You cannot improve it.
If you try to change it, you will ruin it.
If you try to hold it, you will lose it.

Lao Tsu†

The debate on the place of birth is taking place not only in Britain, but also in Europe and the United States and Canada. In the Netherlands, which has one of the lowest mortality rates in the world and where home confinements are still about 50 per cent of the total, the normal environment for birth is thought to be the home. Yet change is taking place rapidly, and many Dutch obstetricians, wanting to use the sophisticated obstetric technology introduced from abroad, and to a large extent from the United States where many receive part of their postgraduate training, believe that labour can be effectively and safely managed only in a hospital setting. Professor Kloosterman is a powerful advocate of home confinements for those clearly not 'at risk', of careful selection for hospital, and skilled domiciliary midwifery.

As everywhere else on this planet obstetric care in the Netherlands was originally given entirely at home. Institutional deliveries were the fate of the homeless, the very poor, and unmarried women. In the middle of the nineteenth century these hospitals were, in spite of the medical aid that was given, the most dangerous places where any woman could have her baby, and as late as 1880 there was a violent debate in the municipal council of Amsterdam as to whether the maternity clinic of the University of Amsterdam should be closed. Statistics were presented to prove that there was no place so dangerous for expectant mothers as this stronghold of medical knowledge.

The discoveries of Semmelweis, Pasteur, and Lister changed all this and at the beginning of the twentieth century hospitals were so much improved that they started to lose their frightening aspects. Since then, as in all other countries of the Western world, the number of deliveries in hospital in the Netherlands has risen regularly and over the same period the medical profession has done what it can to improve hospitals and to make them centres of medical knowledge and technology.

† Lao Tsu Tao *Ching* Verse 29. A new translation by Gia-Fu Feng and Jane English. Wildwood House Ltd., London.

There was only one difference between the Netherlands and many other countries: in Holland the medical profession tried not only to improve hospitals but at the same time the conditions of homes as places in which to be born.

As early as 1904 organizations were founded to train young girls in several cities and villages to take care of a healthy woman and her baby during the lying-in period, and in doing her household chores. In 1925 all these organizations were coordinated and united by the Government and since then we have had a special training programme for *'kraamverzorgsters'* (maternity aid nurses), on a national scale. Their training takes 15 months and includes subjects such as hygiene, bacteriology, theory and practice of mother and child care, cooking, budgeting, and looking after toddlers. In short, the maternity aid nurse can replace the mother in her household and can look after her and her baby.

This allows the midwife (who has a 3-year training in obstetrics) to leave the nursing problems to the maternity aid nurses. The midwife can devote herself entirely to her obstetric task (pre-natal, natal, and post-natal care) and is able to take care of 100–200 pregnant women a year.

In this way a 'home care team' is formed, consisting of the midwife or family doctor and the maternity aid nurse, in the same way as the team formed by the doctor and the nurse in hospitals.

The difference between the two teams was (and is) that the 'doctor–nurse' dyad by training and attitude is oriented towards the institution of curative measures whereas the 'midwife–maternity aid nurse' dyad is happy if everything goes well without interference. The first is meant to care for pathology; the second to protect a healthy woman during pregnancy and childbirth and to give her careful observation and mental support.

The basic idea behind this kind of obstetric organization was that childbirth in itself is a natural phenomenon that in the large majority of all cases needs no interference whatsoever, only close observation, moral support, and protection against human meddlesomeness. Thus a large group of women can deliver their baby by preference where they feel most at ease, and for the majority this was at home. Only a minority was in need of medical interference and this group belonged in the 'sickhouse', the hospital.

The most important objection to this basic idea is that pregnancy and labour are normal only in retrospect and that there always is a possibility that something unexpected can happen. This problem is considered almost everywhere else in the world (and also, increasingly, in the Netherlands) as an absolute condemnation of the Dutch system. Its realization stimulated prenatal care in a way unparalleled in any other country. In Holland every woman, midwife, and doctor knows that only a spontaneous and uncomplicated delivery can take place at home. Therefore everybody is convinced of the importance of frequent and extensive pre-natal examinations. The list of indications for hospital confinements became longer every year and in the last few years we have radically changed our system of indications for hospital delivery. As a precondition for home confinement we ask now for the absence of all indications of abnormality.

A woman is allowed to stay at home (and is entitled to engage a maternity aid nurse) if she is in good health; if there are no features of toxaemia, providing there is no hypertension, if the head of the baby is well engaged, and if there are no symptoms of disproportion. There must not be a multiple pregnancy, nor abnormalities in the medical and obstetrical history. If nulliparous the woman has to be under 35 years of age or if multiparous under 45 years. Labour must start spontaneously after 38 weeks and before the end of the forty-second week (before 295th day after last menstruation). The social circumstances of the expectant mother must be such that there is a bedroom with heating equipment at her disposal, and a W.C. on the same floor. In case of emergency there must be the means to transfer her to the nearest hospital within 60 minutes.

If there is a medical indication for hospital confinement, the costs are paid by 'compulsory insurance' (the Health Service which covers almost 75 per cent of the population, and includes all people earning less than £6000 a year). If there is no indication for hospital delivery the 'compulsory insurance' pays the fee of the midwife and the larger part of the costs of the maternity aid nurse.

If there is no midwife in a district, the family doctor is paid by the insurance company for a 'normal delivery', but if there is a midwife, only she is paid. If the woman prefers her doctor then she has to pay him herself. In this way there exists financial protection for the midwife, a point which is not always appreciated.

Why does an obstetric system with such a large proportion of well-controlled home confinements exist only in the Netherlands?

One explanation is that the Netherlands are the most densely populated country in the world, which together with a good road system and many hospitals allows almost every woman to be transferred from her home to the nearest hospital within 60 minutes if necessary. That there are other explanations to be found in the national character is often suggested, but difficult to prove. The Dutch are very home-orientated. The British sayings 'my home is my castle' and 'be it ever so humble, there is no place like home' are perhaps even more convincing to the Dutch. Some people think that religion has something to do with it. Faith in God and a certain suspicion of man-made institutions are undoubtedly national traits. It may be for this reason as much as anything else that Dutch women tend to feel secure in having babies at home and that childbirth is seen as a process which, whenever possible, should take place in the context of the family.

It has sometimes been suggested that Dutch women represent an ideal set from an obstetric point of view because of their physical build. It is claimed that the Dutch pelvis is abnormally capacious. It is also argued that the high standard of living in the Netherlands produces a population presenting the least obstetric risks. It should perhaps be pointed out that many

Dutch women of the last generation were severely malnourished during the war and that Holland has a large mixed immigrant population of varying physical build, consisting of Indonesians, people from all Mediterranean countries, and from the West Indies. One thing, however, is certain: that in the Netherlands the number of home confinements is declining by 2 per cent every year. Many Dutch doctors advocate 100 per cent hospital deliveries. The pressure of opinion from abroad, claiming that the Dutch system is anachronistic and therefore doomed to disappear, becomes stronger every year. The question is, why are some Dutch obstetricians swimming against the stream, and why do many women in the Netherlands still prefer home confinements (as revealed by a recent survey by Lapré)?

The advantages of home confinements are that in her own home the expectant mother is not considered a patient, but a woman, fulfilling a natural and highly personal task. She is the real centre around which everything (and everybody) revolves. The midwife or doctor and the maternity aid nurse are all her guests, there to assist her. This setting reinforces her self-respect and self-confidence. The modern hospital very often functions in an opposite way. The woman is the guest of the doctors and nurses in *their* home. She becomes a patient, dependant on people who like to mother her. The security of the hospital, so important in situations where interference is necessary, is of no use for women who do not need any interference. The atmosphere in the hospital on the other hand weakens her self-confidence. This explains why in many hospitals (and in many countries with total hospitalization) the percentage of artificial deliveries is rising to such an extent that it is inconceivable that it occurs for good medical reasons.

To summarize, we can say that 100 years ago hospitals were the most dangerous places for healthy young women to have their babies. The enormous improvement in medical science has changed this picture completely, and from a purely bacteriological point of view many hospitals have now reached such a level of safety that they equal or better the situation at home.

What has happened in the field of bodily hygiene can perhaps happen in the field of mental hygiene. It is possible to imitate in a hospital the atmosphere of home, with facilities for the husband to stay with his wife in a situation that combines all the psychological advantages of a home confinement with all the security of a big hospital. That, however, would be extremely expensive. At present it seems worthwhile to preserve a system that makes home confinements possible. The very fact that they exist provides a challenge to the hospitals. Only when hospitals can offer to the completely healthy woman the same advantages as are inherent in giving birth at home should we do away with home confinements. Personally I doubt whether this will ever happen.

The perinatal mortality rate (at present still one of the best yardsticks by which to measure obstetric care) in the Netherlands is low. As can be seen

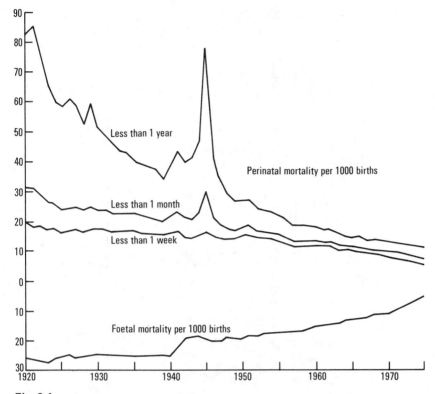

Fig 6.1

from Table 6.1 and Fig. 6.1 it was 13·5 per 1000 in 1975. The perinatal mortality rate for home confinements in the Netherlands has come down from 14·0 in 1960 to 4·5 in 1973 and down still further to 4·2 in 1974. This is comparable with the rate for home confinements in Britain in 1970 of 4·9 per thousand. The perinatal mortality rate for hospital births in the Netherlands was 60·0 in 1960 and went down to 28·1 in 1973 and then still further down to 22·7 in 1974. It is still, as can be seen, a good deal higher than the perinatal mortality rate for home confinements. Only Sweden and Finland have had slightly better overall results over the last 10 years. The results from all other countries computed over the same period have been inferior, and among them there have been many countries with total or almost total hospital deliveries which lagged far behind the results in the Netherlands.

Another argument that the degree of hospitalization is not of paramount significance in improving the results in obstetrics is the fact that in the Netherlands cities with almost total hospitalization show results that are inferior to other cities with less than 50 per cent hospitalization (Centraal Bureau voor de Statistiek, monthly reports).

On the other hand our very low figure for artificial deliveries is certainly due to the philosophy behind the Dutch system. For example, the Caesarean

Table 6.1 Some data about obstetrics in the Netherlands (Population 1974: 13 599 000 inhabitants)

Year	1958	1960	1968	1969	1970	1971	1972	1973	1974	1975
Number of births	240 874	242 407	239 811	250 340	241 500	229 516	215 969	196 745	185 982	177 760
Birth-rate	21·3	21·1	18·8	19·4	18·5	17·4	16·2	14·5	13·7	13·0
Infant mortality (first year)	18·5	17·9	13·6	13·2	12·8	12·1	11·7	11·5	11·3	10·3
Mortality first month	13·2	13·5	10·4	10·0	9·5	9·1	8·8	8·4	8·0	7·1
Mortality first week	11·2	11·7	8·9	8·6	7·9	7·5	7·4	7·2	6·6	5·8
Foetal mortality rate	16·7	14·9	11·3	11·0	10·7	10·2	9·2	9·1	8·8	7·7
Perinatal mortality rate	28·0	26·6	20·2	19·6	18·6	17·6	16·6	16·3	15·4	13·5
Maternal mortality per 1000 confinements	0·41	0·38	0·21	0·19	0·13	0·13	0·10	0·09	0·08	0·07
Percentage of home confinements	74	72	62	60	57	55	53	50	48	47

Source: Centraal Bureau voor de Statistiek, Den Haag.

section rate in the Netherlands in 1971 is 2·0 per cent as compared with one of 6·9 per cent in the United States, 6·4 per cent in Canada, and 4·6 per cent in England and Wales. The same explanation holds for the very low use of anaesthetics and analgesics during labour. A recent investigation by the University of Amsterdam in cooperation with the Ministry of Public Health (van Alten 1976) proved convincingly that it is possible by rather simple but consistently applied means to select a group of women who can deliver at home in a responsible and probably ideal way. In this investigation there was a group of 916 women who were pregnant with their second child and who showed no abnormalities (in accordance with the Dutch list of medical indications for hospital confinements). From this group 24 women (2·6 per cent) were transferred during labour to the hospital. In this group of transferred women there was one artificial delivery (vacuum extraction) and one case of perinatal mortality (foetal blood loss by rupture of a chorionic vessel at the beginning of labour. This case was classed as unpreventable. In the hospital the diagnosis was made after delivery). Of this group of 916 women, 892 delivered at home or in a simple home-like unit where only midwives or family doctors were present and where no hospital facilities for artificial delivery or blood transfusion were available. In this group of 892 women, 893 children were born (one unrecognized twin pregnancy) without any case of perinatal mortality or serious morbidity. Analgesics, for example pethidine, were not used at all. Apgar scores of below 8 at 1 minute were found in less than 1 per cent. In all cases the father was in the bedroom or delivery room and assisted his wife. How many interventions in the normal course of labour were avoided in the above-mentioned group it is impossible to say, but it is highly probable that this figure was by no means negligible.

References

Alten, D. van (1973). 'Het Verloskundig Centrum te Wormerveer'. *Medisch Contact* **28**, 817.

—— (1975). 'Obstetrics in the Netherlands'. Tunbridge Wells Meeting, British Spastic Society.

—— (1976). 'Perinatale sterfte 1970–1973'. Verslag kraaminrichting en Verloskundige huispraktijk van het Verloskundig Centrum te Wormerveer, Amsterdam.

——, Kloosterman, G. J., and Treffers (1976). Letter to the Editor. *British Medical Journal*, 771.

Centraal Bureau voor de Statistiek, Den Haag. Monthly reports. (Data on perinatal mortality, obstetric care, and hospitalization.)

Geneeskundige Hoofdinspectie van de Volksgezondheid, Den Haag. (Data on maternity home help.)

De Haas, J. H. (1954). 'Perinatal mortality and maternity home help in the Netherlands'. *Etud. Neo-natal* 3–71.

—— (1962). 'Perinatale sterfte in Nederland'. Van Gorcum-Assen, The Netherlands.

Kloosterman, G. J. (1968). 'Obstetrics in the Netherlands'. Charter Lecture, Dublin.

—— (1975*a*). 'Obstetrics in the Netherlands; a survival or a challenge?' Tunbridge Wells Meeting, British Spastic Society.

—— (1975*b*). 'De voortplanting van de Mens'. *Leerboek voor Obstetrie en Gynaecologie*, 3rd edn. Uitgeverij Centen, Bussum.

—— (1972). *Vers une naissance sans risques*, p. 530–3. L'organisation obstétricals en Hollande, Monaco.

—— (1976). 'Zur Förderung der Mutter-Kind-Bindung in der modernen Geburtshilfe'. *Monsch–Kinderheilk*, p. 124–566.

Lapré, R. M. (1973). 'Maternity care: a socio-economic analysis'. Tilburg University Press, The Netherlands.

Verbrugge, H. P. (1968). 'Maternity home help and home deliveries'. Wolters-Noordhoff, Groningen, The Netherlands.

The outcome of home delivery research in the United States

In the United States the practice of midwifery is illegal in many states, and prison sentences may be, and in California were, served on people without obstetric qualifications who delivered women. Yet more and more women are having their babies at home. This appears to be partly because of the high cost of medical treatment, but also because increasingly couples are questioning the quality of the emotional experience in many hospitals. The home birth movement in the United States started on the West coast and was then picked up on the East coast. It began with drop-outs and those living in the alternative society of communes, but quickly spread so that now more and more ordinary middle-class Americans are asking for home births.

Obstetricians are not trained to attend home births and are very concerned about possible litigation resulting from them (which has not, in fact, occurred), and nurse—midwives are few and far between. One result is that lay midwives are often delivering babies, and another is that new training schools in midwifery are opening.

In this chapter Professor Mehl examines the home birth movement in the United States and questions its safety.

Before 1940 over half the deliveries in the United States were at home, but by 1960 this had diminished significantly—to the point where home deliveries were rare exceptions (Seiden 1976). In recent years, however, there has been a tremendous increase in the number of home deliveries occurring in the United States for reasons which have been described by many (Hazell 1974, 1975; Arms 1975; Ward and Ward 1976; Sousa 1976; Lang 1972). We began our studies on the statistical outcomes of home delivery because of this increase and the lack of any available data on their relative safety. We had hoped to provide data which parents and professionals could use on their individual scales of relative value along with the experiential data on the emotional aspects as they weighed the risks and benefits to determine what kind of delivery they would choose.

The population choosing home confinement

Hazell (1974, 1975) describes the ethnographic set of those planning home delivery as 'composed of quite average people'. In her ethnographic study of 300 San Francisco Bay Area home deliveries, she found that 90 per cent of the informants lived in a single-family dwelling, father gainfully employed, one or two cars, not a member of an ethnic minority, not on welfare, and with no household servants. One of the characteristics of the group which she noted was a hard-to-define level of self-awareness which manifested itself in an individual concern for nutrition, philosophy, positive health, humanistic psychology, ecology, and the survival of mankind as a whole. Typically both members of the couple had attended university, but neither had graduated. The occupations represented were as varied as from violinist to auto-mechanic or from doctor to lawyer to subsistence farmer (although all came from typically middle-class backgrounds). Hazell presents an attitude profile based on 20 guided-association interviews and an attitude confirmation based on 14 in-depth interviews. In summary, she found that the home birth couples did not fear potential damaging physical consequences of birth at home (relating that they had acknowledged the low level of probability and would have to accept such events were they to occur), but rather expressed the idea that hospital birth had disadvantages from a psychological stand-point and also could cause unnecessary physical trauma in the name of pre-vention. They related that labour was hard work, but not to be feared, and most couples found the experience of labour a peak experience. They accepted death as being not a horror, but a part of life, and related that, for them, the responsibility for the outcome of their birth was their own and did not lie within the province of the hospital. Most expressed deep anger at the medical profession for what they felt was usurpation of the management of normal labour.

Home delivery attendants

The groups we have studied (Mahl, Peterson, Shaw, and Creevy 1975, 1976b; Mehl, Peterson, Whitt, and Hawes 1976a) and reported data upon thus far consist of combinations of lay midwives, nurse–midwives, and/or general practitioners (family practitioners). The six groups studied consisted of the following:

1 A rural-based family practice in Western Marin County, California, com-posed of three family practitioners and three nurses trained as midwives, attending both home and hospital deliveries since 1970 as a part of a com-prehensive family practice.
2 An urban-based family practice in Mill Valley, California, composed of two family practitioners and two registered nurses—one a maternity nurse practitioner—attending both home and hospital deliveries since 1973.
3 An urban-based group in Berkeley, California, consisting of one physician with postgraduate training in pediatrics/neonatology and two nurse–midwives affiliated with a women's health cooperative. This group did not have hospital privileges and attended only home deliveries, referring women needing hospital care to local obstetricians. This group had been functioning since 1974.

4 Ten lay midwives from Santa Cruz County, California, functioning in both urban and rural settings, without medical supervision and with poor obstetrician back-up, attending deliveries at home since 1971.

5 A rural lay midwife from Sonoma County, California attending home deliveries since 1970 with good physician back-up, primarily by family practice residents at the Community Hospital at Santa Rosa.

6 A nurse–midwife in urban Palo Alto, California, supervising and training lay midwives since 1975 and, in turn, supervised by a local obstetrician.

The attitudes and philosophies of these practitioners towards birth and towards the indications for obstetrical intervention were remarkably similar from group to group and were very different from hospital practitioners. Uniformly the home practitioners' criteria for indications for intervention were more rigorous and exclusive than the hospital practitioners'. Interventions were made less often by the home practitioners and unusual labours classified more frequently as normal variants by the home practitioners than by the hospital practitioners. Clearly the hospital practitioners believed that their aggressive technological approach improved outcomes, whereas the home delivery practitioners believed that much of this was unnecessary and occasionally even dangerous.

The format of pre-natal care was the same for both home and hospital practitioners, and followed that recommended by the American College of Obstetrics and Gynecology, with some exceptions in content. The home practitioners placed more emphasis on nutrition, the avoidance of pre-natal medication, and the psychosocial aspects of pregnancy than the hospital practitioners. Visits to the home birth groups typically lasted 20–60 minutes compared to 5–10 minutes for the hospital practitioners.

There was no limiting of the mother's weight gain by the home practitioners. It was felt that every woman should gain at least 25–35 lb (11–16 kg) during pregnancy, and the average weight gain was in the 30–35 lb (14–16 kg) range. Women were also counselled as to their diets and given iron-containing compounds when necessary to give a haemoglobin of greater than 12·0 mg per 100 ml. The home delivery practitioners were not bothered by weight gains of as much as 50–60 lb (23–27 kg), provided the woman was eating a high-protein, low-carbohydrate diet. It was felt that such weight gain was often necessary to prevent toxaemia of pregnancy in a woman with a protein-deficient diet prior to pregnancy. Blood pressures of greater than 140/90 were considered abnormal.

For the most part, the home delivery practitioners did not exclude a woman from being attended by them at her home because of a previously bad obstetrical history. It was felt that in most cases, complications occurring with previous pregnancies were due to or exacerbated by iatrogenic factors such as the limiting of weight gain, prescribing of diuretics, and providing of little or no nutritional counselling for toxaemia with prior pregnancies; accoucheur impatience or unwillingness to wait for previous low or mid-forceps deliveries; too many hospital interventions (inductions, medications) for previous still-born infants; excessive traction on the cord to deliver the placenta for previous haemorrhages, and the like. With very rare exceptions for women planning such deliveries regardless of who attended, they would not attend women with previous Caesarean sections at home. This primarily occurred when the woman could not find a hospital-based physician who would supervise a vaginal delivery after Caesarean section and decided to take her chances at home, regardless of who would come. The home practitioners also attended breech deliveries at home, believing that not all breeches were abnormal. One group used a combination of sonography and pelvimetry to make their decision. When there was 0·5 mm clearance on either side of the head when the biparietal diameter was subtracted from the smallest pelvic measurement, this group would attend the woman at home (provided she understood the increased theoretical risks and still planned to deliver at home). Another group used the Zatuchni–Andros breech scoring criteria and attended women at home who met the criteria for vaginal delivery, referring women to the hospital who met the criteria for Caesarean section. The lay midwives initially would not attend breech deliveries, but began doing so in response to the rising Caesarean section rate for the breech presentation in the United States.

Labour prolongation beyond a specified length of time was not defined as pathological and requiring intervention unless Friedman's (Friedman and Greenhill 1974) criteria for arrest of dilatation had been met or uterine inertia was diagnosed. Uterine inertia was usually treated initially with buccal oxytocin by the physicians at home, cautiously and in low concentrations, and, if results were not forthcoming, the woman was transported to the hospital for intravenous oxytocin. Neither was simple prolongation of the second stage of labour treated as a condition requiring intervention unless Friedman's criteria (Friedman and Greenhill 1974) for arrest of descent had been met or uterine inertia was diagnosed. The home delivery practitioners preferred a longer second stage lasting 2–3 hours or more to a shorter second stage characterized by an intense pushing effort on the part of the mother. It was felt that a gentle, longer delivery was preferable to a more intense, shorter delivery for both baby and mother. Intravenous oxytocin was not administered at home, nor were analgesics or anaesthetics. Forceps were not used in the home either. The midwives used a herbal mixture of cohosh, shepherd's purse, and liquorice root, which they felt was as useful as buccal oxytocin, for the initial treatment of uterine inertia at home.

The foetal heart-rate was followed closely throughout labour using a foetal stethoscope or an ultrasound foetoscope, and it was felt that, as Haverkamp, Thompson, McFee, and Cetrulo (1976) have confirmed, any change in heart-rate necessitating intervention would be noticed. Depending on the rate, regularity, and downward or upward trend, the heart-rate was auscultated from after every contraction (if an ominous pattern were suspected) to after every 20–45 minutes. During second stage, the foetal heart-rate was auscultated from after every contraction to after every 20 minutes, depending again on rate, regularity, downward or upward trends, and the rapidity of descent of the foetal head. Foetal distress was usually defined as a foetal heart-rate less than 105 per min during first stage, less than 100 per min during descent of the head to the perineum, and, with the head on the perineum, less than 80 per min during a contraction or less than 90–100 per min between contractions. Blood pressures were checked approximately every 1–3 hours during labour. The foetal heart-rate was occasionally listened to during and after a contraction to determine the presence or absence of any abnormal patterns.

Meconium-stained amniotic fluid was not considered evidence of foetal distress without a falling foetal heart-rate pattern. Meconium staining alone was not treated with intubation and lavage of the infant after delivery unless there had been a significant foetal heart-rate drop sufficient to stimulate breathing *in utero*. Rupture of membranes longer than 24 hours was followed at home if labour was progressing but if rupture of membranes had persisted for 24–48 hours without labour, the woman was usually transported to the hospital for induction of labour. It was felt that within the less bacteriologically pathogenic atmosphere of the home, intervention within 24 hours was not necessary to prevent infection assuming middle or better socio-economic status women with good hygiene. It is interesting to note that, for full-term infants, Sacks and Baker (1967) and Lebhery (1962) found little indication for aggressive intervention among a middle-class population whereas Russell and Anderson (1961) and Ekvall (1962) found that aggressive intervention improved outcome among a lower-class population (all delivering within a hospital).

Initially the midwives (but not the physicians) attending home deliveries taught the parents perineal massage and stretching exercises to prevent tearing. These exercises were usually begun 8 weeks prior to delivery and practised 5–15 minutes daily. As time passed, all groups began using these methods. It is felt by all that these exercises reduced the incidence of lacerations and obviated the need for episiotomy.

The room in which the delivery occurred was kept warm and the baby was given to the mother immediately after delivery to hold and nurse with blankets placed around the infant to prevent heat loss. The efficacy of this has been demonstrated by Phillips (1974) and Dahm and James (1972). The umbilical cord was not clamped and cut until it ceased pulsating except in Rh-negative mothers in whom it was clamped immediately. Silver nitrate ophthalmic drops were not routinely applied to the infant's eyes unless there had been a past history of gonorrhoea or one or both parents were unsure of the other. Virtually all infants were fed *ad lib* by breast without glucose or formula supplementation. It was felt that this *ad lib* feeding situation prevented neonatal hypoglycaemia.

The home birth practitioners did not feel that the risks introduced by age (women 17 years or under or 40 years or older) were sufficient to preclude a home delivery, although these labours were followed more closely than their mid-age-range counterparts. Likewise, gestations up to 44 weeks were not thought to preclude a home delivery. By 44 weeks or more, the woman would still be attended at home if weekly stress tests (done in the hospital) were negative.

Primigravidae were routinely attended at home (unlike in Britain). It was felt that the home was the ideal place for the primigravidae, since these labours tended to be longer and needed the comfort of family, friends, and the home environment more than shorter labours. It was also felt that the hospital practitioners tended to intervene more often with primigravida labours and that this could be avoided in the home. The physicians also attended the birth of twins at home, assuming the parents understood the theoretical risks and planned a home delivery regardless. Women with systemic medical disease such as cardiovascular disease, diabetes, hypertension, renal disease, and the like were not attended at home. The distance from home to hospital ranged from 1 min to 90 min, and transport was by car.

Home visits were made each day for the first 3 days by a nurse, midwife, or physician. Physiological jaundice was usually not treated unless levels were greater than 16–17 mg per 100 ml, and then, occasionally, by using Gro-lights at home, rather than with phototherapy in the hospital. The infants and mothers were observed for signs of other complications at the home visits.

Studies of medical outcomes

The initial studies of the medical outcomes of home delivery in the United States were all descriptive and suffered from the absence of a comparable hospital population from which to draw conclusions. Mehl et al. (1975) studied the medical outcomes of the 287 home deliveries attended from 1971 to 1973 by the 10 Santa Cruz County lay midwives described earlier. It was felt that, if there was to be a significant complication rate associated with home delivery, it would be apparent in this group whose clients were of a somewhat lower socio-economic class, and tended to be more from the counter-culture, than the remainder of the home delivery population. Their attendants also tended to have less medical training than the other services. The results were favourable, with a neonatal mortality of 0·0 per 1000 and a perinatal mortality of 3·5 per 1000. There were 3 post-partum haemorrhages, one neurologically abnormal infant (the average length of follow-up was 4·0 months), and lower levels of foetal distress, labour dystocia, meconium staining, and the like, than are usually reported in the literature for hospital deliveries.

In a study of a larger population of home deliveries comprising 1146 deliveries of the first five services already described, similar good results were obtained (Mehl et al. 1976a). Although suffering from not having a hospital comparison population, this study is of value in that it details the rate of occurrence of complications among a large group of home deliveries attended according to the philosophies of the practitioners already described, in order that parents contemplating home delivery could make a more informed choice regarding risks and benefits, as could professionals potentially planning to attend home deliveries. Table 7.1 presents the statistics on the presentations and deliveries. Of the 21 breech presentations, 10 delivered successfully at home by choice, and 11 were unsuspected by lay midwives and were transported to the hospital without mishap. Six sets of twins were planned to deliver at home and did so without mishap.

Table 7.1 Characteristics of presentation and delivery

	Number	Per cent
Presentation: total	1146	100·0
Vertex	1125	98·2
Brow	(3)	(0·3)
Shoulder	(3)	(0·3)
Breech	21	1·8
Delivery: total	1146	100·0
Caesarean	28	2·4
Vaginal	1118	97·6
Analgesia, only	14	1·2
Anaesthesia, only	3	0·3
Both	6	0·5
None	1095	95·5
Oxytocin		
First and second stage labour	85	7·4
Third stage labour	235	20·5
Low forceps	11	1·0
Mid forceps	6	0·5
Lacerations requiring repair	148	12·9
Episiotomies	89	7·8

It is also interesting to note that the incidence of perineal tears was 5 per cent among home births attended by lay midwives and 40 per cent among those attended by physicians. As the physicians gained experience and adopted the gentle head delivery techniques of the lay midwives and the pre-natal massage techniques, their incidence of lacerations and episiotomies significantly dropped.

Interestingly (and contrary to the British supposition), the total number

Table 7.2 Reasons for transportation to the hospital and therapy applied

Complication†	Physicians N = 58	Midwives N = 78	Statistical significance‡
First stage complications			
No prenatal care			
Dehydration → IV hydration	1	0	NS
Severe toxaemia → Caesarean	0	1	NS
Prolonged rupture of			
membranes → induction	0	4	$p < 0.01$
Dystocia 1st stage (excluding CPD)			
Uterine inertia → oxytocin	7	19	$p < 0.001$
Labour prolongation with ↓ FHT →			
internal monitor and oxytocin	1	0	NS
Arrest of dilation			
Involving ↓ FHT and uterine			
inertia → internal monitor and			
oxytocin	1	0	NS
Brow presentation → oxytocin and			
low forceps	1	0	NS
Arrest and uterine inertia →			
oxytocin low forceps	0	2	NS
Arrest → CPD, Caesarean	10	7	NS
Arrest → FHT nuchal cord × 4 →			
Caesarean	1	0	NS
Hypertension: Treated with			
Magnesium sulphate	1	0	NS
untreated	5	0	NS
Bleeding during labour → no treatment	1	0	NS
Amnionitis → antibiotics	1	0	NS
Fear, desire for hospital	2	6	$p < 0.05$
Desire for anaesthesia			
Anaesthesia given	3	0	NS
Analgesia only	1	0	NS
Hyperemesis → IVs and compazine	1	0	NS
Dropping FHTs			
No therapy, monitor applied	0	4	$p < 0.001$
Caesarean section	0	1	NS
Cord prolapse → Caesarean	0	1	NS
With meconium → intubation	0	3	$p < 0.025$
Psychotic reaction to labour →			
Caesarean	0	1	NS

Complication†	Physicians $N = 58$	Midwives $N = 78$	Statistical significance‡
Second stage complications			
Protracted descent			
Treated with low forceps (1 FHT↓)	4	2	NS
Treated with mid forceps with FHT↓	2	1	NS
Treated with oxytocin	5	9	NS
Arrest			
CPD, Caesarean section	4	2	NS
Abnormal presentation, mid forceps	1	1	NS
Brow presentation, low forceps	0	1	NS
Dropping FHTs			
Low forceps	1	0	NS
With meconium → oxytocin, intubation	0	2	NS
Mid forceps	1	0	NS
Bleeding → oxytocin	0	1	NS
Third stage complications			
Retained placenta → manual removal	2	5	$p < 0.05$
Haemorrhage → oxytocin, meth., blood	1	4	$p < 0.025$
Cervical laceration → suturing	0	1	NS

† sums of complications
‡ based on total Ns (685 and 461, respectively)
FHT = foetal heart tone
Meth. = methergin (Methylergonovine)

of complications of labour and delivery found in this study were comparable for primigravidae and multigravidae. The incidence of labour dystocia, foetal distress, meconium staining, post-partum haemorrhage, and post-partum depression were all low compared to the literature (Eastman and Hellman 1966; Friedman and Greenhill 1974; Klaus and Fanaroff 1973; Friedman 1973). There were significantly few differences between the outcomes obtained by physicians and lay midwives, the minor exceptions being related to training and the paucity of emergency equipment which the lay midwives brought to deliveries. Table 7.2 lists the reasons given for transporting women to the hospital with broad categories of therapy applied.

There was no maternal mortality or residual morbidity. Infant morbidity and perinatal outcome are summarized in Tables 7.3 and 7.4. The total

Table 7.3 Infant morbidity

Condition	Number	Rate per 1000 live births	Delivery	Complications	Outcome
Congenital defects	6	5·2			
PDA			Home	None	Repaired surgically at 1 year
Coarctation of aorta			Home	None	Repaired surgically at 2 years
Omphalocele			Home	None	Repaired surgically at 15 hours
Myelomeningocele, thoracic			Home	None	Mental and motor retardation at 18 months
Multiple minor anomalies			Hosp.	$FHT\downarrow,\bar{c},\bar{s}$	No mental or motor retardation at 1 year
Down's syndrome			Home	Meconium	Mental retardation
Cerebral palsy	2	1·7	Home	Meconium$+++$ $FHT\downarrow$	Motor retardation
			Home	None	Mild spastic with slow verbal development
Surgical conditions	2	1·7	Home	None	Pyloric stenosis repaired at 5 and 8 days
Low birthweight	15	13·1	Hosp.	Second-trimester bleed	1·332 kg, in hospital 1 month, no problems
			Home	None	1·729 kg, in hospital 2 weeks, mild RDS
			Home	Breech	2·154 kg, in hospital 12 days, mild RDS
Others			Home	None	No problems

PDA = patent ductus arteriosis
RDS = respiratory distress syndrome

prematurity rate including mothers screened out earlier was 3·0 per cent. Forty infants (3·5 per cent) had 1-minute Apgar scores of 4–6 and seven infants (0·6 per cent) had 1-minute Apgar scores of 3 or less and required resuscitation. At 11·5-months-average follow-up of all the infants, four (0·3 per cent) were neurologically abnormal: 2 with cerebral palsy and 2 with mental retardation. Over 80 per cent of the infants were followed to 6 months. Table 7.5 lists the causes of perinatal death. The average cost for physician-directed deliveries was $325.00 for mother and baby; the comparable hospital figure was $1450.00.

Table 7.4 Perinatal outcome

	Number	Study rate	California rate —1973
Total births†	1152		
Live births†	1147		
Foetal deaths‡	5	4·3	10·2
Neonatal deaths	6	5·2	10·3
Total perinatal deaths‡	11	9·5	20·3
Low birthweight (< 2·501 kg)	15	1·3 per cent	6·4 per cent

† Includes 6 sets of twins
‡ Foetal and perinatal death-rates are based on 1000 total births; neonatal death-rates on 1000 live births.

Cox, Fox, Zinkin, and Mathews (1976) studied 155 home deliveries in the West Middlesex area of Great Britain. For the entire area, the perinatal mortality was 21·7 per 1000, for which 1745 were born in the hospital and 155 attempted delivery at home. Cox noted that 39 per cent of these 155 women had one or more recognized 'risk' factors and that 15 should not have been accepted for home confinement: six were primigravidae, seven grand multiparae, and one had a previous intrauterine death at 24 weeks. It is interesting to note that all of these women would have been accepted by the United States home delivery practitioners. Cox et al. also suggest that 46 of these mothers (30 per cent) should have been referred for a hospital delivery during pregnancy: nine had diastolic blood pressure readings of 90 mm Hg or over on more than one occasion, two had a haemoglobin level of less than 9·5 g per 100 ml, one had an ante-partum haemorrhage, eighteen were more than 42 weeks' gestation, and six women had low weight gain between 32 and 36 weeks (less than 900 g). With the exception of the woman with the ante-partum haemorrhage, all these women would have been attended at home by the California groups provided their haemo-

Table 7.5 Causes of perinatal death

Age at death	Number	Delivery	Complications	Cause of death
5 months estimated gestational age	1	Home	None	Rh incompatibility, insisted on home delivery
35 weeks estimated gestational age	2	Home	None	Intrauterine death, unknown cause
During labour	1	Hosp.	Amnionitis: IUD in place	Overwhelming intrauterine sepsis
During labour	1	Home	None	Unknown cause
2 days	1	Hosp.	None	Macrosomia, single umbilical artery, bilateral adrenal hemorrhage, numerous congenital anomalies
7 days	1	Home	None	Cystic fibrosis, meconium ilius, post-operative perotinitis and sepsis.
7 days	1	Home	None	Coarctation of aorta
10 days	1	Home	None	Cor biloculare
2 weeks	1	Home	None	Sudden infant death syndrome
3 weeks	1	Home	None	Post-surgery for tetralogy of Fallot

globins rose and their blood pressures did not rise above 140/90. Fourteen mothers had induction of labour at home (which the California practitioners would not have done), five for hypertension (also not done in California). Cox *et al.* (1976) were also concerned with first stages of labour lasting longer than 12 hours and with one primipara who had a second stage of 110 minutes. These were well within the ranges of the California practitioners. Cox *et al.* objected to the delivery of nine women at home with the occiput posterior presentation, because of the greater need for forceps and medication —the avoidance of which for this same presentation caused the California home delivery practitioners to feel that the occiput posterior presentation usually did better at home. These discrepancies between what Cox *et al.* consider high-risk mothers needing the benefits of hospital care and the ways in which home delivery practitioners define the abnormal are illustrative of the basic philosophical differences between most home and hospital practitioners.

Cox *et al.* (1976) report the neonatal outcomes of these 155 deliveries. There was one case of foetal bradycardia (0·6 per cent), seven cases of meconium-stained amniotic fluid (4·5 per cent), and two infants requiring resuscitation (1·3 per cent). Three women were transported to the hospital during labour (1·9 per cent)—one because of a compound presentation, one because of a breech presentation, and one unspecified. Cox *et al.* also criticize the home delivery practitioners for not referring one infant with a birthweight of less than 2·500 kg and seven with a birthweight below the tenth percentile for gestational age to special-care hospital neonatal units. This would not have been done either by the California practitioners, their reasoning being that the babies could be observed at home and were better off with their mothers and families away from the hospital with its high tendency towards intervention, unless intervention became clearly necessary. This also highlights Cox *et al.*'s criticism of the West Middlesex home delivery practitioners' failure to carry out serum bilirubin determinations on five babies which Cox *et al.* considered deeply jaundiced at the end of the first week. Again, the British home delivery practitioners, seemingly, as the California practitioners, appeared to have higher thresholds for intervention. There was no reported maternal or infant mortality or residual morbidity among the 155 deliveries.

On the basis of these findings Cox *et al.* (1976) conclude that efforts should be increased to achieve 100 per cent hospital confinement. It is clear from their bias why they would conclude this, although it does not seem to necessarily follow from their data. The real question is if the occurrence of all these 155 deliveries, or of the 1146 California home deliveries, within the hospital would have improved the medical and psychological outcome for these mothers, babies, and families. For answers to these questions, carefully matched comparison studies are needed.

Fryer and Ashford (1972) have stated that, although the perinatal mortality rate in Great Britain fell until 1967 with increasing hospital delivery, this trend had reversed itself since 1967. They maintained that there was no objective evidence that more than a few deliveries taking place in hospitals enjoyed services substantially better than could be provided in the patient's own home by an effective home birth service. In Cardiff, Wales, recent data suggests that a change in the past decade from largely home- to largely hospital-delivered babies has had essentially no effect on maternal or neonatal outcome (Chalmers, Zleshih, Johns, and Campbell 1976).

Other studies have reported low levels of complications associated with home deliveries, including a prospective series of 465 deliveries in the Washington, D.C., an area attended by an obstetrician and nurse–midwife (Brew 1976), 100 deliveries in Oklahoma City, Oklahoma, attended by an obstetrician (Taylor 1976), a report of 25 years' experience with both home and hospital delivery by a Chicago family physician (White 1976), 300 home deliveries in the San Francisco Bay Area attended by a lay midwife (Hazell 1974, 1975), and a series of deliveries from Los Angeles, California supervised by a nurse–obstetrician team (Berman 1976). Palu, Bennett, Mehl, and Creevy (1976) in a study of the last year of operation of the Chicago Maternity Center's supervision of home deliveries suggested that the utilization of common obstetrical practices at home such as the administration of analgesia or anaesthesia, the use of forceps or intravenous oxytocin augmentation, and artificial rupture of membranes tended to increase risk beyond acceptable limits for a home delivery. Their conclusion was that hospital practitioners with an interventionist tendency could probably practice safely *only* in the hospital, and that a non-interventionist mental set was required of a good home birth attendant.

Home–hospital comparison studies

The first home–hospital comparison study was one by Mehl *et al.* (1976*b*) which compared 200 women attended in the hospital by a group of practitioners also attending home deliveries to the larger California home sample. All these women met the criteria for home delivery had they desired to do such. The populations were very similar in attitudes towards childbirth, desire to avoid labour medications, and the like, although the planned hospital group tended to be less staunch advocates of these positions, to have more education, and to be of higher socio-economic status.

Table 7.6 presents the statistics on the comparisons between the two groups' presentations and deliveries. It is important to note that these women's attendants had the same philosophies as the home delivery attendants, so that a difference in obstetrical orientation was not the cause of these differences, although it is possible that simply being in the hospital environment with its atmosphere and felt expectations skewed these practitioners towards making more pathological judgements and/or interventions. Other possible causes for these differences speculated upon included the increased use of analgesia, anaesthesia, and/or oxytocin, the effects of the hos-

Table 7.6 Characteristics of presentation and delivery

	Total		Home		Hospital		Statistical significance
	Number	Percentage	Number	Percentage	Number	Percentage	
Presentation							
Vertex	1146	100.0	1125	98.2	167	93.8	$p < 0.005$
Brow			3	(0.3)	0	—	—
Shoulder			3	(0.3)	1	0.6	—
Breech			21	1.8	9	5.1	$p < 0.01$
Delivery							
Caesarean	1146	100.0	28	2.4	10	5.6	$p < 0.025$
Vaginal			1118	97.6	168	93.8	$p < 0.025$
Analgesia only			14	(1.2)	9	5.0	$p < 0.025$
Anaesthesia only			3	(0.3)	3	1.7	—
Both			6	(0.5)	1	0.6	—
None			1095	95.5	154	86.5	$p < 0.001$
Oxytocin							
1st and 2nd stage labour			85	7.4	29	15.3	$p < 0.001$
3rd stage labour			235	20.5	54	30.3	$p < 0.005$
Low forceps			11	1.0	7	3.9	$p < 0.001$
Mid forceps			6	0.5	2	1.1	$p < 0.001$
Lacerations requiring repair			148	12.9	26	15.6	NS
Episiotomies			89	7.8	42	25.1	$p < 0.001$

Table 7.7 Perinatal outcome

	Home		California State 1973	Statistical significance	Hospital	
	Number	Rate			Number	Rate
Total births	1152†				180‡	
Live births	1147†				180‡	
Foetal deaths	5	4·3§	8·2§*	NS	1	5·5§
Neonatal deaths	6	5·2¶	10·3¶	NS	1	5·5¶
Total perinatal deaths	11	9·5§	20·3§	NS	2	11·1§
Low birthweight (2·501 kg)	15	1·3¶	5·3¶*	NS	3	1·7¶
Mean length of infant follow-up	11·5 months			NS	11·6 months	
S.D. length of follow-up	±10·3 months			NS	±10·4 months	
Percentage of infants followed to 6 months	83·4 per cent			NS	82·2 per cent	

† Includes 6 sets of twins
‡ Includes 2 sets of twins
§ Per 1000 total births
¶ Per 1000 live births
* For white, non-Spanish surname, age 20–29

pital environment on labour, poor matching between populations, and/or a clustering effect which would diminish differences between the two groups with a larger series of hospital deliveries. Table 7.7 presents the comparison complication figures for the perinatal outcome data.

The most recently completed study of home delivery (Mehl *et al.* 1976c) does begin to answer more of the questions regarding relative safety of home versus hospital. In this study, 1046 home deliveries were compared with 1046 hospital deliveries, matched on a case-by-case basis for maternal age, risk factors, gestational length, parity, education, and socio-economic status. As has been true for all the studies previously discussed, the home delivery sample included all those women planning to deliver at home immediately prior to the initiation of labour, rupture of membranes, or emergence of

Table 7.8 Characteristics of the mothers

	Home		Hospital		
	Number	Percentage	Number	Percentage	Statistical significance
Mother's age					
20	23	2·2	23	2·2	
20–34	1004	96·0	1004	96·0	
35	19	1·8	19	1·8	
Mean age		25.2		25.2	
Parity					
0	611	57·7	611	57·7	
1	263	24·3	263	24·3	
2	118	10·4	118	10·4	
3	33	2·2	33	2·2	
4	9	0·9	9	0·9	
5	4	0·4	4	0·4	
6	1	0·1	1	0·1	
Years of education		13·5		14·6	$p < 0·10$
Length of gestation					
Average (weeks)		39·8		39·8	
38 weeks	54	5·2	54	5·2	
42 weeks	91	8·7	91	8·7	
Birthweight, mean		3·518 kg		3·439 kg	NS
Labour length					
parity 0, 1st stage		14·5 h		10·4 h	$p < 0·01$
parity 0, 2nd stage		94·7 min		63·9 min	$p < 0·05$
parity 1, 1st stage		8·5 h		5·9 h	$p < 0·01$
parity 1, 2nd stage		48·7 min		19·0 min	$p < 0·005$
parity 2, 1st stage		7·7 h		6·6 h	NS
parity 2, 2nd stage		21·7 min		15·9 min	NS
3rd stage		21·0 min		4·6 min	$p < 0·005$

a complication necessitating immediate hospitalization and delivery.

Table 7.8 presents demographic and labour characteristics of the two populations. Education attained and socio-economic status were matched so that the hospital group had the same educational and/or socio-economic level as the home birth group or higher. Some significant differences in labour length emerge, too, in that for women of parity 0 or 1, the length of first and second stage were significantly longer for the women delivering at home. Third stage was also significantly longer for women delivering at home.

Table 7.9 presents a summary of risk factors and a distribution of the types of practitioners attending deliveries in the two groups. The average risk score was 1·6 and 9·2 per cent were considered high risk in each group by the Nova Scotia criteria. Data are presented up to 4 days of age for each group, the time of hospital discharge. In work in progress, we are attempting to extend the follow-up of both populations to 1 year of age.

Table 7.9 Pre-natal risk factors

	Home		Hospital		
	Number	Percentage	Number	Percentage	Statistical significance
Presentation					
Vertex	1022	97·7	1022	97·7	NS
Brow	1	0·1	1	0·1	NS
Arm and head	3	0·3	2	0·2	NS
Breech	19	1·8	17	1·6	NS
Transverse lie	0	0·0	2	0·2	NS
Face presentation	1	0·2	2	0·2	NS
Twins	5	0·5	5	0·5	NS
Pre-existing hypertension	5	0·5	6	0·6	NS
Pre-eclampsia, mild	2	0·2	2	0·2	NS
Previous Caesarean	1	0·1	1	0·1	NS
Obstetrician attended	0	0·0	783	74·9	$p < 0.0001$
Family physician attended	696	66·5	263	25·1	$p < 0.005$
Lay midwife attended	322	30·8	0	0·0	$p < 0.0001$
Nurse–midwife attended	28	2·7	0	0·0	$p < 0.005$
Average risk factor score	1·6		1·6		NS
High risk (risk factor 3)	96	9·2	96	9·2	NS

Table 7.10 presents a summary of the procedures used during the deliveries of each of the two groups. The hospital practitioners used significantly more oxytocin, both before and after delivery. In home births, buccal oxytocin was administered for uterine inertia, and, if no results were forthcoming, intravenous oxytocin after hospital transport. Many more forceps deliveries were performed by the hospital practitioners, as well as more Caesarean sections. Despite a nine-fold greater incidence of episiotomies, the hospital delivered women sustained significantly more second, third, fourth degree, and cervical lacerations. Analgesia and anaesthesia were also used much more frequently. No caudal anaesthesia was administered in the hospital group, however. (Analgesia, anaesthesia, and forceps deliveries were given or performed only after transport to the hospital for the home-birth group.) The

Table 7.10 Intervention procedures used

	Home		Hospital		
	Number	Percentage	Number	Percentage	Statistical significance
lst stage oxytocin	69	6·6	159	15·2	$p < 0.0001$
2nd stage oxytocin	38	3·6	159	15·2	$p < 0.0001$
Total pre-partum cases	76	7·3	173	16·5	$p < 0.0001$
3rd stage oxytocin	251	24·0	993	95·0	$p < 0.0001$
Mid (low) forceps†	10	0·9	205	19·6	$p < 0.0001$
Low (outlet) forceps†	3	0·3	115	11·0	$p < 0.0001$
Mid forceps rotations	3	0·3	40	3·8	$p < 0.001$
Manual rotations	0	0·0	5	0·5	NS
Caesarean sections	28	2·7	86	8·2	$p < 0.05$
Episiotomy	103	9·8	914	87·4	$p < 0.0001$
1st degree lacerations	18	1·7	18	1·7	NS
2nd degree lacerations	136	13·0	56	5·4	$p < 0.0001$
3rd degree lacerations	8	0·7	44	4·3	$p < 0.001$
4th degree lacerations	5	0·5	73	7·0	$p < 0.0001$
Cervical lacerations	3	0·3	32	3·2	$p < 0.0005$
Pudendal anaesthesia	0	0·0	655	62·6	$p < 0.0001$
General anaesthesia	2	0·2	96	9·2	$p < 0.0001$
Paracervical block	1	0·1	52	5·0	$p < 0.0001$
Manual removal of placenta	15	1·4	15	1·4	NS
Analgesia	14	1·3	555	53·1	$p < 0.0001$
Caudal anaesthesia	32	3·0	0	0·0	$p < 0.0005$

†Forceps definitions are based upon American College of Obstetrics and Gynecology definitions. From observation it was determined that outlet forceps (not defined by the American College of Obstetrics and Gynecology) were equivalent to low, and low equivalent to mid (see text).

incidence of manual removal of the placenta was the same in both groups.

The differences in the indications for oxytocin for the two groups were seen to emerge from greater use of oxytocin in the hospital group for rupture of membranes without labour, first stage uterine inertia, and for elective induction. More oxytocin was used in the home group for second stage uterine inertia than in the hospital group. Typically, the home birth group waited longer, occasionally longer than 24 hours, before initiating oxytocin therapy.

The majority of the hospital practitioners used the criterion of a second stage of labour longer than 1 hour as an indication for forceps delivery. The home birth practitioners typically accepted any length of second stage as long as some progress was evident and there were no signs of foetal distress. This difference in approach is reflected in the greater number of forceps deliveries in the hospital for 'prolonged second stage'. The hospital practitioners used occiput posterior as an indication for forceps rotation and did not permit any patient to deliver occiput posterior, whereas the home birth practitioners did not intervene in the occiput posterior labours and deliveries unless signs of labour arrest or foetal distress were present. This is reflected in the higher number of mid forceps rotations in the hospital group. The two groups of practitioners also defined the same type of forceps delivery by different terms. For the home group, a low forceps delivery was equivalent to a hospital practitioner's outlet forceps delivery and a mid forceps delivery was equivalent to a low forceps delivery. The home birth practitioners' definitions were the same as the American College of Obstetrics and Gynecology definitions and those of Friedman and Greenhill (1974). There were also significantly more forceps deliveries in the hospital delivery for foetal distress.

The hospital group did many more Caesarean sections for first stage arrest, cephalopelvic disparoportion, and/or non-progressive labour than did the home birth practitioners, and did more Caesarean sections for primigravida breech presentations and for foetal distress. From the table, it is also evident that the indications for Caesarean section were more liberal for the hospital group than for the home group.

Of the complications of labour and delivery for the two groups, the hospital group had significantly more intra-uterine foetal distress, elevated blood pressure during labour (from a non-elevated pre-labour baseline), meconium staining, and reported shoulder dystocia. The home group had more second stage labour dystocia, bleeding during labour, and occiput posterior deliveries. The hospital group had significantly more post-partum haemorrhages.

Turning to neonatal complications: the hospital group experienced significantly more birth injuries and neonatal infections: the baby received significantly more oxygen for 2, 3, 4, and 5 or more minutes, had more respiratory distress lasting 12 hours or more among full-term infants, and more total non-congenital neonatal complications. The hospital group neonates required more resuscitation, and had lower 1-minute and 5-minute Apgar scores than the home group. There was no significant difference in the incidence of foetal, intra-partum, or neonatal deaths, or in the incidence of neurologically abnormal infants. 113 mothers and/or infants were transported to the hospital from home either to complete their delivery or for resolution of a post-partum problem. 101 of these were for problems relating to delivery, 6 mothers for post-partum problems, and 6 infants transporting to neonatal intensive-care units.

Given two matched populations, Mehl *et al.* (1976*c*) concluded that outcome differences should accrue from the events occurring during labour and delivery, and that, for the home delivery population described, one could expect an outcome for baby and mother essentially as good as that resulting from a medically matched population delivering in hospitals providing high standards of medical care. In fact, for certain parameters of outcome, the home birth group fared better than their hospital counterparts. To explain this, it could be said that the hospital environment may alter the perceptions of the birth attendants so that the normal is perceived as pathological. Most of the aggressive management encountered in the hospital, including forceps delivery after one hour in the second stage, liberal Caesarean section, routine episiotomy, liberal use of oxytocin augmentation to labour, and so on, is thought by many to improve outcome, but this study showed that this may not be so, and speculated that aggressive management may tend to increase risk. As regards this, Friedman (1973) has noted increased mortality following elective mid forceps delivery. As an example of the possible superfluousness of some aspects of hospital procedure, the incidence of maternal infection was the same in the two groups and the incidence of neonatal infection was higher in the hospital. In the hospital surgical asepsis was maintained, whereas in the home the only sterile protection used were gloves worn by the attendant along with clean (non-sterile) towels or pads beneath the mother. The hospital's emphasis on asepsis did not seem to change the incidence of infection over the home born infants.

Mehl *et al.* (1976*c*) continued to conclude that, for low-risk women, home delivery is an alternative that cannot be dismissed as contra-indicated because of unacceptable high risk to maternal and infant health, and that pilot projects for out-of-hospital deliveries should be planned and encouraged.

Psychological outcome studies

Very little data has been reported for the psychological effects of childbirth on women, infants, and families. Peterson, Mehl, and Leiderman (1976*a*, *b*) studied the role of prenatal attitude, birth experience, birth environment, anaesthesia, and parent–infant separation on maternal and paternal attachment among three different childbirth experiences—anaesthetized childbirth, natural childbirth in the hospital, and home delivery. For mothers, the most important variables in determining attachment were birth experience, presence or absence of separation, and anaesthesia. For fathers, birth experience tended to be all important. The higher quality the birth experience—that is, the more the father touched the mother during labour, participated in labour and delivery, and felt involved—the more attached he was. For the mothers, this held along with avoidance of separation and anaesthesia.

The contribution of birth experience as an important variable increased as one progressed in the continuum from anaesthetized hospital delivery to home delivery, leading Peterson *et al.* (1976*a*, *b*) to conclude that, as the couple became more involved in taking control for and planning their own birth experience, in educating themselves for childbirth, and in preparing for the actual delivery, the contribution of other variables such as the parents' own parenting, their prior acculturation, and emotional–personality factors diminished as the importance of birth experience increased. This led them to suggest a model for intervention for individuals and couples at risk of parenting difficulties which used childbirth education to alter expectations, beliefs, and acculturations and to provide new role models and which used interventions into the delivery environment to humanize it and augment the birth experience. In a case report, Mehl *et al.* (1976*d*) reported the use of these techniques to help a woman, both pre-natally and during labour, work through guilt feelings regarding the prior adoption of an unwanted pregnancy. These interventions were carried out within the framework of a hospital delivery.

In another study, Peterson *et al.* (1976*c*) examined the effects of delivery on the self-esteem of women. Anaesthetized hospital delivery was found to have a humiliating effect with decreases in self-esteem, whereas natural hospital, and more so, home delivery, tended to increase self-worth and self-esteem, and in several cases, resulted in major increases in creativity and in breakthroughs in resolving personal problems. More symptoms of post-partum depression were present in the anaesthetized hospital deliveries and decreased in the continuum from an anaesthetized hospital to home delivery. All of these studies were carried out among 60 middle- to upper-middle class families in the Palo Alto to Santa Cruz area of California.

Conclusions

It is interesting to speculate about what may be responsible for good outcomes of childbirth from any perspective, but what is clearly apparent is that we are just beginning to uncover the important factors, and, however important this process may be, it should remain secondary to the parents' right to use whatever data is available to make an intelligent, informed choice about the kind of childbirth experience they will have. The studies reviewed here have indicated that a number of childbirth options are safe medical alternatives. The final decision must always remain the parents', for they live the rest of their lives upon that choice—not for an instant as do obstetricians, family physicians, midwives, researchers, and statisticians; and clearly, if parents had to wait for researchers to prove their own personal values and needs, attachment would have never occurred. Both options, then, must be viewed as an existential decision-making process wherein benefits and risks, and issues regarding quality of experience are weighed as they relate to the personal values of that individual/couple.

It is interesting to speculate on some other additional factors which may bear on perinatal outcome. Kennell *et al.* (1976) recently found that immediate post-natal mother–infant contact decreased the rate of neonatal infections over controls. Haverkamp *et al.* (1976) have shown, for high-risk patients, that nurse auscultation provides slightly better outcomes than foetal monitoring, with more patient satisfaction. Newton, Foshee, and Newton (1966) and Newton, Peller, and Newton (1968) have shown experimental inhibition of labour in animals through environmental disturbances. Bergström-Walen (1963) found a significant difference in the average duration of labour between women who attended childbirth education classes and controls matched for education and occupation. Similarly, Davidson (1962) found marked differences between a control group and a group of women who had had hypnosis in labour and hypnotic training sessions during their pregnancy, which sessions had included suggestions concerning the ease of labour with regard to length of labour. Haire (1972) has reviewed the deleterious effects of analgesia and anaesthesia on perinatal outcome along with the disadvantages of common hospital practices. Chan, Paul, and Toews (1973) and Shenker, Post, and Seider (1975) have reported improvements in intra-partum death-rates within their hospitals following institution of routine foetal monitoring which are not statistically significantly different from the intra-partum death-rates obtained in the home delivery series, confirming, as does Haverkamp, the value of an experienced nurse auscultator. Clearly these few examples illustrate that the current technological trend in childbirth does not have all the solutions and that other options such as home delivery need to be examined.

References

Arms, S. (1975). *Immaculate deception*. San Francisco Books.

Bergström-Walen, M. (1963). 'Efficacy of education for childbirth'. *Journal of Psychosomatic Research* 7, 131.

Berman, V. (1976). 'Comments on home delivery'. Paper presented at North American Psychosomatic Obstetrics and Gynaecology meeting, Chicago, 1976.

Brew, J. (1976). 'Outcomes of homebirth'. Paper presented at annual conference of National Association of Parents and Professionals for Safe Alternatives in Childbirth, Washington, D.C., 1976.

Chalmers, I., Zleshih, J. E. Johns, K. A., and Campbell, H. (1976). 'Obstetric practice and outcome of pregnancy in Cardiff residents 1965–73'. *British Medical Journal* i, 735–8.

Chan, W. H., Paul, R. H., and Toews, J. (1973). 'Intrapartum foetal monitoring'. *Obstetrics and Gynecology* **41**, 7–13.

Cox, C. A., Fox, J. S., Zinkin, P. M., and Mathews, A. E. B. (1976) 'Critical appraisal of domiciliary obstetric and neonal practice'. *British Medical Journal* **1**, 84–6.

Dahm, L. S. and James, L. S. (1972). 'Newborn temperature and calculated heat loss in the delivery room'. *Pediatrics* **49**, 504–13.

Davidson, J. A. (1962). 'An assessment of the value of hypnosis in pregnancy and labour'. *British Medical Journal* ii, 591.

Eastman, N. J. and Hellman, L. M. (1966). *William's Obstetrics*, p. 988. Appleton Century Crofts, New York.

Ekvall, L. D., Wixted, W. G., and Dyer, L. (1961). 'Spontaneous premature rupture of the fetal membranes'. *American Journal of Obstetrics and Gynecology* **81**, 848–58.

Friedman, E. A. (1973). 'Patterns of labor as indicators of risk'. *Clinical Obstetrics and Gynecology* **16**, 172–83.

Friedman, E. and Greenhill, P. (1974). *The biological basis of modern obstetrics*. W. B. Saunders & Co., Philadelphia.

Fryer, J. G. and Ashford, J. R. (1972). *British Journal of Preventive and Social Medicine* **26**, 1–4.

Haire, D. (1972). 'Cultural Warping of Childbirth'. *ICEA News* Special Issue, ICEA Supply House, Seattle, Washington.

Haverkamp, A. D., Thompson, H. E., McFee, J. G., and Cetrulo, C. (1976). 'The evaluation of continuous fetal heart rate monitoring in high risk pregnancy'. *American Journal of Obstetrics and Gynecology* **125**, 310–18.

Hazell, L. D. (1974). *Birth goes home*. Catalyst Press, Seattle, Washington.

—— (1975). 'A study of 300 elective home births'. *Birth and The Family Journal* **2**, 11–18.

Kennell, J. *et al.* (1976). 'Immediate postnatal contact and neonatal infections'. Paper presented at the Society for Pediatric Research meeting, St. Louis, Missouri, 1976.

Klaus, M. and Fanaroff, A. (1973). *Case of the high risk neonate*, p. 141. W. B. Saunders, Toronto.

Lang, R. (1972). *Birth book*. New Genesis Press, Felton, California.

Lebhery, T. B., Boyce, C. R., and Huston, J. W. (1960). 'Premature rupture of membranes: a statistical study from 7 U.S. Navy Hospitals'. *American Journal of Obstetrics and Gynecology* **81**, 658–65.

Mehl, L. F., Peterson, G. H., Shaw, N. S., and Creevy, D. C. (1975). 'Complications of home delivery'. *Birth and The Family Journal* **2**, 123–35.

——, ——, Whitt, M. C., and Hawes, W. H. (1976a). 'Outcomes of 1146 elective home deliveries'. Paper presented at North American Society of Psychosomatic Obstetrics and Gynecology meeting, Chicago, 1976.

——, ——, ——, and Creevy, D. C. (1976b). 'Outcomes of Elective Home Birth'. Paper presented at National Association of Parents and Professionals for Safe Alternatives in Childbirth meeting, Washington, D.C.

——, Leavitt, L. A., Peterson, G. H., and Creevy, D. C. (1976c). 'Home versus hospital delivery; comparisons of matched populations'. Paper presented at the annual meeting, American Public Health Association, 20 October, 1976, Miami Beach, Florida.

——, Peterson, G. H., Ruben, D. A., and Creevy, D. C. (1976*d*). 'Childbirth as psychotherapy'. Abstract submitted to American Psychiatric Association.

Newton, N., Foshee, D., and Newton, M. (1966). 'Environmental inhibition of labor through environmental disturbance'. *Obstetrics and Gynecology* **27**, 371–7.

——, Peller, D., and Newton, M. (1968). 'Effects of disturbance on labor'. *American Journal of Obstetrics and Gynecology* **101**, 1096–102.

Palu, M., Bennett, S., Mehl, L. E., and Creevy, D. C. (1976). 'Outcomes of elective home birth: comparisons with the Chicago maternity center and implications for screening'. Paper presented at International Childbirth Education Association Convention, Seattle, 1976.

Peterson, G. H., Mehl, L. E., and Leiderman, P. H. (1976*a*). 'Birth experience and prenatal attitude as predictors of paternal attachment'. Submitted to *Pediatrics*.

——, ——, and —— (1976*b*). 'Birth experience and prenatal attitude as predictors of maternal attachment'. Abstract submitted to the American Psychiatric Association.

——, ——, and —— (1976*c*). 'Effects of childbirth on the self-image of women. Abstract submitted to the American Psychiatric Association.

Phillips, C. R. N. (1974). 'Neonatal heat loss in heated cribs vs. mothers' arms'. *Journal of Obstetrics and Gynecology in Nursing* **3**, 11–15.

Russell, K. P. and Anderson, G. V. (1961). 'The aggressive management of ruptured membrane'. *American Journal of Obstetrics and Gynecology* **83**, 930–7.

Sachs, M. and Baker, T. H. (1967). 'Spontaneous premature rupture of the membranes'. *American Journal of Obstetrics and Gynecology* **97**, 888–93.

Seiden, A. (1976). 'The special psychology of women. *American Journal of Psychiatry*. (In press.)

Shenka, L., Post, R. C., and Seider, T. S. (1975). 'Routine electronic monitoring of the fetal heart rate and uterine activity during labor'. *Obstetrics and Gynecology* **46**, 185–9.

Sousa, M. (1976). *Childbirth at home*. Prentice-Hall, Englewood Cliffs, New Jersey.

Taylor, C. (1976). *Proceedings of the International Childbirth Education Association Convention*. ICEA Supply Center, Seattle.

Ward, C. and Ward, F. (1976). *The home birth book*. Inscape Press, Washington, D.C.

White, G. (1976). '25 years experience with home and hospital birth'. Paper presented at the North American Society for Psychosomatic Obstetrics and Gynecology meeting, Chicago, 1976.

LUKE ZANDER, MICHAEL LEE-JONES,
AND CHLOE FISHER

8

The role of the primary health care team in the management of pregnancy

This chapter deals with the organization of maternity care from the point of view of the primary health care team. In the first part a general practitioner in undergraduate and postgraduate education and a general practitioner obstetrician look at administration from the point of view of the general practitioner, and the second focuses on the changing role of the midwife, its opportunities, and some of its frustrations.

Introduction

Obstetric care has undergone much change over recent years with the introduction of many sophisticated techniques and development of a more 'active' approach to labour. One aspect of these developments has been the marked increase in the proportion of babies now delivered in hospital as detailed in other chapters of this book.

It is important to remember that the care of a woman during her pregnancy involves more than concern for the actual confinement. The manner in which an expectant mother is prepared for childbirth, both physically and psychologically, may well be relevant to how she will cope with the delivery, and similarly, her care during the early post-natal days may be of critical importance to the way in which she adapts to her new role as mother. The antenatal and post-natal stages, together with the delivery itself, form a natural continuum, and this should be reflected in the nature of the management that they receive.

The general practitioner (GP) has been defined as a doctor who provides personal, primary, and continuing medical care to individuals and families (Royal College of General Practitioners 1972). These characteristics suggest that he has an important role to play in the management of his patient's pregnancy. (The needs of the patient and her family should remain the central and overriding consideration of those responsible for her care.)

One of the more significant changes that have taken place recently in primary care in the United Kingdom has been the rapid development of group practices. In 1948 over two thirds of GPs were in single-handed practices, whereas by 1974 over 80 per cent were working either in partnerships or group practice. A direct result of this trend has been to encourage the attachment of paramedical staff, such as district nurses, midwives, and health visitors, with the development of the concept of a 'primary health care team'. Thus, rather than considering the role of the GP in obstetric care in isolation, it is more relevant to think in terms of a closely integrated group of doctors and nurses, with different and complementary expertise, comprising a team with responsibility for the continuing care of the mother, her baby, and the family.

In attempting to define the appropriate role of pregnancy it is important that the essential aspects of care are clearly identified.

Antenatal care

First antenatal visit

The objectives of the initial antenatal visit are:

1 *To make a general assessment of the patient in physical, psychological, and social terms.* It is widely accepted that full consideration should be given to the clinical aspects of the pregnancy and to the past and present medical status of the patient, but less often appreciated that a full assessment also encompasses an evaluation of the patient's state of mind and—of particular relevance—the attitude of both her and her husband towards the pregnancy. All these factors should be seen in the context of her family and home background.

2 *To establish a plan of management for the pregnancy.* It is important that if optimum care is to be achieved, due attention should be given to all relevant factors in the formulation of a plan of management. This necessarily includes the subjective feelings of the patient which may not be clearly formulated at an early stage of the pregnancy, and for this reason, as well as for that of a changing clinical picture, decisions should be provisional and always amenable to modification at a later time.

3 *To establish a relationship between the patient and her doctor and midwife.* The importance of achieving a satisfactory relationship lies in the fact that it is often the nature and quality of this that governs the extent to which the particular needs of the patient are identified and provided for. A doctor–patient relationship can ultimately be judged by the degree of real (and therefore *two*-way) communication that exists between the individuals concerned on issues that each considers to be of importance. One important way in which this can be developed is by encouraging the woman to be involved in all decisions relating to her pregnancy. If the doctor is able to share with her his findings and conclusions she will be able to understand the clinical basis of her ensuing care, and also to make her often very valuable contribution to the decision-making process. If en-

couraged to take a full part in this way it is also less likely that she will harbour fears and anxieties.

Subsequent antenatal visits

The purpose of the subsequent antenatal visits is to monitor the progress of the pregnancy. This includes assessing the physical and psychological state of the mother, the growth and development of the foetus, and the early detection of any signs indicating abnormality. At each visit the doctor and midwife need to check their findings against the initial management plan and be prepared to modify the plan accordingly, keeping the patient informed of the reasons for any change. Women whose antenatal care is being undertaken at the Specialist Clinic may benefit from a few visits to the GP and midwife which are, strictly speaking, clinically 'unnecessary' to maintain contact with those who will have the responsibility for the continuing care of her and her baby following the delivery.

At all visits an important task of each member of the health care team is to assist in the general adjustment of the woman to her pregnancy. We can look at this adjustment from several points of view. It entails a knowledge about pregnancy, childbirth, and early parenthood; the skills involved in the preparation for childbirth and the early post-natal period; and attitudes of both the patient and husband towards the birth, the coming baby, and the experience of pregnancy, all of which may be relevant to the way in which they develop and mature as individuals and as a couple. So that the antenatal care might achieve these objectives it should be organized so that:

1 regular clinical care is provided by professionals suitably trained and orientated to the needs of their patients;
2 the care should be acceptable to and made use of by the patients;
3 there should be a meaningful continuing personal relationship between the patient and her professional 'advisers' throughout the pregnancy;
4 the patient and her husband should be provided during the pregnancy with appropriate instruction classes on preparation for childbirth and parentcraft;
5 during the pregnancy the mother should get to know the setting in which she is to have her baby.

Antenatal care can be undertaken in either the hospital or general practice setting, irrespective of where the delivery is to be conducted. In many ways the two settings present marked contrasts, and yet often the choice of place is arbitrary with little consideration being given as to which is best. Table 8.1 summarizes the comparative advantages and disadvantages of the two settings. These contrasts indicate that there may be many advantages to a patient in having antenatal care given by her own doctor. This will invariably occur when a home confinement is planned, but can also take place when the delivery is arranged for hospital. In these circumstances a form of shared care is instituted, in which the patient attends her own doctor for a certain number of antenatal visits and at intermediate times attends the hospital antenatal clinic. The success of this form of combined management depends to a large extent on the degree of cooperation that exists between the GP and the hospital obstetric team, and the understanding that each has of the contribution that the other can make to antenatal care. If a GP obstetric unit exists in, or is closely related to, a specialist obstetric unit, this combined management is comparatively easy to arrange, but even when this is not the case close cooperation can be established. This is not always easy, however, especially in the large conurbations, and will often

Table 8.1 Where antenatal care takes place: the advantages and disadvantages of general practice and hospital settings

General practice setting	Hospital setting
Familiar surroundings	Unfamiliar surroundings
Likely to be easily accessible	Likely to be further from the home
Likely to have a short waiting time	Likely to have longer waiting time
Patient will usually see a doctor who is well known to her	Patient will see several doctors and midwives
A doctor–patient relationship will already be established at the onset of pregnancy and will continue after its completion	No doctor–patient relationship will exist at the onset of pregnancy and that which is established will be solely for the duration of the pregnancy
The midwife seen antenatally will often or usually be involved in the labour	The midwife seen antenatally will usually not be involved in the labour
A relationship can be established members of the team (the midwife and health visitor) who will later have responsibility for the continuing care of mother and baby	No contact can be established with those who later will have responsibility for the mother and her baby
The GP–obstetrician is also responsible for the general care of the patient	The obstetrician has no responsibility for the general care of the patient
The doctor is likely to be aware of the social background of the patient	The doctor will not usually be aware of the social background of the patient
The doctor will usually be aware of and actively concerned with the needs of the patient's family	The doctor will not be concerned with, and usually be unaware of, the needs of the patient's family
The doctor is not likely to be very knowledgeable about obstetric abnormalities but experienced in the process of normal labour	The doctor will be very knowledgeable and skilled in obstetric abnormalities but may have less personal experience with normal labour

require considerable effort from all concerned. The onus for establishing satisfactory contact usually lies with the GP, but as has been successfully demonstrated by the Professorial Unit of St. Thomas' Hospital (Zander, L., Taylor, R., and Morrell, D. C. M., personal communication), the obstetrician can also 'take the lead' and come out into the district to undertake his antenatal care. Contrary to expectations, instead of this being an extravagant use of resources, it is an arrangement that can allow the obstetrician (together with the mother's own practitioner) to monitor personally the antenatal care of as many patients as he could undertake in the hospital antenatal clinic. Moreover, his time is better used when he sees only patients who need a specialist.

In those cases in which delivery is planned to take place either at home or in a GP obstetric unit, the GP–obstetrician's responsibility in antenatal care assumes particular importance. A significant facet of this is that of the selection of mothers suitable for this kind of care. Much of the criticism that has been levelled against domiciliary obstetrics relates to the issue of the unsatisfactory selection of patients (Butler and Bonham 1963; Cox, Fox, Zinkin, and Matthews 1976), and there is no doubt that this is an aspect of care that is of extreme importance. The criteria of selection, which should not be absolute, but rather provide a useful frame of reference in which the decision concerning selection can be made, should be carefully identified and agreed upon by both the practitioner and the obstetrician, and discussed with the patient. In the ideal situation this should take place at the time of a combined consultation at which the plans for the delivery can be discussed. Such an arrangement, if achieved, will inevitably help to develop a sense of cooperation and mutual understanding that can only be of benefit to the patient under their combined care.

Intra-partum care

We think there is unlikely to be a dramatic and large-scale return in this country to home confinement, but the situation might be stabilized at a point at which there will continue to be a definite, though probably small number of women, who wish to have the experience of childbirth in the setting of their own home.

Those who consider there remains a place for home confinements at a time when it is now possible for all mothers to have their babies in hospital, base this view on the belief that:

1 childbirth is a natural phenomenon that in the majority of cases needs no interference, but careful supervision, psychological support, and protection from meddlesome intervention;

2 that a spontaneous delivery in the absence of detectable abnormality is a form of labour that can rarely be improved upon;

3 that the chances of ensuring an optimal labour are probably increased if

the expectant mother is confident and free from unnecessary psychological stress;

4 that the experience of childbirth may be significant in the emotional development of an individual;

5 that it is possible by good antenatal care to differentiate between the large group of mothers with no detectable evidence of recognizable 'risk' factors, and the much smaller group in which varying degrees of abnormality are present. The latter need to be under the special care of obstetricians working from an appropriately equipped hospital, whereas the former can and should be managed by the expert in the physiological management of childbirth—the midwife—with the appropriate support in case of difficulties.

The main objectives to be achieved in the conduct of a confinement are first and foremost that it will result in a healthy mother having a healthy baby with the minimum of avoidable complications; that the mother will be helped to feel emotionally satisfied and fulfilled by the experience of the birth of her baby; and that it will strengthen the bond between husband and wife and other members of the family by allowing them to share this very personal and deep human experience.

For the family doctor, the achievement of these objectives provides a unique opportunity to strengthen the relationship with the family in a way which can influence very positively his subsequent professional and caring role towards them.

Further advantages of having a home confinement include the informal conduct of the labour, with the opportunity to be up and about during the first stage, and the absence of any particular routine to which the mother feels she must accommodate her wishes and actions. A midwife is continuously in attendance throughout the labour and is often a person with whom the mother has already formed a relationship during her antenatal care. Also her own doctor will usually be present during at least part of the labour. There is a noticeable sense of relaxation and security engendered by being in familiar surroundings, often with the husband and other members of the family present. A home confinement strengthens the belief that 'having a baby' is a normal event, and this can therefore give confidence to the expectant mother. The surroundings are not suitable for medical interference, and this is therefore likely to be discouraged.

It is important that the home should provide a setting in which the mother feels physically and psychologically 'at ease' and should also be reasonably conveniently situated for the GP and the midwife.

The advantages of a home confinement may seem indisputable, but there are also some very real problems in undertaking this form of care in contemporary general practice. First, there is the nature of the commitment for the doctor and the midwife. For both it may mean several hours in the home. The GP's working day has now become much less flexible than it used to be and it is increasingly difficult to accommodate time-consuming emergencies. Administrative arrangements for contacting the doctor and midwife need to be well organized, and with a smaller number of midwives now working over larger areas, some solution such as radio-call systems need to be given careful consideration.

GPs have in recent years, to a large extent, handed over the care of their patients during labour to the hospital. As a result doctors entering practice are less likely ever to have seen a home delivery and therefore have not had the chance to gain personal experience of situations and views that may run counter to those they acquired during their education in the hospital setting. Also, and significantly, many hospital obstetricians sincerely dislike the whole idea of home confinements. This is an important factor, both because they are in a position to influence greatly the attitudes of those training to enter general practice, and because the practitioner is well aware that he may at any time require the services of his hospital colleagues and therefore does not want to practise in a way that is likely to jeopardize this cooperation.

Those arguing for a 100 per cent hospital confinement rate do so from a belief that it is a safer form of obstetric practice. When one removes from consideration the oft-cited problem of poor clinical practice (which can clearly occur in any setting) the obstetric problems of labour conducted in the home relate to unexpected emergencies that might arise at any time. By good pre-natal selection the incidence of these can be minimized but not abolished, although as has been shown by various studies (Cookson 1963; Hudson 1968; van Alten, Kloosterman, and Treffers 1976) they can be kept to an exceedingly low level. It is absolutely essential that the existence and satisfactory functioning of a flying squad is established before domiciliary obstetrics is contemplated. It is important that the practitioner is able to make an early diagnosis of such problems so that critical time is not wasted before assistance is summoned. Also he should be capable of starting immediate treatment from which the patient might derive benefit before more skilled help arrives. Thus he should ensure that he is equipped for all likely eventualities and should be prepared to undertake such procedures as the initial resuscitation of the newborn as well as the suturing of tears and episiotomies.

In a list size of 2500 patients a GP would expect about 30–40 pregnancies each year. The great majority of these will be confined in hospital. Thus it is inevitable that he will have difficulty in maintaining his expertise in such procedures as forceps deliveries. Rather than assuming that such competence is a necessary prerequisite for undertaking any form of intranatal care, and thereby inevitably excluding all but a very small minority of GPs from this role, a more constructive approach is to accept that domiciliary obstetrics means essentially the care of non-intervention, and in those cases in which this is inappropriate further assistance should be sought.

The practitioner who is undertaking confinements in the home may with benefit provide himself with certain items of special equipment, such as an intravenous infusion set with a saline bottle and a laryngoscope (although a spoon is usually quite adequate to visualize the larynx of the 'flat' baby). Other items that may be useful include a portable neonatal resuscitation trolley and also some form of stirrups to make the positioning for suturing more satisfactory.

The question of a practitioner's care for the delivery of his patients has been discussed in terms of domiciliary confinements, but a more common situation is that in which a delivery is conducted within a GP obstetric unit, either in a separate cottage hospital, or in a unit closely attached to the obstetric department of a general hospital. The advantages of such a situation clearly lie in the close proximity to obstetric colleagues, but it is important to remember that the selection of cases for delivery in such units should be much the same as for confinements conducted in the home.

No doctor undertaking home confinements should do so with a false sense of complacency. But on the other hand if he feels that, in the interests of his patients, this is the right setting for the confinement to take place, he should be reassured that with good clinical obstetric care it is a justifiable and appropriate decision.

Post-natal care

The post-natal period is one of transition, marking the end of one important state—that of pregnancy, and the start of another—that of motherhood. If the concern of those providing care is primarily orientated towards the former it is likely that emphasis will be laid on identifying pathology, excluding any post-partum abnormalities and complications, and ensuring that both mother and baby are essentially healthy individuals. If, however, this period is seen in the more dynamic terms of marking the start of a new life and relationship—rather than the end of a physiological process—the orientation of care will be directed towards helping adjustment to these new roles and responsibilities.

Early post-natal care should include:

1 specific management relating to the delivery, e.g. monitoring the involution of the uterus and the vaginal blood loss, care of the breasts, and detecting early signs of physical complications such as infection, thrombophlebitis, etc.;
2 providing general management of the mother who needs rest and emotionally supportive nursing care;
3 conducting the initial examination and observation of the newborn baby;
4 monitoring the satisfactory establishment of feeding;
5 assessing and monitoring the general mental state of the mother during this initial stage of readjustment;
6 monitoring and helping, where appropriate, the establishment of the maternal role and encouraging the mother in the early development of a bonding relationship with her baby;

7 facilitating and encouraging the father in his supportive and paternal role.

It is important that regular professional surveillance is available and that the mother is under the care of those whose advice and support is both helpful and minimally conflicting with that of others; that supporting care is available for allowing her to have adequate rest; and that she is in an environment in which she feels relaxed and removed from unnecessary stress; and any restriction on the father's contact with his wife and baby are kept to a minimum.

In comparing the hospital and home setting for the early post-natal period the factors laid out in Table 8.2 may be of particular relevance.

Following delivery at home, or early discharge from hospital, the care of the mother and baby become the responsibility of the midwife, GP, and the health visitor. Statutorily, it is necessary for the midwife to visit twice a day for the first 3 days following delivery, and then daily up to a minimum of 10 or maximum of 28 days. During this time she plays a most important role in helping the mother to adapt to the new and very often anxiety-provoking responsibilities that she faces. As a result of the increasing mobility of the population, and the decreasing size of families, the young mother with her new baby is frequently very isolated, with little real support available to her from others with previous personal experience of childbirth.

Although there are certain physical aspects of post-natal care which occupy the attention of the midwife, probably the most important aspect of her role is in the psychological field of guiding and encouraging the mother in the way she begins to handle and feed her baby. It is most important that both she—and those who are responsible for organizing her schedule of work—fully appreciate the importance of this function if adequate time is to be allowed for her to carry it out. Much of the success of her care will depend on the nature of the personal relationship that she has been able to establish with the mother, and therefore there is much to be gained if only one or two midwives are involved in the post-natal care.

The GP probably visits the mother at home during the first days following delivery if she has had a home confinement or an early discharge following hospital confinement, largely to ensure that the mother and baby are progressing satisfactorily and that the care described above is indeed being carried out. The day-to-day support in the first 2 post-partum weeks is given, however, by the midwife. In the following section we shall consider her role in more detail.

After about 2 weeks the family is visited by the Health Visitor, and it is her responsibility to help the mother in any non-clinical problems that she may have in her new mothering role.

The GP will probably arrange a post-natal examination after about 6 weeks. Apart from the usual physical examination, the value of which is

Table 8.2 Where early post-natal care takes place: the advantages and disadvantages of home and hospital settings

Home	Hospital
Familiar setting	Unfamiliar setting
Baby unlikely to be separated from mother	Baby likely to be separated from mother for varying periods of time
Mother and baby are surrounded by the family	Mother and baby are separated from the family
Physical rest may be restricted by household demands, especially if there are other children at home, but on the other hand may be very attainable	Mother can often rest well having no responsibilities for house-keeping, but her rest may be disturbed by the ward routine and the presence of other babies
Opportunities for comparison with other mothers and babies are not present	Mother may feel influenced by comparing the performance of herself and her baby in feeding, sleeping, etc., with that of others in the ward
Mother is under the care of those with whom she has already established a personal relationship	The mother is under the care of professionals with whom she has had little previous contact
Mother can do what she likes when she likes	The patient tends to have to conform to the ward routine
No inherent conflict between mother and midwife, who will tend to be orientated to the needs of each mother whom she tends to regard as an individual rather than as one of a group. Mother is also much less likely to be viewed as a 'patient'	Potential conflict exists between nursing staff and the mother (a) over 'who knows best' about what is right for mother and baby, (b) because the post-natal ward does not fit into the usual model of the hospital in that the patient does not see herself in a 'sick role'
Advice is usually only given by one or few advisers and, therefore, less likely to be conflicting.	Advice is often given by several advisers and, therefore, is frequently conflicting.
Medical advisers (general practitioner and health visitor) tend to see this as the start of their continuing care for the mother and baby	Medical advisers (midwives and obstetricians) tend to see this time as the end of the process of childbirth following which they will have no continuing care for the patient

often rather minimal, particular attention should be given to the recognition of any signs of a developing puerperal depression which has been shown to be quite commonly present. This is often masked, and may have serious long-term effects (Dominian 1974). It is also a suitable occasion to ensure that the couple have received appropriate family planning advice. Thus, in the setting of general practice the management of a pregnancy merges imperceptibly into the care of the mother and child. Also the fact that the bond of the doctor–patient relationship may have been strengthened by the shared experience of the pregnancy can have considerable relevance in the practitioners continuing caring relationship for that family.

Training general practitioners

Undergraduate medical education has moved far from the time when its objective was to produce a 'safe doctor' and it is now generally accepted that the clinical course can do no more than to introduce the student to the various principal specialties and to provide a foundation on which the vocational orientation of the early postgraduate years can later be built. An important recent development has been the establishment of organized vocational training as a preparation to starting in general practice, and it is likely that this will become a necessary prerequisite in the near future. This training programme comprises 2 years in various hospital posts which usually includes a 6-month post in obstetrics, often with responsibility also for gynaecology, and 1 year in a training practice.

In 1971 the number of hospital confinements was less than 80 per cent of the total number of deliveries in only 15 out of 168 Area Health Authorities, and the widely held and often-stated view of obstetricians was that they would welcome a continuation of this trend until all but very few confinements take place within the hospital setting. A joint working party of the representatives of the Royal College of Obstetricians and Gynaecologists, and the Royal College of General Practitioners (1974) expressed the view that in the future nearly all confinements would take place in a fully equipped maternity department with 24-hour cover by a resident obstetrician. Their recommendations for training were as follows:

1 *Doctors who propose to offer full obstetric care to their patients in their homes or in the general practitioner obstetric unit.* The minimum training should be a 6 months' resident appointment in a recognized obstetric post. Except for practitioners working in maternity hospitals, subsequent special periodic refresher courses would be required.

2 *Doctors who undertake routine antenatal and post-natal supervision of their patients, but not intra-natal care.* Such doctors should have a comparable basic training to that of those who undertake full obstetric care, i.e. a 6-month resident appointment in obstetrics, as it was felt that this type of supervision should not be undertaken without previous training in intra-natal care.

3 *Doctors who do not intend to engage in obstetric work of any type.* It was felt that the experience gained by undergraduates in medical schools was not enough even for this group, in view of the fact that they may be faced with emergency obstetric problems or medical problems arising in any of their patients who happen to be pregnant. Therefore, it was advised that the basic postgraduate vocational training scheme for general practice should include at least 2 months' training in obstetrics and gynaecology.

The D.Obst.R.C.O.G. is an examination that can be taken at the completion of a 6-month obstetric appointment, but it was not felt that all GP obstetricians should necessarily hold this diploma.

Any registered practitioner—whatever the limitations of his postgraduate training—is now able to undertake the obstetric care of his patients, but he will receive the full payment for this only if he has been admitted onto the Obstetric List of the local Family Practitioner Committee. To achieve this he must have fulfilled certain criteria, the most demanding of which is the 6 months' full-time residential hospital appointment.

It is interesting to note the change in the attitude of practising doctors to the requirements in obstetric experience that they expect from new entrants to their practices, as judged by the advertisements for partnerships in the *British Medical Journal* (Lloyd 1975). Between 1961 and 1971, in spite of an increase in the availability of GP maternity beds, there was a marked fall (from 41·9 per cent to 19·8 per cent) of requests for any previous obstetric experience.

The control of quality of care, or audit, is now receiving increased attention. The most satisfactory way of approaching the problem is by developing ways of self-audit, in which the provider of care participates in his own continual clinical assessment. For this to be successful it is important that he is motivated to do this and does not feel threatened by its outcome. Ideally, a close relationship, based on mutual trust and respect, should exist between the practitioner and his obstetric consultant colleague, and this provides the basis on which a constructive form of critical clinical assessment can be built. If it is missing it is the care of the patient that will ultimately suffer.

The midwife

A midwife is a person who is ... trained to give the necessary care and to advise women during pregnancy, labour, and the postnatal period, *to conduct normal deliveries on her own responsibility*, and to care for the newly born infant. At all times she must be able to recognise the warning signs of abnormal or potentially abnormal conditions which necessitate referral to a doctor and to carry out emergency measures in the absence of medical help. She may practise in hospitals, health units or domiciliary services. In any of these situations she has an important task in health education within the family and the community. In some countries her role extends into the fields of gynaecology, family planning and child care. (WHO 1966)

One result of the considerable increase in the rate of hospital confinements over the last 10–15 years is that British maternity care has become more and more obstetrician-orientated. Obstetricians are not trained to deal primarily with normal labour; rather, how to manage dysfunctional labours which require their special skills. At present, a large proportion of women are being confined in specialist units although they do not need this type of care. The management of physiological childbirth is a separate and often undervalued skill. The midwife with specialist training in physiological child-birth is, *par excellence*, the person who can best support the mother in the process of natural childbirth.

It may be significant that in the West it is the midwife, not obstetrician-orientated services that have achieved the lowest perinatal mortality rates. Norway, Denmark, Sweden, Finland, and Holland all rely on midwives to conduct normal labours and, as is seen in Table 6.1 on p. 90, they have the lowest perinatal mortality rates in the world. It is difficult to understand the logic behind the current trend in Britain towards a service in which all labours, normal or abnormal, will be managed by obstetricians.

The latest edition of one of the most popular midwifery textbooks (Myles 1975) extols the virtues of midwives being part of a team in the hospital, and states that it would be a retrograde step for a midwife to take sole charge of an expectant mother because this would deprive her of the scientific care that only the obstetric team with its sophisticated technology can provide. But an advanced technology is no guarantee of good care. Though we talk much about the desirability of continuity of care for the child-bearing woman, we have in fact become highly successful in segmenting care —and both the mother and the midwife are losers under such a system. One team manages the antenatal phase, another the intra-partum, and yet another the post-partum period.

Modern interventionist obstetrics can have subtle effects on the psychology of the midwife. When an obstetrician takes over, the relationship between the midwife and the labouring woman is immediately effected. The midwife is expected to carry out the instructions of the obstetrician even though, with her previous knowledge of the woman and her labour, she may believe there is no justification for them. It is not surprising that many midwives protect themselves by not becoming emotionally involved or committing themselves to the woman in labour. The midwife may well feel that she has been relegated to the role of an obstetric technician.

A pioneer in the use of oxytocin for the induction of labour, commenting on the superiority of normal physiological labour subsequently stated that 'The spontaneous onset of labour is a robust and effective mechanism which is preceded by the maturation of several foetal parts, and should be given every opportunity to operate on its own' (A. C. Turnbull, unpublished). If there is to be a trend towards recognition of the importance of normal labour, then it is the responsibility of the NHS to ensure that there are skilled midwives trained to be able to conduct these labours.

Britain trains more midwives than any other developed country—but one wonders how, with the present patterns of care, they can ever be experienced enough to practise with confidence and accept responsibility for both mother and baby. Many are sent forth to practise in under-developed countries where there is no technological help and even minimal availability of drugs. We are also training midwives who are unable to appreciate the advantages of home confinements because they have not had the opportunity to assist at any. To have a comprehensive maternity service it is essential that all students training as midwives should have experience of home confinements.

The new 1-year integrated training scheme for registered nurses, which will soon be the only one available, can be seen as a corollary of the official policy of aiming at 100 per cent hospital confinements. The student midwives spend 3 months in the community after an initial 17 weeks in hospital—and some may not deliver any babies during this time. They then return to hospital and spend the remaining 6 months concentrating on abnormal obstetrics. Such a pattern of training results in midwives losing any confidence they previously had in the normal mechanisms of physiological labour and they emerge with a strong bias towards hospital-based midwifery and interventionist obstetrics.

The community-based midwifery services are being fragmented by administrative changes which reduce the scope of the individual midwife's work and destroy continuity of care. The National Health Service was reorganized in 1974. Many parts of Britain, even in 1976, are still struggling to complete their new plans. In many there will be a Midwifery Division run by a Divisional Nursing Officer responsible for all midwives in her area, whether practising in hospital or in the community. The majority of divisional officers are hospital-orientated, because it was from the hospital field that most were selected.

Because, for the first time, community midwifery is being administered separately from the other community nursing services, i.e. health visiting and district nursing, the combined role of joint District Nurse/Midwife has now ceased in all but the most remote areas. There are thus many fewer midwives practising in the community, and in rural areas they are very few and far between. One result of this is that couples seeking a home confinement are now told that there are not enough midwives to provide adequate cover. Midwives now also receive on-call payment at night, so attempts are made to restrict the number of staff by instituting a rota system. Although officially the new Area Health Authorities inherited from the former Local Health Authorities the responsibility for providing an adequate service for those wishing to be delivered at home, this is often conveniently forgotten.

While all these administrative changes have been taking place, the need for experienced midwives has been highlighted by the new surge of interest in breastfeeding. Today midwives who can give adequate support are rare, whereas 20 years ago it was an important part of the midwife's task to help initiate a satisfactory feeding experience for mother and child. In its recommendations in the report 'Present day practice in infant feeding', the Department of Health and Social Security (1974) states that:

1 Because we are convinced that satisfactory growth and development after birth is more certain when an infant is fed an adequate volume of breast milk, we recommend that all mothers be encouraged to breast-feed their babies for a minimum of two weeks, and preferably for the first four to six months of life.

2 We are concerned that women do not receive adequate advice and encouragement to breast-feed their babies, and we recommend that steps be taken to remedy this situation.

It is now recognized that the post-natal period is of major significance to the physical and mental well-being of the mother and her baby. As the importance of breastfeeding is accepted, so the midwife's role during this period becomes even more vital.

The future

Could not the community midwife be encouraged to be the expert in normal midwifery? A very good case for this is made by Willmott (1976):

We give personal care and attention throughout labour, indeed through pregnancy and the postnatal period as well; we have a first-class maternity service; our midwives have been attracted to the community service and retained; the turnover of community midwives is minimal. . . . Ours is a specialist service, requiring skills and experience associated with meeting mothers in their homes with their families and other individuals in the house, and an accurate knowledge of a large borough, its general practitioners and many other community workers. Our work, with its daily mixing of antenatal care, deliveries and postnatal care, enables us to use our knowledge and skill to the full, giving us great 'job satisfaction'. This concentrated care includes invisible, preventive care at the primary level through continuity and one-to-one knowledge of mothers and babies. The community midwives are anxious to continue working in this way as practitioners of normal midwifery in their own right, and as members of the team which includes their hospital colleagues, to whom they turn in the case of any abnormality and for specialist care and investigations. We are concerned that the community midwifery service, in some parts of the country, is becoming very limited, at a time when it is being recognised in other fields that the emphasis should be on primary care in the community, with hospital stays as short as possible. . . . In order to keep a good team of community midwives, with high morale, they must not be restricted to pre- and postnatal care only. In our view they must be encouraged to do the deliveries as well, if they are to retain their skills and enthusiasm.

What then is the community midwife's role to be? She would deliver both at home and in GP units. She would be the expert in normal labour and lactation. She would play an important part in the training of student midwives, and possibly help hospital-based midwives to understand early neonatal behaviour a little better. An important aspect of her work is to 'mother' the women who come under her care—an element missing so frequently in today's nuclear family, and one which is essential during the early puerperium when the woman is full of self-doubts about her own ability to mother.

In the United States (e.g. Brown, Lesser, Mines, and Buryn 1972; Lang 1972) there is increasing public dissatisfaction with the quality of institutional maternity care (see Chapter 7). There are now signs of growing consumer protest in Britain as well. It is doubtful if this can be met by providing flowered wallpaper and television sets in maternity wards. What is required is a humanized caring service, every member of which treats the pregnant woman with respect.

Can we allow the British midwife to disappear as a vitally important member of the primary health care team?

Conclusion

In this chapter an attempt has been made to underline the important and unique role that the GP and midwife can play in childbirth.

The trend is for the hospital to take over an increasing responsibility for obstetric care, and unless a critical reassessment is made soon of the relative benefits to be derived from the community and hospital-based services, there is real danger that the organizational structure on which domiciliary obstetrics is dependent will become irreversibly run down, and this before research has been done to show whether, in fact, hospital is the 'best' place for all babies to be born. It is the responsibility of those who believe there is value in the primary health care team's continuing participation in obstetric care not only to ensure that this does not happen, but also to provide the means whereby it is encouraged to realize its full potential.

References

Alten, van D., Kloosterman, G. J., and Treffers, A. (1976). 'A place to be born'. *British Medical Journal* i, 771.

Brown, J., Lesser, E., Mines, S., and Buryn, E. (1972). *Two births*. Random House, New York; The Bookworks, Berkeley.

Butler, N. R. and Bonham, D. C. (1963). *Perinatal mortality. First report of British perinatal mortality survey*. Livingstone, London.

Cookson, I. (1963). 'Family doctor obstetrics'. *The Lancet* ii, 1051.

Cox, C. A., Fox, J. S., Zinkin, P. M., and Matthews, A. E. B. (1976). 'Critical appraisal of domiciliary obstetric and neonatal practice'. *British Medical Journal* i, 84.

Department of Health and Social Security (1974). *Present day practice in infant feeding*. Report on Health and Social Subjects 9. H.M.S.O., London.

Dominian, J. (1974). 'Marital pathology'. *Proceedings of the Royal Society of Medicine* **67**, 780.

Hudson, C. K. (1968). 'Domiciliary obstetrics in a group practice'. *Practitioner* **201**, 816.

Lang, R. (1972). *Birth book*. New Genesis Press, California.

Lloyd, G. (1975). 'The general practitioner and changes in obstetric practice'. *British Medical Journal* i, 79.

Myles, M. (1975). *Textbook for Midwives* (8th edn). Livingstone, London.
Royal College of General Practitioners (1972). *The future general practitioner. Learning and teaching.* B.M.A. House, London.
—— (1974). Report of Joint Working Party. 'Training general practitioners of obstetrics'. *Journal of the Royal College of General Practitioners* **24**, 355.
Willmott (1976). *Midwives Chronicle and Nursing Notes* **89**.
WHO (1966). *Technical Report Series* **331**.

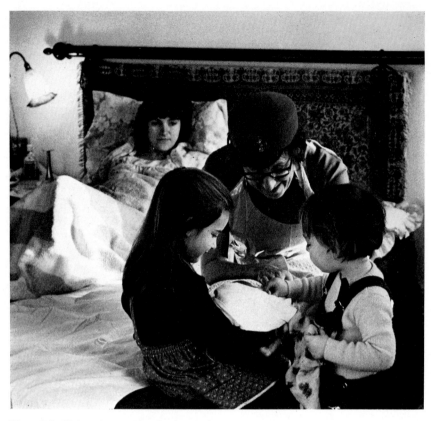

Plate 9.1 Birth at home. Introducing the new arrival. See Chapter 9

Women's experiences of birth at home

The Department of Health and Social Security has stated that 'it has never been our intention that health authorities should refuse a home confinement to a woman who wishes to have one',† that it 'would not expect pressure to be placed upon the woman to accept hospital confinement against her express wishes',‡ and that it is willing to look into complaints received from those who are having difficulties in arranging a home confinement. It is extremely difficult, however, for women in some areas to obtain a home confinement. Yet some continue to seek one even when told that this is impossible and that there is nobody willing to deliver them.

This chapter looks at what women say they liked about birth at home and some of its problems. It examines also the previous hospital deliveries which they described and the way in which these were related to their determination to seek birth at home next time.

So in this chapter we see the maternity services from the consumer's point of view. But here the economic model is inappropriate because it must be remembered that mothers are not just consumers, but also the people who actually have the babies. It can be seen that one of the things women got from having a baby at home was the feeling that they were active creators, not passive patients. They also believed that birth in the setting of the home had far-reaching effects, not only for themselves and the baby, but also for the family.

Some expectant mothers want to have their baby at home even when many difficulties are put in their way or when home confinement is flatly refused them. Why do women wish to give birth in their own homes? This chapter is based on an enquiry designed to find out whether women who had attended antenatal classes preferred home or hospital confinements, and for what reasons. In a National Childbirth Trust newsletter sent out in 1975 to all members, those who had views about the best place for confinement were invited to write about their experiences. There were 65 responses. Of these, 23 were primiparae and 42 multiparae. Three women had four or more children, 5 had three children, and 34 had two children. There were 74 accounts of hospital confinements and 55 of home confinements. Although 3 of the women had experienced only birth at home, and although 8 had had hospital births only, all the others (54) had had experience of both home and hospital births.

Members of the Trust may have different attitudes from the population

† Letter to Society to Support Home Confinements, 12 July 1976.
‡ Letter to Society to Support Home Confinements, 17 September 1976.

as a whole. They tend to be middle class, to have stayed at school after the age of 16, and to be articulate. It must also be remembered, however, that these women may express with clarity some of the things which other women feel, too, but find difficult to put into words. A forthcoming study (in press) by Maureen O'Brien of the Institute for Social Studies in Medical Care, with a random sample of just over 2000 mothers in different areas of the U.K. indicates that this is so. In presenting an analysis of these letters I wish to emphasize that this is not a statistical survey but is material which may allow some insight into criteria relating to the place of birth which these women bore in mind when they made their decisions, and into their personal experiences of labour.

Only three respondents said they preferred hospital confinements. Some respondents appreciated the need for hospital confinement with a specific birth, but if they planned to have another baby wished to have the next one at home. Because of the open-ended nature of the question (simply asking how they felt about the place of birth), respondents gave their own reasons for their preferences, but there was remarkable uniformity in the attitudes expressed.

The four most marked reasons for wanting a home confinement were:

1 Objections to routine hospital practices and to hospital 'atmosphere' which creates an impersonal context for birth and lying-in.
2 Wanting a natural birth, avoiding interventionist obstetric practices, e.g. induction and acceleration of labour, and concern to avoid drugs.
3 Concern about difficulty of emotional bonding with the baby in hospitals where infants are removed at night, and sometimes for long periods during the day as well. Concern of this kind was expressed by more than half the respondents.
4 Wanting the birth to be presented as a normal part of living to other children in the family, and to avoid separation from toddlers.

Other reasons were also given, and these included:

5 Continuity of care and a personal relationship with a midwife who is a trusted friend.
6 Wanting the husband to participate fully and share in the labour.
7 Belief that breast-feeding is most easily established at home.
8 Wanting the delivery to be as gentle as possible, and post-natal care to be sympathetic, for the baby's sake. This included statements by mothers who had read about the Leboyer method.

One interesting aspect was that when informants reported on a home delivery, where there was a choice between the definite article and the personal pronoun, they tended to talk about 'my' labour. When they reported on a hospital delivery, however, they usually spoke of 'the' labour. Twenty of the women who talked about their hospital labours referred to 'the labour' and 16 of those who had home confinements spoke of 'my labour'. In fact, although two mothers who had home deliveries spoke of 'the' labour, not one single woman spoke of 'my' labour in hospital. It seemed that labour at home might be a more intensely personal experience. (The numbers are small here, because other terms and phrases were often employed.)

Home as a place of safety from interventionist obstetrics

Nearly all the respondents indicated that they wanted to manage labour themselves, so far as possible, and to avoid, for example, 'frequent internal and external examinations without regard to discomfort caused', 'pethidine given when not desired', 'indiscriminate use of drugs', and 'timing to suit staff'. They also said they hoped to avoid admission procedures of shave, enema, and shower which some saw as 'humiliating' and which many found uncomfortable.

Some women whose previous labour had been induced felt that it had been unnecessary: 'There was nothing about the baby or the placenta to indicate that she was in the least overdue'. They also disliked being 'confined immobile by the dread bottle of chemicals to the radius of my hose'.

They were often critical of the effect of pain-relieving drugs given in a previous labour; pethidine in particular came under criticism for producing distressing effects: 'Immediately I lost touch, kept feeling sleepy and distant, then coming to in the middle of a contraction!' 'I wasn't involved in the idea of giving birth. The pethidine made me feel as if my mind and body had separated.'

Pethidine was often given without realizing that the woman was about to go into the second stage.

'I was given pethidine without being asked if I needed it, although I knew I was right at the end of the first stage, and it had no pain-relieving effect, but made me feel very nauseous.' 'The midwife was standing by with a needle', but 'I had no pain or discomfort whatsoever. I think that staff tend to allow themselves to become too nervous, but it must be hard for them when they have such a responsible job.'

Respondents also queried the need for routine episiotomy and often remarked how pleased they were that they did not need an episiotomy at home.

It appears that midwife's and obstetrician's distress occurs no less frequently than foetal and maternal distress. The over-riding impression with the hospital births described is that this often complicated the second stage, leading to a rushed and desperate second stage for the mother. Women having home births are usually, of course, multiparae, so that there is less likely to be a sense of urgency about getting the patient to bear down when it is known that she has already delivered a baby vaginally, and it is true, too, that some domiciliary midwives and doctors allow the woman little time in the second stage, and cajole and exhort from the moment that the cervix appears to be fully dilated. But it was the women in hospital who were most likely to feel that bearing down involved a race against time and was a matter of life or death for the baby. This could mar an otherwise happy labour. It resulted in uncoordinated and often ill-timed efforts to bear down, and excessive straining which produced exhaustion in the mother. Some women commented that it was much easier to let the process of birth unfold naturally at home, and emphasized above all that they were not hurried. Writing of a first birth, one mother said that she had been told by the midwife that the second stage was not permitted to last longer than 30 minutes (from mothers' accounts a frequent practice in this particular hospital):

The bright light, the half hour, shocked me. I thought, my God, this is it now, 30 minutes while I push this unreal child into reality. Suppose it's no good. . . . The urge to push receded while I lay in terror. Either the midwives were in a hurry or they didn't trust me. . . . My eyes hardly left the clock. 3.20. God help me. Episiotomy. I asked if the baby's heartbeats had slowed down—no they hadn't, but they might soon. I said I felt very strong and could go on pushing for much longer. I wanted to cry. I was giving birth anally. I was a complete failure. I just pushed and pushed, with or without contractions. I didn't push very efficiently because I was feeling so miserable.

Unhappy hospital experiences

There were 52 descriptions of distressing labours in hospital (i.e. over half the hospital confinements described). Negative hospital experiences related primarily induction and acceleration of labour. One woman who had had a happy, easy pregnancy, for example, said, 'I was very reluctant—wanting the labour to be as natural and spontaneous as the pregnancy', but ultrasound indicated that the baby was probably at term and she was induced for reasons of 'hospital policy', although she obtained what she called 'a reprieve' for 4 days. Her mood changed to become 'sombre, thoughtful, low, and apprehensive'. 'I couldn't sleep at all and felt like a small frail boat about to set out across the great waters.' The next morning she left for her 'appointment with fate'.

Women complained that the 'corset' from monitoring equipment is far too tight ('I couldn't even wriggle') and caused them unnecessary pain. Respondents also found that they were often interrupted during contractions by doctors, nurses, and students talking, or wanting them to turn over and lie flat on their backs to be examined.

The labours experienced by those who were induced seemed to be unusually painful. Accounts often include statements like 'I'm afraid all breathing techniques had gone by the board', 'I mashed R's hand through the contractions', 'I felt desperate', and 'Contractions were thick and fast and very painful', and they even talked about 'long minutes of pain which are too horrible to remember'.

One respondent said that when a syntocinon drip was set up 'we got under way with a vengeance', and added that her consultant said, in front of her, 'Hit them hard in the beginning and keep upping the dose every 15 minutes'.

Negative hospital experiences were also often associated with the use of what mothers called 'artificial aids' generally, and with feelings of constraint about their own roles in labour. Some very unhappy letters came from husbands. One man explained his anger as a reaction to the hospital's attempt to persuade his wife and himself 'to dissociate from the experience, to deny natural spontaneous feelings (such as wanting to cuddle the baby, or to surrender to the rhythm of the second stage rather than compulsively push)' and wrote about his conflicting feelings of joy and anger as he left the hospital after the delivery.

We are not happy about the way the birth was. I don't think we are clinging on to some romantic idealization of how it could have been. Those who describe so cheerfully what seem often like small atrocities done to them are idealizing their giving birth and discounting what they must somewhere feel as a violence to their experience and their integrity.

His wife had been allowed half an hour in the second stage, and this time limit worried her. Midwives and medical students encouraged her by saying: 'Push, push harder, go to the toilet, in the back passage', and they felt that this forcing had been unnecessary. 'They simply weren't going to let us do it in our own time.' He asked:

Was our baby in danger? Was she more in danger of swallowing fluid than other babies who take longer than half an hour in the second stage? Was it because she had the membranes ruptured artificially soon after we came into hospital? (They thought us very strange for questioning this and said, 'You'll have a long labour otherwise.')

One woman described:

lying on the hard table in the delivery room, listening to piped Muzac, while a woman having her sixth child gave birth with a vast grunt and a squeal and I wondered if it would be like that for me. I was left alone much of the time with only the occasional 'assault' of the internal examination and prods and pokes by cool midwives who made no attempt to explain anything to me. My husband had been sent home, as they informed me I had 'hours' to go. In fact the second stage came and I have vague memories of calling out 'for someone, anyone to help me' and being proffered a mask and injections and wheeled away in a state of utter panic. They gave me a drug which made me feel rather like Alice, falling, falling down a never-ending rabbit hole, while I still retained enough awareness to be bothered by the glaring lights of the delivery room and, it seemed to me, hundreds of little men in white coats. My first awareness of having given birth was having a telephone thrust into my hands, on the delivery table, and being told to tell my husband that I had a son. My husband said later he was horrified to see how grey and drugged I looked. When I finally came to I felt weak and exhausted and hurt from the episiotomy. When people asked me about the birth I said, 'Oh, it was quite an easy one.' In actual fact I had little memory of it, but later on I realized it had not been an enriching experience—it had been too full of panic and unknowingness, and the numbed feeling that drugs leave behind.

In reports of straightforward labours, there were frequent irritations which interrupted the woman's concentration in handling contractions and were associated with poor staff–patient relations. One multigravida went into hospital worried because she had been unable to find anyone to care for her toddler other than a stranger. Contractions which had been coming every 7 minutes, stopped for 20 minutes on admission (and from many of the accounts a slowing-down of labour on admission to hospital is a frequent occurrence). The mother was in a new unit, with flowered paper on the wall facing the bed and an armchair for the husband; but she found the room 'soul-destroying' because it had no window. Many mothers like to watch trees or other scenes outside while in labour, and it seems that a room without a window can lead to a sensation of being trapped. This woman had backache but made herself comfortable lying in the front lateral with her upper knee raised slightly on a pillow. But sister came in, sent her husband out of the room and 'forbade me to have a pillow there—"pillows go under your head, and will give you thrombosis under your knee". Nothing I said would alter her view, and as she remained in the room I was unable to make myself comfortable again.' She asked for Pethidine, and passed the rest of the first stage 'in a haze of discomfort'. In the second stage, progress was slow at first: 'and the sister was cross and said I had just been wasting time and energy for the past half hour, which I thought was most unreasonable'. After delivery she was just about to drink a cup of tea, when an obstetrician appeared to suture the perineum. 'This was singularly unpleasant, and he appeared to take a sadistic delight in causing pain, and was most resentful that he was being kept from his dinner. Even the midwife said afterwards she thought he had been a butcher.'

Women also disliked being separated from their husbands shortly after delivery, a time when they especially wanted to be together. Although heavily drugged women were able to drift off to sleep and did not mind that their husbands had gone, others, particularly those who had found their husbands a great support in labour, felt isolated once the husband had left: 'I longed to be alone with Tom, just talking over the experience we had been through and looking at our child asleep. It seemed a real deprivation being separated just now. I felt terribly unsure of myself, lonely and tearful.' She discharged herself early, and: 'As soon as we got home without nurses who seemed so efficient and other mothers with all sorts of complications, I felt my strength returning, until Tom and Rachel and I began a sort of honeymoon period. I feel frightened to think how easily I could have spent this time in hospital, like most other women.'

The mother–baby bond

For 34 of the respondents (i.e. about half), bonding with the baby was the primary factor in wanting a home rather than a hospital confinement. In letters written during pregnancy, *none* of the primiparae who wrote of their wish to have a home confinement mention this as being important, but *all* the multiparae who had previous experience of a hospital confinement referred to it. And most did not just refer to it, but wrote several hundred words on the subject.

After a home confinement, informants described with pleasure how the baby was handed to them immediately and then put in a cot beside the bed:

Later that night, when I was too happy to sleep, I took the baby from his cot and held him against my shoulder for the rest of the night. I seemed to breathe in his very essence and he I believe mine, too. I heard a psychologist once remark that a mother feels a sense of loss when her baby is born. I felt quite the opposite. Every part of me seemed to fill with what I can only describe as 'a loving ecstasy'. This intense communication (for I am sure it was two-way) was never possible in hospital immediately after birth as the babies were not beside me. But I wonder too if there it could have taken place. It was something so special I think it needed exactly the right receptive conditions on both our parts for it to happen.

One informant, comparing the birth in hospital of her first child and that of her second child at home, wrote of the hospital experience: 'I remember one glimpse of my red and sleepy little son who had been whisked away and put behind glass.' Later the baby was brought to her:

I had an uncontrollable curiosity to find out about him—watch his funny little movements, take his clothes off and examine all his fingers and toes. I think this process of getting to know your baby in the physical sense is underestimated in the very beginning—that women do in fact need long periods of privacy when they can be allowed just to watch their baby and to explore his or her body. I remember the feeling of never wanting to let him go from my bed. I wanted him to be with me, and I felt it a terrible deprivation when he was taken away to the nursery. I resented the fact that nurses were changing his nappy, picking him up, etc. when he was a part of me, and I couldn't wait to leave the hospital and have him to myself!... I longed to get home to total involvement with my baby.

Another woman described how the baby was brought to her:

... wrapped up in what looked like a little strait jacket, and I was ordered not to unwrap her to look at her or to try to change her, and to keep her on the outside of the bed-linen.... Like any mother, I longed to take off all her clothes and see how she looked, and hold her warm little body against my bare skin, but the nurse kept coming in or sat at the foot of the bed watching, so I didn't dare.... I had to convince myself that she really was my baby. When you've waited around for nine months to see your baby, it's very hard to be told you can see it only on schedule and it really won't be yours to take care of for a few more days.

Women saw closeness of mother and baby not only from the point of view of the advantages to the baby, but also in terms of having a more restful post-partum experience when they could care for the baby themselves:

... no separation—even temporary—between mother and baby after the birth. He's by your bed from the start. In my opinion this is a more restful situation (contrary to hospital theory and practice) than having to listen to him yelling his head off in a distant nursery. Although this seems an awesome responsibility when the door finally shuts behind the midwife and you're on your own, it does help you realise that it's *your* baby and *your* job to love and look after him, not some expert's. Gordon Bourne states that the newly delivered mother can only get the rest she needs in hospital. I found the total opposite to be true.

Many mothers said they slept badly in hospital, sometimes because they were afraid their babies would not be brought to them when they cried if the mother were sleeping: 'I did not dare sleep and was a terrible nuisance about not letting the baby out of my sight.' Some disliked the routine taking of sleeping pills because they might not hear their babies. Although most of the mothers who were parted from their babies were in consultants' units, this also applied in some general practitioner units. One woman wrote:

I think here I encountered all that is worst in hospital care. The babies were kept in the nursery except for an exactly timed 30 minutes at each feed. There were constant injunctions 'not to touch that baby', 'put it down', and so on. Consequently I left hospital with a strange baby. I had no idea whether she cried between feeds always, sometimes or never. It took me at least six weeks to like her at all, which I feel can be attributed to the GP unit rules. It certainly left me feeling totally inadequate as a mother, and really unused to physical contact with my baby.

Babies were often removed from their mothers not only at night, but for long periods of the daytime, too, including visiting hours, the times when doctors' rounds were made, when paediatricians were visiting the nurseries, when physiotherapists were giving mothers exercises, and when meals were served. In some hospitals babies are still only brought to mothers at feeding times, and then only during the daytime: 'I found I couldn't hold my daughter unless I was actually feeding her (2 minutes each side, 5 times a day). I knew I'd got to go my own way or go crazy.' These women often commented on their separation from the baby as leading to a failure of nerve as mothers. One remarked: 'I didn't feel a mother properly until the fifth day, when he was allowed in the ward with me', and even then she said, 'It's hard to visualise it was him growing inside me, it was he who was so rudely born.'

In contrast, women saw home birth favouring a situation in which 'the experts did not take over and thus inhibit spontaneity, the expression of feeling, and the unfolding relationships between mother, father, and child': 'Psychologically there is a real advantage for a woman to give birth in her own home territory, where the doctor is a visitor, rather than in his territory, the hospital, where she feels deprived of dignity. Her positive attitudes may affect her confidence in her ability as a mother, which will, in turn, affect her relationship with the baby.'

Difficulties in being allowed to have a baby at home

It was after negative hospital experiences such as these that women decided that they would do everything they could to get a home confinement next time. Many of them had a long, hard struggle through the ensuing pregnancy to get a home birth, and seemed to be subjected to quite severe emotional stress as a result. 'I was appalled to find that there were absolutely no facilities for home delivery in our area. A fruitless search for a friendly doctor or midwife drew a complete blank', one couple wrote, who later went on and delivered their baby themselves.

Respondents were worried about the safety of a home confinement, especially since they were frequently warned of the dangers by obstetricians: 'I spent several months in an agony of indecision between my very sincere wish to give birth at home and my fear that I was being romantic and irresponsible where my child's life was involved', wrote a woman expecting her third baby. Many women were told by their doctors that they might cause their babies' deaths.

A man whose wife was expecting their second child wrote:

My wife and I both want to have the child born in our own home. This is especially important to us since my wife's first experience in hospital was extremely upsetting and we have worked and practised together for the event. Last time the birth was quite normal and quick, but in the second stage forceps were used, and because of this the same consultant who made my wife's experience a cold clinical lesson for his medical students is now putting tremendous pressure on us through two doctors and the midwife to have our child in hospital. We would both be most grateful for some objectivity as we realise that unless we get some human communication on the subject we are in danger of giving in or else absolutely refusing to give in to this dictatorial treatment. It would be a pity if we just agreed, because we so much want to have the child at home. It would also be a pity if we refused to go to hospital when the advice is real and should be accepted however badly it has been expressed to me.

Some women stopped using contraceptives only after they had discussed the possibilities of a home confinement with their general practitioners, having believed that they would be allowed one. One woman booked for a hospital confinement asked if her husband would be allowed to be present for the birth, and was told that he would. She made a 48-hour booking and 'felt very happy and confident'. But then the trouble started:

It transpires that they meant quite literally for the birth, not for the first stage. The labour wards have 3 beds and the theory is that other women might get embarrassed if a man is present. In the second stage I will be taken to a private room, and here 'if Sister agrees' and 'if we aren't run off our feet' I will be allowed to phone for my husband. We have no car, so he could be too late. And I do not feel confident that I will be aware enough to phone at this stage, and certainly do not feel that the staff are likely to help me to do so. In any case, I want to be with him for the first stage when I know his presence would help me.

When I ask doctors and midwives about this they are quite sure that he will be sent home while I am in the first stage, and they refuse to be committed about the second. I have written to my consultant assuring him of co-operation, not interference, but so far he remains sympathetic but unbending about the first stage. I am really disappointed and cannot see the birth in the same positive way if it is not to be shared with my husband. Can I insist on having the baby at home?

One respondent who very much wanted a home confinement obviously was not going to be allowed to have one. Her reasons for wanting to be at home were mainly associated with an induced labour which she found a 'frankly terrifying experience'. She wrote: 'Our first child was born at home, which we found a deeply satisfying experience.' A year after, however, she had an antepartum haemorrhage 10 weeks before term, and was induced 'without any explanations to us.... Immediately after the delivery I was left alone for 4 hours, semi-drugged, without being attended to at all. They had apparently "forgotten" me because of the rush to get the baby into an incubator. During that time I didn't know whether he was dead or alive.' A year later she was pregnant again and asked for a home confinement because 'both my husband and I have strong views about being together, if at all possible, during the birth of our children, and we had been denied this in hospital.'

Even in areas where home confinements are permitted, arrangements to have one take a long time. One couple kept a diary, which started in December when the woman saw her GP and asked him and the midwife if she might have a home confinement. In late January the midwife called and said it would not be possible 'for administrative reasons', and asked which hospital she wanted to go to. The woman said she still preferred the idea of home. In early February she and her husband together saw the GP and the midwife, and followed this by writing to the Community Physician. The GP also wrote, saying that he had agreed to a home confinement. A reply came in late February saying that the matter was being investigated, and then in early March a letter from the Divisional Nursing Officer giving tentative approval if it could be arranged administratively was received. In mid-March the midwives met and decided to take on the case.... So it took the best part of 4 months, and one wonders what unnecessary stress it added to this particular home confinement; the woman was anxious until 8 weeks before the birth because she did not know where she would be having the baby.

Although some midwives are very positive about home confinements, increasingly it seems that younger ones, who have in many areas had little or no experience of home confinements, are worried that they lack the skills for delivering outside hospitals, and in some cases opposition has come from the midwife even though the GP has been willing to take the case. This sometimes leads to bizarre reasons being given for refusing a home confinement. One woman was surprised to be told by the midwife: 'You have fitted carpets in your home so you can't have your baby there. You've got to have floor boards!'

Many obstetricians did not take women's fears, or their reasons for preferring a home confinement, very seriously. In discussion with her consultant, a woman said that she wanted to avoid Pethidine because of the possible deleterious effect on the baby, and that she felt that she might reduce the need for drugs if she had a home birth. He said, jokingly, that Pethidine must be acceptable as he had it when he was born, and if the current thinking that it impaired development was right, then he would have been an absolute genius, instead of an ordinary genius. 'When I pressed him further about home confinements, and about some people's fear of being in a strange institution, he asked me if I would want to die at home, seeing I was so keen on giving birth at home. He was genuinely surprised that I said, "Yes, I would like to die at home, surrounded by loved ones."' And she concluded: 'I think it worrying that these men have so much control over birth, and yet seem to understand so little about life.'

A woman wrote that because there was a policy of 100 per cent hospital confinement in the city where she lived, she and her husband had put off having their second child, since 'hospital is in my opinion for people who are ill, and I don't believe that labour is an illness'. Some women moved out of areas where there is such a policy, to stay in another area where home confinements are still permitted, and had their babies in rented rooms or at friends' houses rather than go into hospital. Where there is still a domiciliary midwifery service these women can be catered for. When and if that midwifery service no longer exists, these women will be delivering themselves, or being delivered by friends or husbands, as is now happening not only among hippie and rock groups and in communes in California, but in many parts of the United States. Although some of these young parents are those who have opted out of society in its more traditional forms, by no means all the people having babies at home and with untrained assistance in the United States belong to such fringe groups, and an increasing number are middle class and in many ways conformist. One woman expressed it in these terms:

I am a citizen of the U.S.A. and am expecting my third baby. I am not a hippy. I want to have my baby at home. My first child was born naturally, with no medication whatsoever, and everything except what the hospital did to my baby and me was absolutely normal. My second baby was born in England; he was born at home with the attendance of my husband, a midwife and our GP. I do not accept pregnancy as a state of illness, but as a state of health.

She described how she had booked a trained midwife but state law made it illegal to be delivered by her and went on to say that she could not understand 'how anyone has the right to say what I do in my own home and whom I invite into it. My neighbors commit adultery openly in their home, which is offensive to us and against the law, and they are not prosecuted.'

It is reasonable to assume that what is happening in the United States today may also soon be happening in the United Kingdom, unless something is done to reassert the status and skills, and the supporting services available to, the domiciliary midwife.

Midwives

All but 3 of the letters and labour reports had positive things to say about the help and friendship of the midwife. Women valued her cheerfulness and encouragement, the reassurance she gave, her patience, resourcefulness, and 'quiet understanding'. 'I never felt like a case, but a person. My questions were answered sympathetically and everything explained carefully.' 'One of the best things about a home confinement is the friendship of a midwife who has grown to know you over the weeks and with whose help *you* can plan your labour, instead of following rigid hospital procedure.' 'The midwives were like old family friends, which made me feel relaxed and confident.' Again and again the women used the word 'friend'. In many cases this was obviously a reciprocal sense of comradeship which must have been emotionally satisfying for the midwife, too. One woman said of her midwife: 'She said that she felt like one of the family and I, in turn, felt very loving towards her. We established a very good relationship.'

Mothers appreciated the individual, skilled attention of the midwife at home and often contrasted this with hospital experience, saying, for example, 'I don't think I got more than five minutes' individual attention, as distinct from passing comments'; 'Frequent changes of staff in the middle of my labour began to get me down'; 'It's much easier to discuss problems when the midwife is alone with you'; 'The attention that I received from the midwives [at home] was excellent'. A woman whose midwife arrived with her knitting found this confidence-inspiring as 'I knew she would be with me, and only me—throughout the labour—very comforting.' Yet another knitting midwife 'sat on the end of the bed doing her knitting for much of the time, pausing to murmur "beautiful" as I breathed my way through the contractions.' Emotional support of this kind is all that many women need when they give birth in the security of their own homes, and it is precisely this support which is so often lacking in the busy modern hospital.

Women appreciated the way in which one midwife cared for them not only during the labour itself but for 10 days after the birth, and many stressed the sense of luxury and contentment that resulted from being given 'constant, individual attention continuously' through the labour and the post-partum days. If our hospitals are to be made anything approximating women's homes this is one aspect of care which it may be very difficult to incorporate in the administrative system of large institutions.

'Trust' was also very often stated as an important part of the patient's relationship with her midwife: 'I trusted her completely'; 'I had a midwife whom I knew and liked and trusted'; 'I was very confident at being in the capable hands of my midwife'. One respondent defined the quality of the care she received as 'professional support on a basis of equality'. The manner in which this support was given was sometimes idiosyncratic but remarkably effective, as with the midwife who when her patient entered the second stage and 'bellowed like a cow, not with pain but with effort', remarked drily that this 'would not make him fly, much less birth him'.

One obvious factor with all of the midwives who had good relationships with the families they were helping was their flexibility. Domiciliary midwifery evidently appeals to the kind of woman who is able to adapt quickly and gracefully to whatever circumstances she encounters. One midwife, discovering that the future father was down with 'flu, did the shopping while her assistant stayed with the woman in the early first stage. Acts of friendship such as these gave the home births a special quality of human warmth. The labours were not without their amusing moments: as one woman reached 10 centimetres 'a legacy in the form of a large black piano arrived', reported the baby's father. 'Other back-rubbers took over and I was able to assist Jim and Ben the moving men (really!) to manoeuvre the monster through our diminutive door. As he left, one man glanced at the labouring woman and commented, "I 'ope as 'ow your missus 'as a better time delivering of that chiel than we 'ad delivering this ruddy piano!"'

Midwives were particularly appreciated for regularly explaining the progress of labour to both husband and wife, and women liked it when the midwife managed to avoid any sense of rush or the stress that results from harassing the mother to push the infant out at speed:

The midwife was with me from 8 a.m. till midnight (the baby was born at 10 p.m.) —never did she try to hurry things or force me to accept drugs or gas and air, which I wanted to try to do without. The atmosphere was calm but exciting all the time. Though she must have delivered many babies, she never treated us as though she'd 'seen it all before'.

She was compèring the final stage with the colour of the hair and so on. She must have been very tired but she didn't rush at all.

This relaxed attitude helped the woman in labour to relax: 'I had an exceptionally humane and considerate midwife. What struck me most about it all was the sheer simplicity. A few flowers, a sweet midwife, and I had a rewarding birth experience. With Ray's [her husband] encouragement— and the midwife's guidance it all seemed so natural and certainly there was no pain.'

Many women praised their midwives for help in establishing breast-feeding, as did one woman who said that 'she helped me against all the odds to be successful at breast-feeding'. The midwives were admired not only for their knowledge about lactation, but also for their flexible approach to the subject. Some women emphasized that both midwife and doctor behaved as guests in the house: 'It's so much more conducive to conversation and communication when you can receive the midwife from your own bed, with your toddler sitting on it, and you can offer her a cup of coffee.'

Midwives were also praised for the way in which they related to other children. One mother said:

It was such a family affair. Emma and James had got to know the midwife well during the previous nine months and looked forward to her visits. They were able to come and see the baby about five minutes after he was born and in fact helped the midwife to bath and dress him. I'll never forget seeing them rushing backwards and forwards with soap, talc, hairbrush, etc.—they were so pleased that at last this much-talked-about baby was a reality.

In hospital the baby always seemed to belong to 'them'.

One woman commented,

... at home it was always and exclusively ours as a family. The midwife asked us every day how the baby was, and the children delighted in telling her all that had happened since her last visit. These may appear to be trivial details. But when I read of the break-up of families perhaps they are not so trivial, but vitally important factors instead.

The general practitioner

The success of any home confinement hinges on the skills and personality of both the midwife and the GP, whether or not he is actually present at the delivery, and the tone is set by the relationships established during the antenatal period and the quality of care received then. Women commented on the advantages of 'consistency of care' and of seeing the same person at each antenatal clinic visit: 'You feel they're genuinely interested in you; my GP always asks "Any worries?" and answers them, and I don't feel I'm wasting his time because there's no long queue of expectant mothers outside the door.'

It may be interesting to note that the GPs who did home deliveries come over not merely as non-authoritarian, but as relaxed and flexible in their attitudes and opinions. They are never described as 'fatherly'. Nor, it must be admitted, is there much mystique. The home birth reports contrast with the reports of induced births in hospital which I was studying at the same time, in which one woman, for example, said of her doctor, 'Mr. F is not an obstetrician only. He is a saint.' None of the GPs even approached being described as saints. The relationship between doctor and patient is more nearly one which social psychologists describe as *reciprocal*.

What one father admiringly called 'a low-key approach to medicine' contrasts strongly with the situation in a hospital delivery which the patient and her husband obviously saw as near chaos:

One of the factors which to my mind demands a return to home delivery is that we experienced conflicting medical opinion from no less than 7 doctors and in the five hours at the hospital were attended by 6 midwives at different times who also conflicted as to my wife's progress. We were really psychologically on our own, but it was sad to hear two women hysterical on either side being told not to be 'silly'.

Individual GPs were compared favourably with some relatively anonymous hospital doctors, who were described as 'the tall, handsome, cold fish', 'a robot', 'this important, very busy man', 'the consultant fate had awarded me'. One

seemed annoyed at the inconvenience of there being a human inside my pregnant body—and on such a busy Saturday.... He came in, and without observing me push through one contraction announced that I would have to have a low forceps delivery. I suppose he just happened to have half an hour free. I was taken completely by surprise and it took several minutes to realise just what was happening. I was speechless with hatred, disappointment and futility.... As my legs were being strapped into the stirrups I said to the consultant, 'I suppose there is nothing for me to do but submit.' His response: 'Submit to what? Sex?' ... In the eternal retrospect I wish I had mentioned to him that submission is not my chosen response in sex either.

The head was delivered by forceps, 'and then he didn't even let me push the rest of the baby out'. This woman felt she had been 'most terribly violated' by the consultant, and much preferred the personal relationship with her GP.

Labours at home

In describing their labours at home women emphasized reduction in stress, and in particular the normality of their activities during a large part of the first stage, during which they undertook everyday activities in the house or garden. One woman planted runner beans, stopping only to relax and 'breathe deliberately' with each contraction. 'When labour starts', said one woman, 'there is no upheaval, having to rush out into the cold night, find somewhere to park the children, etc. You can carry on as normal and go to bed when you feel like it.' There were statements such as 'one's home is usually more comfortable than a hospital room and can be adjusted to suit personal needs', and 'It is harder to standardize care in such individual surroundings.' Another woman described how after the waters had begun to leak and she had had contractions at 10-minute intervals for 4 hours which then died away, she went out to supper with her husband, and then to bed for a 'good few hours sleep' before labour began in earnest. Many women referred to the advantages of being in one's own home and one's own bed, in familiar, comfortable surroundings. 'Labour seemed much shorter', one woman commented, 'because I didn't go upstairs until I got to the stage of feeling if I didn't go up soon I wouldn't manage the stairs'. A woman who said, 'There is no need for the expectant mother to change her usual daily routine or to go to bed until she feels like it, so that birth seems a much shorter process', added that: 'It may actually be shorter, if the relaxation possible in the comfort and security of one's own home allows physical processes to proceed with less interference.'

Even where the situation was not easy, when for example there was a posterior presentation with a long backache labour, or in one case where the woman had a bad relationship with her midwife, the women who had had home confinements said they preferred them to previous hospital births. The one who disliked her midwife who, she said, 'agitated us all by flapping around' largely because she was inexperienced with home deliveries, still summed up the labour in very positive terms:

My daughter was born in a very peaceful, happy atmosphere, and was a very peaceful, contented baby. I felt much more rested [than after a previous hospital delivery] and had no postnatal depression. I was in control, I was in my own bed (where I had been born, in fact!) in my own home, and I didn't feel 'taken over' by a vast body of people in white masks. Traditionally birth was never a mysterious activity to be carried out in hospitals under the supervision of men. It was an essential part of the role of women which took place in the baby's home amid the comfort of friends and relations. Certainly we do not want to return to the days of high infant and maternal mortality, but surely we are now able to strike a balance between the old mysticism and the new.

All the letters describing the experience of home confinement referred to the pleasure of the post-partum days, and the mother's feelings of well-being and contentment then. One attributed 'getting off to a splendid start' with the baby to the fact that her midwives and doctor had 'much more interest in mother and baby as a unit' than when she had her first child in hospital where, she added, 'there was the feeling that *they* had produced and were caring for the baby, and "Mother" was an extra.' Another woman said, 'The next days were really almost a holiday.' One woman contrasted the atmosphere of home with that of the 'sixth form dorm' in which she had had to spend the post-partum days after a previous hospital delivery. A husband wrote, 'I particularly noticed the relaxed atmosphere at home after the baby was born, contrasted with the very tense time (for me) when she came home from hospital after our first son was born. We went to bed with a sense of joint achievement, having acquired a delightful addition to the family with a minimum of fuss and disruption.' This couple wrote when the baby was 2 weeks old, saying that they were still 'in a honeymoon mood a fortnight after Timothy's arrival'.

The displaced sibling

Multiparae invariably drew attention to the advantages to the toddler of a home confinement and especially, as we have seen, when the midwife related well to the older children: 'Family life carries on and the mother can still keep in touch. It is better for the other children'; 'Sam was able to see the baby when she was just half an hour old'; 'Paul accepted Christopher very rapidly, and now, two weeks later, seems to accept him as a fact of life'; 'The older children came in with great joy and excitement in the morning. I helped them to get dressed as usual and together we admired the new baby'; 'The older child slept through everything, and woke to find a new baby with whom he was allowed to play immediately, and as I was at home he did not feel he had been pushed out at all, being able to come into my room and bed as and when he pleased.'

Mothers told how the informal atmosphere of home, and birth within the normal context of family life, allowed the toddler to accept the new baby more easily, saved the older child from the trauma of maternal absence, and also educated the toddler in positive values in relation to birth, instead of making him infer that having a baby was something a woman went to hospital for in order to be 'made better'. Women also said that birth at home meant that *they* did not have to worry about the inevitable upset involved for a toddler whose mother has to leave him, and that this meant that they were more rested and a good deal happier.

One problem occurred because of the presence of a toddler in the house during a home confinement: no-one could use the telephone to call the doctor —'Needless to say it was Toby who had lifted the receiver off downstairs.' Fortunately the doctor arrived 'just in time for the delivery', and 'after a bit of tidying up, Paul brought Toby to see his sister for the first time. His reactions were touching: he grinned from ear to ear and kissed her very gently—a real honour since he is only prepared to kiss his teddy bear, no-one else—and a minute or two later he switched his attention to his new book and forgot all about her.'

Problems occurring in home confinements

Four women told of difficulties when confronted with home confinements. In one case the baby had respiratory problems and mother and baby were moved to hospital on the first post-partum day.

One couple had faced financial difficulties with the home confinement and said they thought that help should be provided to cover basic equipment and the costs of a domiciliary birth.

A woman who had a very poor relationship with her very authoritarian midwife during labour found the post-natal visits upsetting too. Some women had felt the midwife was coming in to take over and reacted negatively to her first appearance, occasionally when their own midwives were away and a replacement whom they had not previously met arrived. But in each case the woman, her husband, and the midwife had adapted to each other within the facilitating domestic atmosphere, and it was clear that as the midwife began to relax, the patient relaxed too, and a positive relationship was able to develop.

Only one woman said she found it difficult to get sufficient rest at home, and it was generally felt that mothers had far more chance of rest at home than in hospital.

Need to share the experience of birth with the husband

Most women relied on their husbands to help and support them in labour. For these women it was usually not simply a question of the husband's physical presence, but of hoping that he would be able to guide them and to play a central part in the birth and the days afterwards. They described how their husbands timed and monitored contractions, helped them with breathing and relaxation, propped them up and held them in their arms when pushing, and constantly encouraged and praised them. Except in the most enlightened hospitals where husbands are accepted as a matter of course and are important members of the labour team, many men feel awkward intruders in the hospital, and that they are there on sufferance rather than by right. Moreover, the routines and obstetric practices of a busy maternity unit may in themselves prove inhibiting to the husband and challenge his role as labour 'coach'.

Even in those hospitals which encourage husbands to be present, it is frequently the practice to send the husband out of the room while the woman is examined and for forceps deliveries, and respondents often said that this is when they would have particularly valued their husbands' presence. Interventionist practices, including the giving of drugs, were sometimes performed while the husband was absent, and he came back to find his wife drowsy with pethidine and unable to use her breathing techniques effectively. In one case a woman in the late first stage had been asked by the professor to 'help with my research' and had been given valium and pethidine which together appear to have caused maternal disorientation and some paediatric concern about the baby's condition. The paediatrician explained to the mother that she was there because 'your baby may be sleepy ... because of the valium'. Some of the husbands missed the delivery because staff did not realize how far advanced in labour the woman was—a problem encountered when a woman has been to good antenatal classes and is handling her contractions quietly and happily, especially in hospitals where pain and distress are anticipated and taken as a measure of progress. Then there was a last minute rush: 'My husband was left in the waiting room and didn't see the baby born, something we've both regretted ever since.'

Some of the domiciliary midwives were excellent at fully involving the husbands and were sensitively aware of the significance of the experience of birth for the couple. 'A final push and there it was, this little navy blue head,' wrote one woman. '"Touch it, touch it, both of you," said the midwife, and it was a thrill to feel it.' It is impossible to estimate the effect that this kind of experience can have on the relationship between husband and wife, but one writer, who had had marriage problems in pregnancy, tried to assess it in her own case:

We have all gained something more than a baby. Our relationship was sorely tested during the more difficult later months of the pregnancy, but so much was shared at the birth, and now in the joint caring for our children. I feel as if an extra dimension has been added, and that this is the beginning of so much. I have learned a great deal about myself and have gained a greater sense of awareness of relationships with family and friends.

Three quarters of the women who described home births mentioned how they valued sharing the immediate post-partum days, and they sometimes compared this with their loneliness when their husbands went home leaving them in hospital. At home 'the involvement with my husband made us a family from the beginning', wrote a woman whose husband, a parish priest, announced the birth of a daughter to his congregation by hanging a variety of pink garments on the washing line. Twelve women specifically referred to the emotional bonding of the father and his child: 'My husband felt a greater bond having seen this baby born and handled him from the beginning in a happy relaxed way, something which took a long time to achieve with the first baby.'

Breast-feeding

We have seen already that women often mentioned breast-feeding. Of the 74 accounts of hospital confinements only 9 women felt entirely happy about the support and assistance they had with breast-feeding. Although approval, and even enthusiasm, is expressed for breast-feeding in hospitals, and although individual midwives and nurses are skilled at giving encouragement and advice, the overall picture is one of muddle, of contradictory instructions, unbending rules, and reiterated suggestions that a woman does not have enough milk or is not going to succeed. In contrast, those having their babies at home usually found domiciliary midwives helpful, relaxed and permissive in their approach to breast-feeding, and if they were not, it did not really matter, since the mothers were left to get on with it instead of being constantly and critically supervised in this intimate relationship. Women saw attachment between mother and baby, and privacy to 'do their own thing', as important for successful breast-feeding:

I feel that establishing breast-feeding is very much easier without the structure of hospital routine to fit into. There is current medical opinion that more is needed to be done to help mothers breast-feed. I think it is sad that it has got to this, though I suspect it is true, as feeding should initially be a physical relationship between mother and child, and I think the 'help' offered must sometimes come between the participants. You wouldn't make love, even for the first time, *especially* for the first time, with someone standing over you telling you where to put what.

Some mothers discharged themselves because of 'bad and contradictory advice' about breast-feeding and strict routines which permitted babies to be fed only every 4 hours.

A husband contrasted the difficulties in establishing lactation after a hospital confinement with the ease of doing so after a home delivery:

Oliver was given glucose and water and brought to Jane some 8 hours later. Until Jane's milk came in he was given 4 oz evaporated milk at each feed after his sucking at the breast. When she enquired if this was necessary, she was told it was completely standard practice—'You can't let him go hungry'. On the third day her milk came in and she immediately made it clear that he should have no more bottles from anyone. However, for the rest of Jane's stay in hospital her confidence was continually undermined, as Oliver cried every evening and the nurses said that it was because she didn't have enough milk. He weighed 8 lb 1 oz at birth and 8 lb 11 oz at 8 days. She was also constantly woken up by nurses for routine procedures when trying to nap between feeds, and there were a host of minor irritations stemming from the fact that the nursing staff treated all the mothers as totally lacking in brain. At 9 days she was suffering from lack of sleep and discharged herself. It took her mother and me a week of fairly intensive care to restore her to her usual happy state.

After the home birth, however, 'Jane put the baby to the breast straight away, without any other foods being given him.' The wife said: 'After Jeremy had had another suck we went to bed in our own bed with our new son asleep in his crib beside me. My milk came in in 48 hours, Jeremy slept and fed well, and I recovered very quickly indeed.'

Home birth and the handicapped or still-born baby

Many of the writers mentioned their concern during pregnancy that they might be harming their babies by choosing a home confinement, and said that this anxiety was often reinforced and magnified by remarks made by obstetricians. Some mothers were worried that if they had a handicapped baby the hospital would insist on trying to save its life come what may, and this was one reason they gave for preferring to have the baby at home: 'If the deformity were so severe that only special machines and heroic measures could keep the baby alive, I don't think I would want it to live. I would also prefer being spared the decision that can only take place in hospital, of whether or not, and if so when, to cut off the machine.' One who was herself a nurse had visited an intensive-care unit:

There were 15 children. I have nursed small, very ill children, but I was seeing it now as a mother, and as part of a Community Health Council. The Sister, a charming woman, came to one cot and announced with great, and no doubt justifiable pride, that here was a babe who had threatened to abort several times, but that it had been saved, and when it was born, very prematurely, there had been a struggle to keep it alive. 'But it has survived.' It has, poor wee thing. It is one of these children neither male nor female, and it is going to have and give problems probably for the rest of its life. In my lay view there were three children in that ward who would probably have to be supported entirely for their lives, and others that will probably be emotionally impaired by having spent the first weeks of their lives in incubators. The mothers were allowed down twice a day to see them. These cases obviously make statistics of perinatal mortality look more respectable, but I question the highly technical medical ability that enables life to continue in these cases, if on no other than long-term economic grounds.

One woman had experienced a still-birth at home, and yet believed strongly that home was the best place to have a baby. She explained exactly what was done by the midwife and her assistant to try and get the baby to breathe, having observed it all closely herself, and then said, perhaps significantly: '*We* rang for the doctor and ambulance.' The GP and a colleague arrived in 3 minutes and intubated the baby, but without success. 'After half an hour it was obviously no use, and we accepted that the baby was dead. This may seem to be an indictment of home deliveries. Obviously we asked ourselves whether this might have been avoided or more might have been done in hospital. I think the answer is not', and then she went on to say:

The great advantage of this situation arising at home was that we were able to feel part of the fight for our baby's life, and of her eventual death. She was lying on my bed where I could see her and everything that was happening. We were able to feel useful by ringing for the doctor and the ambulance. It was a great comfort to me that I was not lying in the formal atmosphere of the hospital, shut away with soothing words, probably given valium, not allowed to see what was happening, not allowed to see the baby. As it was, the fact that she was not going to live dawned on us gradually. With my husband, my own G.P., a midwife whom I had grown to trust, it was rather more bearable than it might have been. I was able to refuse tranquillisers, and to stay in my own family. I was obviously not with other women who had had babies. In these special circumstances I definitely prefer home deliveries. I would think that home delivery with a happier outcome must be equally good.

This woman's third baby was born in hospital, and it was a very happy experience. The interesting thing from the point of view of this enquiry is that her conclusion is that 'everyone should be able to have a home delivery if they wish' and that 'there are enormous advantages psychologically, not only for the mother, but also the rest of the family.' 'If there has to be a hospital confinement for reasons of safety', she wrote, 'then the more human and informal and understanding the hospital, the better. Certainly the fact that the hospital saved my third baby's life, and obviously cared for the psychological well-being of mothers and families almost converted me to hospital deliveries. Almost, but not quite. Obviously in an ideal world home deliveries would be as safe as those in hospital. I do hope that you are able to bring that a little nearer.'

Conclusion

The views expressed by these women should be set alongside those voiced by obstetricians. It may be that advances in the care of mothers and babies before, during, and after childbirth will come not only from technical developments which contribute to obstetric knowledge, but also from a concern with the quality of the environment in which women give birth and into which babies are born. Is pregnancy an illness of which a woman must be 'cured' by an obstetrician? Or is it part of a developmental process in which a couple grow to be parents and a family welcomes a new member? Decisions made now about the quality of maternity care and the options available to women when they have their babies which can have far reaching consequences in the future should be the concern not only of professional experts in obstetrics and paediatrics, but of society as a whole. For these are not exclusively, nor even primarily, medical decisions, but ethical ones. They involve a responsibility which cannot be delegated to doctors, but which we all must share.

One of the mothers wrote: 'I feel very strongly that "there is no place like home"' and went on to quote from a book which describes a major community health care project in the 1940s, The Peckham experiment (Pearse and Crocker 1943): 'In biology there is no basis for the relegation of the pregnant woman at the time of delivery to the position of "patient" to which modern civilisation has condemned her. Neither is there any basis for the conversion of the natural crisis of birth into the catastrophic crisis that delivery at the present day is tacitly accepted to be—above all by the health authorities.'

Perhaps that is a lesson that we need to learn today.

Reference

Pearse, I. H. and Crocker, L. H. (1943). *The Peckham experiment: a study in the living structure of society.* Allen & Unwin, London.

JOEL RICHMAN AND W. O. GOLDTHORP **10**

Fatherhood:
the social construction of pregnancy
and birth

The expectant father has too long been neglected or regarded facetiously.

Weiner and Steinhilber, 1961

The only justification for a husband's presence during labour is to support and comfort his wife, and this can best be done during the first stage. If an ideal relationship exists between the husband and wife, he must be moved by her condition in the second stage; in such a state, he can only be an added burden to his wife and an embarrassment to her attendant.

Matthews, 1961

Babies have fathers too, and men are increasingly wishing to share in the birth of their children. Obstetricians and midwives either simply tolerate their presence, or can make them welcome and support them in their roles.

In this chapter a sociologist and a consultant obstetrician together look at the organization of the maternity unit to see what fathers feel about being present during labour and what can be done to help make childbirth a positive experience for them.

The present surge of professional and lay interest in birth has made many people cease to take for granted the way in which it takes place in our society. Birth is now a theme politically fused at all levels and presents a challenge to the established medical ideologies. The major opposition to some modern obstetric practices has come from the Women's Movement, who present their struggle as one of freeing their bodies and minds from male domination. Another impetus for the recent interest in birth has been generated by the rapidly declining birth-rate (1976–7 was the lowest rate ever recorded), which has placed a higher social premium not only on the decision to reproduce, but also on the social milieu of birth. In such debates the expectant father has often been culturally submerged. Although, for example, his presence is increasing in delivery wards, his role has been accorded only token recognition; often as 'unpaid comforter' alleviating staff shortages.

Our concern here is to acknowledge, primarily from the sociological perspective, the father's role in pregnancy and focus upon a number of salient points: first to explain why there has been this cultural conspiracy against fatherhood in modern times; second to collate and evaluate, briefly, the existing studies related to fathers' responses to pregnancy (these are sparse, and are heavily influenced by findings from ethology, Freudian psychodynamics of personality and late nineteenth century anthropology); thirdly to try to present findings from our ongoing research of fathers' construction of pregnancy careers (see p. 166) and their conceptualizations of hospital delivery. Finally, some policy recommendations will be made to facilitate the visible incorporation of fathers into the birth drama.

The conspiracy against fathers

The overt dominance of motherhood has its origins in the rise of the Christian ethic and was reinforced by the institutional division of labour between male and female activities and values accompanying industrialization. Today the sex stereotyping still explains motherhood as 'natural' and 'instinctive' behaviour, a view endorsed by the church, medical profession, and other sections of society. Symbolically and by social action this is demonstrable in a number of ways: religious art forms inevitably portray the Madonna and child, rarely Joseph and child. In this context, Macintyre (1976) has shown how married women who do not want children find their motives suspected and their normality questioned by medical practitioners. Married men are not subjected to similar questioning. Maternity as a career is fostered by commercial interests and buttressed by public and private rules. The woman is channelled into new client relationships with other knowledgeable mothers, often forming a subculture, and with the health services. An expectant father is often a peripheral appendage to such relationships. The Employment Protection Act (1976), guaranteeing her job after leave of absence for pregnancy, is a further endorsement by the state of the increasing significance of motherhood. Also, only in 'exceptional' circumstances (e.g. lesbianism) will the courts consider a father suitable to have custody of young children.

Pregnancy for the woman is matrixed in a pattern of ritual forms and sequences. The mathematical calibrations indexing her obstetric progression (Richman and Goldthorp 1976) imprint a heavy, cultural tattooing. White (1957) has also described how the 'mental illnesses' associated with childbearing, with their confusing terminology, ritualizes the woman's pregnancy: puerperal insanity; gestational psychosis; confusional insanity; insanity of pregnancy, of puerperium, and of lactation; toxic and infectious exhaustive psychosis; etc. Fathers-to-be are granted no similar, 'scientific' recognition and statistical frequency. Significantly, medical explanations for the above genre of 'depressions' pivot largely on the mother's attitudes, or hormones; rarely is her condition attributed to the father's responses to her pregnancy.

The cultural subordination of fatherhood can be elaborated, more specifically, in Parsonian terms (Parsons 1952): men are expected to play instrumental–adaptive roles, whereas women are allocated expressive–integrative ones. Fathers are presented primarily as the economic providers for the family unit and are seen as the coupling linking the family to the occupational statuses of the market economy. Being the economic provider has the further connotations of virility and rationality. Women, conversely, are portrayed as being the providers of emotional support *within* the household. Women do engage in outside work activities, but many of these jobs mirror their domestic, supportive roles. The bulk of psychiatric theory and philosophy of child care lends direct support to this accredited male–female dichotomy. Expressions like 'unmarried father' and 'tenderloving father' lack common usage. Since Freud placed the mother in the heliocentric position of the child's universe, linked concepts of 'maternal-deprivation' have long constituted part of the vocabulary of social work. The father is invoked in mental health schema as a subsidiary to the mother–child relationship when drastic deviations are recognized. The father appears, 'normally', only at a 'later' stage, in developmentally based themes of child psychology, and then as an 'object' of identification. Howells (1970) suggests as child psychiatrists are frequently women this may introduce a bias by their empathizing with the mother. To express 'fatherliness' in its own right risks the danger still of it being labelled effeminate behaviour. Josselyn (1956) has even argued that for fathers to be involved in 'baby affairs', without taking on the guise of being temporary and expedient mother-substitutes, exposes them to 'symbolic castration'.

However, conjunctive societal and familial changes are blurring the formerly held role definitions and these cannot but feed into the psychosocial attitudes to the many facets of birth. Although the achievement of sexual equality within the home is still much exaggerated and banners such as 'democratic', 'egalitarian', or 'symmetrical' hoisted optimistically are slogans more of normative expectations than being fulfilled realities, men are becoming more child-centred. There are many exceptions, of course, for example the absentee middle-class husband (Cohen 1975) engaged in long-distance commuting. For many, work is ceasing to be the central interest in life; home is becoming more a private refuge from increasing alienation. Studies by Neuloh (1959) in Germany, and Faunce (1959) in the United States, as well as British examples, show the trend that when hours at work are reduced the released time is used within the home participating in domestic activities and family outings. Marriages are no longer maintained by the husband's economic and legal bonds; new, intimate divisions of labour are appearing based more on mutual reciprocities, but to some extent still dependent on emergent crises.

The father's response to pregnancy and birth

A primary component of these exchanges is the husband's new input of increased emotional support. Within this context the father's involvement with pregnancy and birth is more apparent. Pregnancy holds a high degree of ambiguity, merging both social and medical implications. Rosengren (1962) was the first to show clearly the social–structural conditions facilitating enacting the sick role during pregnancy; e.g. women who are mobile between class positions and experiencing status ambiguities tend to have difficult labours; women whose antenatal care is punctuated with quarrels with their physicians do likewise. Thus, it is obvious that the father, as a part of the social network encapsulating the birth, must have an influence on the course of events.

The effects of the social parameter of the father are still not clear. The few empirical investigations made to date show that the husband's presence at birth has a desirable effect on the quality of the woman's birth experience. Henneborn and Cogan (1975), testing Tanzer's findings, state that the 'social–emotional component provided by husbands present for labour and delivery was important in affecting reported pain during labour'. It must be noted that the study used a sample of couples who had undergone Lamaze, or psychoprophylactic, pre-natal education classes and the husband acted as a 'labour coach' throughout. They also indicate that prior attitudes towards birth are not changed by the Lamaze classes. Those husbands who wished to be present only for the labour did not change their minds as the classes proceeded, in fact they chose a hospital which did not allow husbands to be present at delivery. Sassmor (1972), from the United States, again claims that in 'over 45 000 documented cases, fathers have proved they can be a valuable asset to the obstetrical team without untoward sequelae'; she argues that the presence of a 'prepared' father complements the quality of obstetrics. There is no evidence, however, to give warranty to the unbounded optimism of the proponents of the psychoprophylactic movement who suggest that the father's presence, per se, is a panacea for the future success of the family. Forbes (1972) has argued, 'it gives him confidence to face future problems, support his wife and care for his children.'

One British study (Goldthorp and Richman 1974 a, b) made of 65 mothers' evaluations of the maternity services when, during a hospital strike, they were compelled to have a domiciliary delivery, showed, again, that one of the reasons for their favourable responses to home delivery was the husbands' presence at birth: in some instances it was an absolute necessity. Although only 22 per cent had indicated their prior willingness to be present at the hospital delivery (many in fact do drop out), 48 per cent were present at home. The husband's presence had neutralized the potentially disruptive situation caused by the hospital breaking its client relationship with the mother. The mother's favourable response to domiciliary delivery was not influenced by whether the birth was difficult or easy.

In this section we shall focus more directly on fathers and briefly review the main findings pertaining to show how childbirth affects their beliefs and behaviour. The researchers, from different discipline areas, emphasize one point in common: that very little is known, even though our secularizing society is ostensibly diminishing its sexual taboos. Significantly, very little energy has been expended in discovering the sociological overtones of fatherhood, one of the great biological and social universals. For example Hartman (1966) writes: 'explanations offered are largely impressionistic, sketchy and embarrassed by the limited empirical data.' Existing knowledge on fatherhood is atypical in a number of ways. One strand still relies on extrapolations from nineteenth century tribal 'exotica' in which interpretations of the couvade† are prominent. Another strand, Freudian theorizing, developed by Reik (1931), drawing upon the same source, relates how birth activates the father's Oedipus complex with its fear of incest, and portrays the child as a phallic competitor, or makes the husband experience womb envy. Many of the studies are in the clinical mould of deviance and pathology, based on small numbers of patients and are unrepresentative of the population at large. Others use highly selected categories of the population, as found in the total institutions of prisons and army camps.

Some of the characterizations of fathers' responses to pregnancy have been portrayed as follows. Zilboorg (1931) directly attributed the depressive reactions and mental illness of both parents to childbirth. Another post-Freudian, Jarvis (1962), in a study of four patients follows a similar tact arguing that childbirth always has a psychological effect on the father; pregnancy precipitating a shift in the mental equilibrium of the psyche. He develops the interesting insight that men can react to childbirth with conditions that can resemble post-partum psychosis in women. However, one of his patients had a dog phobia; another never completed his psychoanalysis and the details were gleaned from his wife!

Towne and Afterman's study (1955), at the Veterans Administration Hospital of Palo Alto, California, of 28 patients suffering from psychosis induced by parenthood, causing some to attempt infanticide, locates the nub of their illness in the form of marriage they undertook. Their wives were the dominant partners who perceived their husbands as children and themselves as 'mother–sister–confidantes'. The arrival of the children was therefore regarded by the husbands as a total negation and betrayal of themselves. Two studies have concentrated on the relationship between the more 'physical' symptoms and pregnancy. Inman (1941) makes the case for styes tarsal cysts, and infections of the glands of the eyelids being often associated with 'thoughts and fantasies' about childbirth. He traced the connection through folklore and the bible, finding that gold wedding rings (symbolizing birth?) were an old cure for styes.

Trethowan and Conlon's research (1965) is distinguished methodologically

---

†The word is said to derive from the Basque *couver*, to sit or hatch, i.e. as on eggs. Tylor first introduced the 'couvade' as a technical anthropological term in the 1870s. All writers on the subject seem to agree that the term does not represent the vast array of male birth practices: dietary prohibitions, restrictions on travel, adoption of correct body posture, e.g. not crossing the legs, special language usages, or taking to bed and simulating delivery.

by being the only study to have a control-sample against which to juxta-pose their findings. In a sample of 327 fathers, whose wives had just con-ceived, they discovered: (a) the expectant fathers had experienced more toothache, nausea, and loss of appetite; (b) the peak incidence of symptoms occurred in the third month, with a secondary rise in the ninth; (c) in just under a third of the cases the symptoms cleared before labour started, with another third becoming symptom-free immediately after the birth. Another interesting feature revealed that the expectant fathers aged 45 and over exhibited less symptoms than their comparable age group within the control sample. The gastrointestinal complaints have clear linkages with anxiety states but toothache, which has long figured in pregnancy myths, is more difficult to explain medically.

Studies that make clear the subjective feelings fathers hold about birth, attributing 'conscious' motives for their desire for children, an attribute ex-tensively covered in the literature on mothers, are almost totally absent. One notable exception is Benedek's (1946) account of parenthood in wartime. She describes how soldiers' desires for children can be interpreted as a strategy for overcoming the strangeness engendered by active service. The baby is wanted as a means of reinforcing one's ties with normal life and developing a 'maturity' denied by the military hierarchial structure. When demobbed the baby represents the means of restitution, the possibility of becoming again a 'good man' and atoning for one's wartime evils. In sum, these cameos on fathers reveal two things. Fathers do not associate their symptoms with pregnancy and, equally crucial, their family doctors are also not aware of the possible connections.

In tribal society fatherhood was more readily acknowledged by a series of customs loosely grouped under the heading of the couvade. Strabo, Didorus, and other classical writers have commented earlier on its occurrence in ancient Europe and regarded it as a rite for propitiating ancestral spirits for the child's benefit. Interpretations of the couvade are still the source of much speculation. One notion, completely untestable, relying on nineteenth century evolutionary biology considers that the couvade commemorates the period when society was allegedly transitional between matrilineal and patri-lineal obligations. Frazer (1910) regarded the couvade as a magico-protective rite transferring pain from the mother and deflecting evil spirits from the baby. Restrictions on travel during the pregnancy and birth fixes the father to the birth event. His behaviour is believed to affect the baby's progress: e.g., the Caribs of Honduras (Coelho 1949) do not permit the father to en-gage in physical exertion since his perspiration will cause the baby's navel to bleed. Malinowski (1927) also argued that the couvade fulfilled the 'func-tion' of legitimating the child's need for a father and in so doing em-phasized the family as society's supreme, moral unit. Levy-Bruhl argued that the couvade was additional evidence that the mind of primitive man was pre-logical and therefore unlike that of modern man.

It has been proposed (Freeman 1951) that the occurrence of 'symptoms' among expectant fathers is due to modern man cocooning himself from the crisis of fatherhood. Symptom formation, having the characteristics of private rituals, and so being the equivalent of the couvade, provides prescribed patterns of behaviour for coping with the problematics of birth. However, such a notion contains the unwarranted assumptions that the couvade was widespread in tribal society and when practised was efficacious, but, according to psychoanalytic theory, its practitioners were deluded neurotics.

The father's construction of the pregnancy role and his concepts of delivery

In this section we draw together some of the threads already discussed, often meagre and speculative, which have been attached to the father's pregnancy role. We examine, more specifically, some of the ways in which they have constructed their social reality of birth, both as a symbolic and practical event. The analysis is based upon the first stage of research designed initially at attempting to distinguish the social parameters influencing the father's decision to attend the birth at the hospital.† It was soon apparent from observations that fathers who attended the birth and fathers who attended the labour only were not fixed categories. There was a process of 'drift' (Matza 1969), encouraged, in part, by some staff, primarily from the 'original' labour-only attenders.

In examining the social composition of the two groups there was little to distinguish them overall. Table 10.1 shows that 50 per cent of the birth-attenders had white-collar socio-economic status, compared with 52 per cent of the labour-only group. When the wife worked outside the home during pregnancy there was a slight tendency for those with labour-only husbands to engage in more white-collar jobs, 54 per cent as opposed to 43 per cent. Neither the wives' nor the husbands' age was of significance in distinguishing the two groups. In terms of the husband's work routine no factor was apparently critical: 23 per cent of the birth-attenders stated they were losing money by being there as opposed to 24 per cent of the labour-only group.

Of those attending birth 73 per cent were doing so for the first time. In 50 per cent of the cases the birth-attenders were present for a first child, as opposed to 66 per cent of cases for the labour-only fathers. Forty-two per cent of the birth-attenders had previous children, compared with 34 per cent of the labour-only fathers, suggesting for some, at least, a prior sensitizing process to the nuances of birth can be operative influencing

† The data was collected by a variety of techniques. A sample of 100 birth-attenders and 50 labour-only fathers were surveyed. Nineteen were interviewed in depth, and these interviews were tape-recorded. These fathers welcomed the opportunity of discussing their attitudes and feelings towards pregnancy not only as a break from their wives' labour, but also because they never had a previous opportunity of attempting to clarify some of their beliefs and expectations they had erected around pregnancy. Due to their fatigue and state of high emotional arousal much of the data resembled that often associated with therapeutic interviews. Other data was collected by indirect interviews and participant observation on walk-arounds.

Table 10.1 Socio-economic status (Registrar General's classification) of parents (figures are percentages)

	1	2	3a	3b	4	5	6†
Fathers attending birth (total 100)	5	23	22	39	9	1	1
Fathers attending labour only (total 50)	8	26	18	38	6	2	2
Wives‡ of fathers attending birth	–	11	32	7		2	39
Wives‡ of fathers attending labour only	2	10	42	8	16	–	22

† no data supplied, not in paid employment
‡ in paid employment at the time of pregnancy

attendance decisions. Decoding, in retrospect, the allocation of responsibility for the 'initial' husband–wife decision regarding attendance practice is very difficult. However, there was some evidence to suggest that the decision made by the labour-only fathers was one they took more by themselves, whereas the birth-attenders tended to involve others: they made the decision in conjunction with their wives and to a lesser extent involving friends, relatives, and midwives.

The birth event, climactic though it may be, is but one part in pregnancy. Thus, in attempting to understand the meaning of birth for the father, it is essential that his pregnancy career *in toto* be outlined. The concept of 'career' is offered not in its 'objective' usage for occupational line but in its more 'subjective' content as 'any social strand of any person's career through life' (Goffman 1959). A pregnancy career is but one of many in which he can be engaged simultaneously. We have referred elsewhere (Richman, Goldthorp, and Simmons 1975) to the interplay between occupational and pregnancy careers. For example, some manual workers recount how becoming a father will make them more 'responsible'. Fatherhood provides the legitimation for escaping from one's stereotype at work for being hotheaded or militant. Birth provides the justification for initiating a series of new practices. The woman's status passage to birth is biologically and culturally visible. Men's pregnancy careers are primarily opaque, often more diffuse, but are still capable of producing equivalent attachment to the child-to-be. The general, medical view, as expressed by Pawson and Morris (1972), is, to an extent, a commonsense fallacy: 'Unlike women, they have no hormone changes, no remarkable physical and *emotional* experiences to help them adopt and identify with their new child. It is a secondary form of relationship.'

Generalizing, pregnancy does generate the potential for the husband's disengagement from certain spheres of activities. The wife is strategically positioned to be the arbitrator on the progress of the pregnancy, controlling the information from the medical authorities, as well as self-monitoring the foetus. The decision to go into hospital at the opportune time belongs primarily to the woman. Within the hospital men suffer from an 'entrance trauma', especially with a first birth. In the reception area they describe how their wives are 'taken away from them', or 'disappear' with a midwife who treats them as a non-person. They often feel outsiders in a world geared for women. These features tend to substantiate Pawson's and Morris's pronouncement on fathers' 'secondary relationships'. However, many fathers attempt to create a 'special relationship' with their unborn child. Many male pregnancy careers include an acceleration in the completion of jobs around the home, usually involving the preparation of the baby's room. Delivery can subsume their dominant work roles: fathers plan their holidays around the birth. Approximately one-quarter of birth and labour-only attenders claimed to have taken their wives 'most times' to the antenatal clinic; some risked dismissal for bad time-keeping. A number of pregnancy careers also included the husband's deliberate abstention from sexual intercourse; there is a general diminution of frequency around the fifth month. This was noticeable when there had been a previous, 'unexpected' miscarriage when starting a family. The father's relinquishment of sexual intercourse, signifying 'sacrifice', indicated his special contribution towards a successful birth; also, it was considered as a magico-protective device supplementing the technico-medical practices to overcome the uncertainties of birth.

There are a surfeit of studies showing the complexity of meanings mothers gave their pregnancies. For example, Weiner and Steinhilber (1961) emphasize that conception can represent: an increase in prestige within the family; an escape from intolerable conditions; a means of getting support; a sense of triumph over others, such as an elder sister; a method of dealing with an unsatisfactory marriage, as when a partner is promiscuous or an alcoholic. Again, Crowther (1965) logs the permutations of behavioural pathways related to the mother's perception of her pregnancy. Some from early on regarded the foetus as a separate organism with definite personality traits, and as male or female. These mothers quickly affiliate with their offspring on delivery. Others would defer acknowledging the onset of pregnancy and delay making preparations. Fathers, likewise, invest the foetus with a constellation of values, which groove their responses to the birth. To indicate but a few: the baby is expected to bring the husband and wife closer together; make them happier; make life much fuller; make a real family unit. Thirty-two percent of the birth-attenders stressed these themes compared with 22 per cent of the labour-only fathers. Other significances were attributed to the baby: it would now complete the family unit; it would rectify the sex or age imbalance among the existing children; it would furnish new challenges and ambitions; it will make life more exciting watching the child grow up. For a few, more particular birth meanings were expressed:

it would now demonstrate in the eyes of their mothers they were 'proper men'; they had reached fulfilment by perpetuating themselves giving life to others. However, a minority, 10 per cent of the birth-attenders and labour-only fathers claimed the baby would make no, or minimal, differences to their lives.

It is possible to arrange the dominant pregnancy careers of fathers along four axes:

1 The father denies the existence of the pregnancy and accordingly adopts strategies of disavowal, e.g. abandons the mothers, or engages in new activities, usually outside the home, in attempting to create an alternative identity. This career is exceptional; our sample did not directly detect this pattern; but is prevalent in the psychiatric case studies noted earlier.
2 The father adopts the stance that pregnancy is 'nothing unusual' and is the wife's responsibility. When requested he may supply some instrumental assistance in the home. This pattern reflects the existing segmental roles of husband and wife and is found among the traditional working class and middle classes with absentee fathers.
3 The father wishes to share the pregnancy experience and develops special bonds with the foetus. He will offer increased emotional, as well as instrumental, support. This pregnancy career appears to be increasing, especially in the younger marrieds.
4 The father claims total identification with the foetus, sometimes to the exclusion of the mother's role, and attempts to sterilize her, socially, from everyday activities. This career is rare and can occur when the husband is much older than the wife, or when the wife has conceived for the first time after a long period of infertility.

A pregnancy career is a dynamic process and can branch off in many directions. This polarized scheme does not convey the myriads of variations between the arcs. Each pregnancy unit must also be considered as a unique moral order, producing its own cultural artefacts to solve its own internal dilemmas. The following case study, showing the meshing of work and family with the present pregnancy career and previous uncompleted one, illustrates how dramatic shifts of emphases occur.

A Catholic executive was frantic to start a family after a previous miscarriage. He came from a large family himself and at the last family reunion in Ireland at Christmas time he was the only head of a household who was childless. During the first half of the pregnancy he put his reluctant wife on a pedestal, forbade her to do any housework and each night requested a progress report on the foetus. During the second half he did not enquire, not necessarily because of Freudian-unconscious feelings of rivalry. The baby was most welcome. It was around the twenty-second week the previous miscarriage had occurred and this period was an ominous benchmark to be passed. The privatized taboo on talking about the baby was a strategy of preparing himself for the worst, as well as a means of fooling 'malevolent' forces about the baby's existence. He also froze his work career, refusing to move and accept promotion till after the successful birth.

In sum, to understand the father's response to birth, his pregnancy career, which in ways crystallizes his other careers, must be explained more fully.

When a father attends birth in hospital, especially for the first time, he can experience the conditions resembling Anomie, i.e. the norms in the setting are often contradictory and some sequences appear normless. He is in a culturally alien environment as a dependent in the midst of often nameless and faceless experts. The delivery can be conceptualized as the rites of transition (Gennep 1960) in the life crises of birth. The mother has undergone the prior preparation of the rites of separation, namely the compulsory bathing and pubic shaving to transform her from her everyday status. The father is ritually unprepared and is propelled into the birth setting of the rites of transition, one characterized by a 'sacredness' in which features of the everyday life are reversed. He is surrounded by the institutional rhetoric of the language and apparatus of medicine, which he normally associates with illness and death. The father can be temporally and spatially disorientated. Birth sequences are governed by foetal, mother, medical, and institutional times and exist largely outside his experience. He can be uncertain where to stand or put his hands. Sections of the delivery room are the private territories of the medical staff, but are not publically demarcated as such. The father's rights are not only limited but vague, according to various doctors' definitions of what constitutes a 'medical interlude' during birth. One doctor may dismiss the father during examinations; another will allow him to stay for a forceps delivery. If unprepared, he has never seen his wife as an 'object' of medical involvement and will abrogate his 'traditional' responsibility as 'protector and provider'. In retrospect, 15 per cent singled out from their dislikes about hospital birth their impotence in not being able to help their wives. That he is gowned from head to toe, but without prior medical socialization, does not always mean the husband feels part of the delivery team. The attire can erase symbolically his distinctive relationship with his wife. In Holland where the birth is more 'normalized', the husband is not so garbed and maintains his identity as *the* father. Roth (1957) has described how modern medicine, although newly forged on scientific principles, still maintains elements of magical content; obstetrics contains a powerful continuity of folklore. He pointed out further that the more senior one is in the medical hierarchy the more one is regarded as being 'germ-free'. The father is slotted in at the lowest level of involvement. For instance, the mask, even if worn correctly, maintains its sterile function for only 15 minutes, yet is insisted upon, unchanged, for the father and thereby transfixes him to the medical spectrum. Paradoxically he has a grandstand view of the proceedings, but may be unable, because of his disorientation to transmit a progress report to his wife. She could therefore have more difficulty, particularly if heavily drugged, in synchronizing her efforts.

However, the fathers present at birth still welcomed the opportunity; and

93 per cent stated they would be present for the 'next' one. The birth experience, *per se*, did have the effect of producing responses differentiating the attenders from the labour-only fathers. The birth-attenders tended to perceive their wives as having an 'easier' time (Table 10.2); 50 per cent

Table 10.2 Fathers' evaluation of mothers' condition in labour/delivery (figures are percentages)

	Comfort-able	Difficult	Very difficult	Don't know
Fathers attending birth (total 100)	50	35	8	7
Fathers attending labour only (total 50)	22	52	16	10

considered the labour/delivery as 'comfortable'. Again, this picture partially reappears when fathers were asked about their labour/delivery dislikes; 32 per cent of the labour-only fathers agreed it was 'seeing their wives in pain', as opposed to 20 per cent of the birth attenders. When considering what pleased the fathers (Table 10.3) it can be seen that those present at birth all made some response; 32 per cent of labour-only fathers made none. Furthermore, the birth-attenders displayed a greater range of topics of involvement. The two fathers wanting to learn about the techniques of delivery were an ambulanceman and policeman, who may be confronted themselves with that situation. It may appear incongruous that more labour-only fathers, 48 per cent, than birth-attenders, 35 per cent, were pleased that they were able to give comfort and support to their wives. But by not ex-periencing directly some of the anomic features of the delivery room—power-lessness, disorientation, and isolation—they could still maintain their identity of offering a supportive role. In recounting the moment of birth the fathers waxed allegorically about the wonderment of nature, and in general displayed a sentimentality 'normally' associated with femininity ... the first sight of the baby's head was beautiful; it was a joy seeing the first start in life; the happiness of nine months coming to fruition.

When asked in what ways the hospital could improve the lot of fathers, those present at birth raised fewer complaints; 60 per cent of labour-only attenders said no improvements were needed whereas 40 per cent of birth attenders responded similarly. On a cautionary note, all the surveys made of client evaluation of hospitals show high rates of 'satisfaction'. Everyday users often lack specialist types of evaluative criteria and their gratitude still reflects the high mystical esteem of medicine. None of the fathers had

Table 10.3 Aspects of labour/delivery which pleased fathers (figures are percentages)

	No one died	Learning about birth	Birth produced wanted boy	Support wife	Birth experi- ence	Knowing what was going on	When all over	Baby came so quickly	Helpful staff	Un- answered
Fathers attending birth (total 100)	6	2	2	35	53	4	1	1	12	–
Fathers attending labour only (total 50)	–	–	–	48	2	2	6	–	12	32

experienced prior birth at home and their babies displayed no apparent abnormalities. They were still elated in the baby honeymoon period.

Discussion

In this chapter we have ranged widely in constructing a sociological view on fatherhood and the accompanying responses to pregnancy and birth; across the boundaries of psychology, anthropology, and medicine. This eclectic approach was dictated by the sparseness of concentrated interest previously shown in the theme. We stressed three major points:

1 In Western society the dominance of the cultural stereotyping of mother-hood as being natural and the font of emotional support transformed pregnancy and birth into a female monopoly. Mirroring this historical process developmental psychology and its symbiotic relationship with social policy ideologically reinforced this stance. Obversely, the father is presented as being peripheral; he is accorded the status of genitor and external economic provider supporting the early mother–child bonding relationship. In some tribal societies the couvade, by its prescribed patterns of behaviour, distinguished the special tie, often of a 'spiritual' kind, between the father and unborn/newly born child. Today, the pregnancy careers of fathers are not culturally explicit, or even denied. Yet, as we have shown, fathers do invest the birth event with many different meanings, some general, some complex, and many highly privatized. The pregnancy career must be read in conjunction with the fathers' other careers. For example, 8 per cent of the fathers attending birth indicated that they intended to have a vasectomy soon after; so the birth was also climactic in that it was to be the severing of their fertility capabilities.

2 There is sufficient evidence to demonstrate that the woman's pattern of pregnancy, labour, and initial responses after delivery are very much influenced by the network of social factors surrounding the pregnancy. Pilowski (1972) has shown that women with complications in childbirth tend to fear for the outcome of the child, resent the disruption of their employment, describe their own mothers' health as poor and have many contacts with women who have had complicated pregnancies. The father, logically and empirically, *must* be considered an integral part of the mother's pregnancy network. The mother till now has been burdened with the total responsibility for 'puerperal syndromes'. In one of the few studies made of husbands' personalities Pilowski (1972) has again shown those on the 16-Personality Factor Test (Cattell and Eber 1957) who were socially effective and enjoyed meeting people, with possibly more interests outside the home, are associated with wives with more severe complications. In an unrefined way hospitals are recognizing the beneficial effects of fathers present at birth. Most fathers are unaculturized into the nuances of birth; they cannot participate to their potential in the alien settings of

hospitals. However, 75 per cent had never considered having their baby at home. Half explained that hospitals were 'safe' places; in making sense of pregnancy the most intelligible way was for them to use an illness label. Most of our knowledge of fathers' birth responses is still atypical; it is impregnated in the mould of pathology and locked in the Freudian labyrinth.

3 Fathers are capable of putting a large emotional input into their pregnancy careers. It is possible by cross-cultural analysis and ethological example (Howells 1970) to demonstrate that fathering is as 'instinctive' as 'mothering', but one does not want to enter into the polemics of the typing of sex roles. Suffice to say that there is a cultural conspiracy against 'ostentatious' displays of fathering in its own right at a time when the traditional male roles are being undermined by the proponents of the Women's Movement. The depth of male penetration into the female 'preserve' of child nurturance is blurred. It has been argued that when men start caring for children the decision is usually made not to conceive further offsprings. The issue is by no means clear.

Policy recommendations

The time is apposite for fathering to be considered appropriate in its own right. To this end a number of steps can be considered. The media can air the dilemmas of fatherhood in a frequent and informed dialogue. Conditions of employment can recognize the obligations of fatherhood with paid time allowances. Medical education should incorporate the subject and sensitize e.g. the GP or occupational health nurse, into an awareness of male pregnancy careers. It is possible to restructure obstetric practices to admit the father into the hub of the affair and make antenatal activities less of a woman's secret society. The unprecedented fall in the birth-rate has reduced the obstetric workload. Husbands could also be counselled on joint visits to the hospital. The advantages of training husbands, who so wish, to be labour coaches has been stressed previously. Some husbands may be suitable with training and supervision to participate in the actual delivery, legal considerations aside. It will be to the advantage of the maternity services, which have been subjected to special criticisms, to fuse lay and medical involvements. Fathers present at birth and have witnessed the hospital procedures are generally more satisfied; in the United States they sue less frequently.

References

Benedek, T. (1946). *Insight and personality adjustment*, Ronald Press, New York.

Coelho, R. (1949). 'The significance of the Couvade among the Black Caribs. *Man* **64**, 51–3.

Cohen, G. (1975). 'The absent Husbands in British middle class families'. Paper presented to British Association Conference at Guildford, Surrey, U.K.

Faunce, W. A. (1959). Automation and leisure. In *Automation and society* (ed. H. B. Jacobson). Philosophical Library, New York.

Forbes, R. (1972). The father's role. In *Psychosomatic medicine in obstetrics and gynaecology* (ed. N. Morris). Karger, Basel.

Frazer, J. G. (1910). *Totemism and exogamy.* Macmillan, London.

Freeman, T. (1951). Pregnancy as a precipitant of mental illness in men. In *British Journal of Medical Psychology* **24**, 49–54.

Gennep, A. van (1960). *The rites of passage.* Routledge, Kegan and Paul, London.

Goffman, E. (1959). 'The moral career of the mental patient'. *Psychiatry* **61**, 123–42.

Goldthorp, W. O. and Richman, J. (1974*a*). 'Reorganization of the maternity services —a comment on domiciliary confinements in view of the experience of the hospital strike, 1973. *Midwife and Health Visitor* **10**, 265–71.

—— and —— (1974*b*). 'Maternal attitudes to unanticipated home confinement'. *The Practitioner* **212**, 845–53.

Hartman, A. A. (1966). 'Sexually deviant behaviour in expectant fathers'. *Journal of Abnormal Psychology* **71**, 232–4.

Henneborn, W. J. and Cogan, R. (1975). 'The effect of husband participation in reported pain and probability of medication during labour and birth'. *Journal of Psychosomatic Research* **19**, 215–22.

Howells, J. G. (1970). 'Fallacies in child care: that fathering is unimportant'. *Acta Paedopsychiatric* **37**, 46–55.

Inman, W. S. (1941). 'The Couvade in modern England'. *British Journal of Medical Psychology* **55**, 37–55.

Jarvis, W. (1962). 'Some effects of pregnancy and childbirth on men'. *Journal of the American Psychoanalytical Association* **10**, 689–700.

Josselyn, I. M. (1956). 'Cultural forces, motherliness and fatherliness'. *American Journal of Orthopsychiatry* **26**, 264–71.

Macintyre, S. (1976). 'Who wants babies? The social construction of instincts. In *Dependence and exploitation: process and change* (ed. S. Allen and D. Barker). Tavistock, London.

Malinowski, B. (1927). *Sex and repression in primitive society.* Routledge, Kegan and Paul, London.

Matthews, A. E. B. (1961). 'Behaviour patterns in labour'. *Journal of Obstetrics and Gynaecology of British Commonwealth* **68**, 862–74.

Matza, D. (1969). *Becoming deviant.* Prentice-Hall, Englewood Cliffs, New Jersey.

Neoloh, O. (1959). 'Automation and leisure'. In *Automation and society* (ed. H. B. Jacobson). Philosophical Library, New York.

Parsons, T. (1952). *The social system.* Tavistock, London.

Pawson, M. and Morris, N. (1972). 'The role of the father in pregnancy and labour'. In *Psychosomatic medicine in obstetrics and gynaecology.* Karger, Basel.

Pilowsky, I. (1972). 'Psychological aspects of complications of childbirth. A prospective study of primiparae and their husbands'. In *Psychosomatic medicine in obstetrics and gynaecology.* Karger, Basel.

Reik, T. (1931). *Ritual, psycho-analytic studies.* Hogarth Press, London.

Richman, J. and Goldthorp, W. O. (1976). 'Time in illness: aspects of gynaecological diagnosis'. Paper presented to British Sociological Conference on Sociology, Health and Illness at Manchester.

——, ——, and Simmons, C. (1975). 'Fathers in labour'. *New Society* **34**, pp. 143–5.

Rosengren, W. R. (1962). 'Social Instability and Attitudes Towards Pregnancy as a Sick Role'. *Social Problems* **27**, 371–8.

Roth, J. (1957). 'Ritual and magic in the control of contagion'. *American Sociological Review* 310–14.

Sassmor, J. L. (1972). 'The role of the father in labor and delivery'. In *Psychosomatic medicine in obstetrics and gynaecology* (ed. N. Morris). Karger, Basel.

Towne, R. D. and Afterman, J. (1955). 'Psychosis in Males Related to Parenthood'. *Bulletin of the Menninger Clinic* **19**, 19–26.

Trethowan, W. H. and Conlon, M. F. (1965). 'The Couvade symptom'. *British Journal of Psychiatry* **111**, 57, 66.

Weiner, A. and Steinhilber, R. M. (1961). 'Postpartum Psychoses'. *Journal of International College of Surgeons* **36**, 490–9.

White, M. A. (1957). 'Obstetrician's Role in Postpartum Mental Illness'. *Journal of American Medical Association* **165**, 138–43.

Zilboorg, G. (1931). 'Depressive reactions related to parenthood'. *American Journal of Psychiatry* **10**, 927–62.

An interpretation of
modern obstetric practice

Behaviour in hospitals is not always as rational and scientific as it would seem
Much that occurs in obstetrics is heavily ritualized. Words and actions and
uniforms define an individual's status in the social system of the hospital and
rules and prohibitions dictate and limit behaviour and interaction.
   In the next chapter a psychoanalyst looks at childbirth rituals in our society,
and asks what their meaning may be.

Let me be open at the start and say that I am among those who have
serious doubts about the rationale of modern obstetric practice. I have been
led to this position through my work as a psychotherapist, and in particular
by my attempts to help mothers suffering from post-partum depression. But
although my views on the subject will emerge in what follows, I am, in this
chapter, primarily concerned to understand the phenomenon rather than
write a polemic about it.
   If we view childbirth from the psychological point of view, and are
concerned with the immediate or long-term effects of the way the mother and
baby, considered as persons, are treated by society, then we may query the
legitimacy of the current preoccupation with techniques, may challenge their
presumed necessity, and, to the extent that we doubt their wisdom may try to
understand why behaviour which we consider inappropriate should become
widely accepted.
   As a first approach one must, I feel, draw a distinction between those
elements which pervade our society and colour attitudes not only to
childbirth but to many other areas of living, and, on the other hand
elements that are specific to childbirth itself (while recognizing, of course
that the two cannot be entirely separated). It is clear that, amongst the
former, the phenomenon of current medical practice is of paramount
importance. Childbirth may be subjected to various dominating influences
It could, for instance, be the occasion of a religious ceremony or festival
in which the midwife assumed a secondary role. But in our society childbirth
is first and foremost a medical matter. The doctor and the gynaecologist are
the authorities who, in the main, prescribe the circumstances of the birth
which takes place in their buildings and under their guidance and control.
   Civilization is the process of taming the wild, because the wild is hazardous
and terrifying. We cannot eliminate the terror of living but we can make
some areas more secure than they were for earlier man. Medicine, based on
contemporary scientific principles, helps to preserve life and reduce disease
If it were as simple as that, a critique of obstetric practice could be

straightforward. But, for various reasons (including the following), we cannot take the beneficial influence of medicine for granted.

First, medicine can bring harmful side-effects and illness.

Secondly, despite the medical profession's doctrine of belief that medicine is about the whole person, and even though doctors, nurses and midwives are human beings (rather than mere agents of a scientific viewpoint), who will, by and large, treat their patients as (whole) human beings, medicine tends to neglect the whole person.

Thirdly, there is the effect of monopoly. As with other branches of science, the success of and belief in medical technology ensures ever-expanding boundaries even in the face of its notable failures. We no longer go to the doctor only when we are sick, we consult him in health; and the pregnant woman puts herself under his care. But we have to ask the question: 'Is there a threshold beyond which the influence of medical science is counter-productive?' And to take note of Illich's suggestion (1975) that our capacity to look after ourselves is threatened by the tendency to rely on experts.

Fourthly, medicine is increasingly controlled by a uniform, centralized policy, with an inevitable increase in impersonality. The relevant question here is 'Can such a personal experience as childbirth be adequately managed in a setting that is orientated towards the impersonal?'

Before pursuing the argument further, I would like to present a brief description of modern obstetric practice. In what follows I shall outline a pattern of social behaviour which, although by no means universal, has significance, in most of its elements, for a large number of mothers in the technological society of the mid-twentieth century. As such it represents an oversimplified model and the fact that it has probably by now passed its peak does not invalidate an attempt to understand the phenomenon.

The modern obstetric régime

1 During pregnancy the mother is advised about conduct beneficial or harmful to the baby, laying emphasis on foodstuffs. She may be warned against having sexual intercourse.

2 In many, if not most, cases, arrangements are made for her to be confined away from her home and family. If this does occur the family is excluded from the procedure and its contact with the mother is strictly limited.

3 The birth is medically induced, i.e. the timing is not left to natural physiological processes but is controlled by means of drugs.

4 The mother is confined to bed during the whole process.

5 The birth area is shaved.

6 Drugs are given to relieve pain and to stimulate labour.

7 The mother is moved from the room in which she has been labouring to a different room in the hospital in order to give birth.

8 For the birth to take place the mother is laid flat on her back, with her knees drawn up and spread wide apart by stirrups.

9 Childbirth is expected to be a painful process. The mother characteristically moans or screams, and in general behaves in a rather helpless way, and is spoken to as though she were a child (and often a naughty child.)

10 In many cases the birth takes place under anaesthesia.

11 Pressure is sometimes applied to the abdomen during delivery.

12 In some areas the baby is delivered by instruments as a normal, routine measure.

13 A surgical incision is made to enlarge the vaginal orifice.

14 The umbilical cord is clamped immediately after birth.

15 The expulsion of the placenta is hastened by pulling the cord, pressing the abdomen, and the use of drugs.

16 After the birth and for the length of her stay in hospital the mother is separated from her baby for at least part of the time in many hospitals. He is looked after by the staff, in a room together with other babies, and presented to the mother only for brief periods, primarily for the purpose of feeding.

17 The baby is sometimes weighed before being handed to the mother.

18 Feeding of the baby is delayed. Later he is given modified cow's milk taken from a bottle at scheduled times.

Setting aside the question of the medical usefulness of these measures (a question which will be confronted elsewhere in this book) we can ask 'Is there a pattern or trend in these practices which can help us to understand why they should be performed? Looked at naively, what is happening to mother and baby?' Certain (interrelated) elements quickly reveal themselves.

a Both mother and baby are placed in a very passive position. The mother's contribution to the birth is almost the minimal conceivable; the process is taken out of her hands and her body is manipulated by professionals. The professionals come as near to having the baby themselves as can be managed by proxy. And afterwards even her baby is removed from her.

b The occasion is one of suffering rather than joy.

c The impersonal mode is ascendant; spontaneity is replaced by control; the significance of psychological reality is denied.

d There is a break of continuity in the mother's life: the birth does not take place in her ordinary place of living.

e Great emphasis is put on cleanliness (purity) and order.

f There is a formality which has something of the character of public ritual.

These are the trends that I wish to underline. Even after as much credence as possible has been given to medical justification for this practice, and even when allowance has been made for the effects of rationalistic–technological philosophy, the phenomenon is sufficiently striking to make us wonder about the meanings that may lie behind it. At a period of history when the importance of individual rights and freedom of expression is not in doubt how can an obstetric regime so antipathetic to these rights gain wide acceptance? When the significance of the early mother–baby tie and of the need to allow basic bodily and emotional drives their due consideration is recognized not only by psychiatry but by a large proportion of the educated public, how can the potential harm of intrusive control be overlooked? Why do professional helpers so usurp the mother's function and why does she let this happen? These are questions I hope to leave in the reader's mind. In what follows I shall make an attempt to shed some light on them and in particular, to explore possible reasons for the existence of a cultural attitude to childbirth that is far less positive than we would like to believe.

The meaning of a pattern of social behaviour is always more extensive than the explanation given by the participants; indeed, the anthropologist's work rests on this assumption. But, as Cohen (1974) suggests, research into underlying meanings are too often reserved for the study of 'primitive society'.

The view, implicit in the evolutionary formulations of Weber and others, that modern society is distinct from primitive society in being organised on the basis of contract, in being secular, rational, manipulative and impersonal, has recently been seriously challenged by many students of society. A rapidly accumulating body of evidence indicates that the bizarre and the exotic in the patterns of social behaviour are not the exclusive monopoly or pre-industrial societies. In many situations in modern society custom is as strange and as sovereign as it is in 'primitive' society.

Scholars are now 'rediscovering' in modern society the existence and significance of an endless array of patterns of symbolic behaviour that have been for long associated exclusively with 'primitive' society.

What might these hidden patterns be in relation to obstetric method? We do not regard the practices surrounding childbirth in our society as ceremonial or ritualistic, but may the ritual be hidden from us only because we are so hypnotised by the apparently rational assumptions behind them that we do not even begin to seek a further explanation? Such overt ceremonials as we have available to us—Christian baptism and churching of women—are gradually paling into insignificance in the face of the powers of the doctor and the hospital. It is well known that when a social order is superseded the old customs are not thereby automatically extinguished but will persist in modified forms. For instance, several elements of the Mithraic religion have found their way into Christian ceremony and theology, and much of the spirit of the Jewish sabbath has continued to pervade the Christian Sunday. May this kind of thing happen when the priest is replaced by the doctor, and the church by the hospital? If this is so, then hospitals may be places where propitiation and blessing play a greater part than we imagine.†

†cf. L. R. Twentyman 'The place of homeopathy in modern medicine in the light of history' (*British Homeopathic Journal* **63**, 82 (1974)) 'It would be very superficial also to ignore or underestimate the symbolic elements in modern medicine and surgery and their influence for good and ill in activating unconscious forces. The ritual of the modern operating theatre is an example. There is the sacrificial altar on which the victim priests and priestesses stand round, the temple sleep is induced and the sacrificial knife plunged in.'

But in searching for hidden meanings I would like to draw on psychoanalysis and anthropology in order to make a comparison between 'primitive' society and our own. In looking through the literature on the subject I am impressed by the relative lack of work on the interpretation of childbirth. It seems to me that the two studies of most interest are neither of recent origin: that of the anthropologist Van Gennep (1960) and the psychoanalyst Reik (1914). In summarizing these studies I shall make use of an earlier paper (Lomas 1966).

Van Gennep's interpretation of childbirth

Arnold Van Gennep published *Les rites de passage* in 1909. In this work he attempted to show that the ceremonies which attach to certain life-crises are similar in having the function of easing the transition from one state to the next and he used the term 'rite of passage' to describe the practices which occur when any barrier, physical, biological, or social, has to be crossed. He shows that, to a greater or lesser degree, such ceremonies can be divided into three stages: separation, transition, and incorporation. The ceremonies that are performed are done so with the purpose of separating the person from his previous state, nursing him through a transitional period, and finally incorporating him into the class of persons of which he is to become a member.

In his introduction to the 1960 (the first English) translation of Van Gennep's work, Kimball writes:

Van Gennep, with others, accepted the dichotomy of the sacred and the profane; in fact, this is a central concept for understanding the transitional stage in which an individual or group finds itself from time to time. The sacred is not an absolute value but one relative to the situation. The person who enters a state at variance with the one previously held becomes 'sacred' to the others who remain in the profane stage. It is this new condition which calls for rights eventually incorporating the individual into the group and returning him to the customary routines of life. These changes may be dangerous, and, at the least, they are upsetting to the life of the group and the individual. The transitional period is met with rites of passage which cushion the disturbance. In one sense, all life is transition, with rhythmic periods of quiescence and heightened activity.

Certain features of Van Gennep's interpretation are immediately apparent:

1 childbirth ritual has no distinctive characteristic over and above those to be observed in other rites of passage;
2 the ritualistic feature that his theory is best suited to explain is the segregation of the parturient mother;
3 ritual serves to ease change which is conceived as being extremely difficult for individual and society: it has a directly positive, beneficial function which, although of unspecified origin, is implicitly attributed to the society as a whole;

4 the actors are the individual and society and little mention is made of the needs and aims of the family.

Van Gennep's interpretation has relevance not only to the segregation of the mother but to the notions of purity and pollution which surround childbirth in so many societies, including our own. The explanations given by contemporary medicine for the control of contagion are simply inadequate. In a study of the use of masks and other protective clothing in a hospital for tuberculosis Roth (1957) found that the occasions when staff and patients were required to wear masks had less to do with the actual risk of infection than with extraneous factors, including staff hierarchy. His report gives confirmation to the suggestion I have made elsewhere Lomas (1969) that patients in hospital, whether sick or parturient, are subject to a taboo because they are in an uncertain and ambiguous state which cannot be readily accommodated by a highly ordered society. In that paper I made the further suggestion (relevant to the discussion below) that illness engenders a painful inequality of power which may provoke exploitation either by patient or society, for which crisis taboo is a crude emergency method of control.

Reik's interpretation of childbirth

In contradistinction to Van Gennep—and following where Freud (1913) had led—Theodore Reik is not content to regard rites of passage as practices organized by society for the benefit of the individual but views them primarily as manifestations of ambivalence to the initiate. In reference to couvade he writes:

The prohibition of the realization of hostile wishes towards his wife, which the primitive man has imposed upon himself, exceeds the period of her confinement because his conconscious wishes continue to press towards active expression through the motor system. The temptation to realize these wishes is not overcome; it is merely displaced, and the protective measures against it have also to move with it. This keeping the man in bed has also the object of protecting his wife from his sexual and hostile wishes. Although up to now we have especially emphasized the preponderating share of aggressive tendencies in the building up of couvade, it must not be forgotten that by means of them an inhibition of sexual wishes may arise.... His inhibited libido joins itself to those inborn sadistic instinctual components which the woman's condition brings to the fore and is turned into latent hate against her. Wicked desires now awaken towards the pregnant woman for whose body the man longs and which is forbidden to him.

Reik sees the protective magic which the husband undertakes on behalf of his wife—the warding-off of devils—as an act of reparation, an attempt to counteract his own projected hostility. Dietetic couvade is viewed—in a similar light—as a reaction–formation against the unconscious desire to devour the baby. What is the reason for this unconscious hostility towards the wife and baby? According to Reik it is primarily rooted in the Oedipus complex. The custom of the sacrifice of the first-born male is, in Reik's view, a consequence of the same fantasy; the infant is sacrificed to the father (God) to assuage Oedipal guilt, a procedure which has the added advantage of eliminating the Oedipal rival of the next generation.

The question of envy

Although Reik is convincing in showing us the husband's repressed hostility and his manoeuvres to counteract it, the reasons for the hostility are not so clearly demonstrated. Is the Oedipus complex the only explanation, or even the most obvious one? If the father's fantasy is that 'it is not the mother who has given birth to the child but the father; to him therefore the child's love must go', the simplest explanation for such a wish is that he wanted to create the child himself and to experience the child's love for him.

Crawley (1927) has expressed the view that theories of marriage and birth customs 'show a sympathy with the father and with the child, but forget the mother, and are thus a modern document, illustrating the history of woman's treatment by man'. It would seem that Reik falls into the error which Crawley impugns to his predecessor. His theory is male-centred and this shows itself first in his failure to conceive that maternity could be an enviable state, and, secondly, that he leaves the woman's psychology out of the thesis.

The psychoanalyst Melanie Klein has stressed the envy which exists in relation to female creativity, and although her ideas about the origin and theoretical implications of envy are open to question, the clinical material that she has adduced is convincing. Elsewhere I have brought evidence to suggest that a parturient mother does, in fact, expect to be envied, and that a dread of such envy may contribute to her mental breakdown (Lomas 1960).

In his book *Symbolic wounds: puberty rites and the envious male* Bettelheim (1955) surveys the initiation ceremony of puberty and concludes that a neglected aspect of its meaning centres on male envy. He believes that there is a crucial difference between male and female circumcision: 'That women can bear children is taken for granted—it is demonstrable. Only men have to participate in ritual rebirth drama.' And the wounds inflicted at puberty spring from the wish to menstruate. By contrast there is a 'relative absence of ceremony accompanying female circumcision'. He suggests that female circumcision is imposed by men on girls in order 'to gain understanding of or power over the process of female genital bleeding' and 'as an expression of their anger at and envy of women's ability to bear children when men cannot'. In reference to couvade he writes: 'the man who is envious of the woman's ability to bear children has no "sympathy" for her. She is expected, if not compelled, to resume her work immediately, though she is exhausted from labour and the physiological readjustments. The husband and father, on the other hand, rests. His empathy with the mother is so great that he recreates in himself the need for special care that would be appropriate and that he denies to her.' Bettelheim thereby focuses on a central feature of childbirth ritual, and one that is mirrored in the way in which the ritual has been interpreted by our society; it is Hamlet without the Prince.†

Envy of maternity is now, however, confined to the male. Although the evil spirits which need to be propitiated by various actions performed as part of childbirth ritual are not, for the most part, specifically female; there exists a vast mythology surrounding female beings who do not take kindly to the event of childbirth; namely witches. Witches are said to cause sterility, abortion, and to steal, kill or eat newborn babies; and, although they possess certain phallic features, they are women, and themselves childless— they only have cats. Moreover they are old; perhaps what they envy most is youth (and what is younger than a newborn baby?). It would seem possible that the belief in witches arises first from the fact that such women—even if less exotic than those portrayed in the myth—do exist in reality, and, secondly, from the projections of the parturient mother herself. Such projections in turn probably have a dual origin; the mother's hostile, envious, and condemning mother-image and her own unconscious hostility towards her baby (it is to be noted that the eating taboos of 'dietetic couvade' are not restricted to the male).

The psychology of the mother

It can be seen from the above description that childbirth customs in our society bear a definite similarity in certain respects to the ancient birth rituals, notably in the practice of segregating the mother and transferring the significance of the procedure away from her. In couvade the husband is significant; in our society one sometimes has the impression that it is the doctor; and the degree by which he takes control of her function—even the details of procedure such as ritual shaving and periotomy—put one in mind of female circumcision and Bettelheim's interpretation of this as an attempt on the part of the male to master his envy. And it would seem that, in general, the interpretations he makes about primitive society are equally applicable to our own; moreover, this similarity of pattern, despite the difference in social structure and rationale, adds weight to the interpretation.

I have mentioned that the interpretations of birth ritual so far made have excluded one notable item: the psychology of the mother. Although, as suggested above, this probably in some measure stems from a bias on the part of the interpretors it must be confessed that the reported facts left

† In her paper 'Couvade and menstruation' Mary Douglas (1968) criticizes Bettelheim's thesis on the grounds that, improperly, he interprets public ritual in the light of his experiences with individual psychopathology, and she maintains that the explanation of the former must be in terms of the structure of the particular society in which it appears. This is a criticism with which psychoanalysts must now be familiar. But a way seems open for recognizing that the discrepancy is not so wide as appears, for sexual envy and social imbalance (as Douglas, up to a point, suggests) may both occur in the same society and have a direct bearing on each other.

them little to go on. Because the mother plays an unspectacular part in the events she does not reveal her mind. In studying our own culture we are in a better position because we can ask her about it.

If it is true that the mother has been cast into a passive, even humiliating, role, it is one which she appears to accept readily. The labour and lying-in wards are not scenes of revolt, and the mother accepts the views, attitudes, and commands of her advisors with meekness. She does not violently claim her baby when he is taken from her and left to cry in another room. Many mothers, on the contrary, not only accept the régime but welcome it, preferring to be delivered under cover of anaesthesia, to leave the responsibility of nursing the baby to others and to substitute the bottle for the breast. But we should not be persuaded by her submissiveness or even overt embracement of her situation into believing it is a genuine and natural wish. Not only is she confronted with the problem of opposing a powerful social force, but, if the argument put forward above has some validity, she will be subject to masochistic urges to propitiate.

A source of confusion over this question lies in the tendency to regard the cultural norms as the biologically necessary. Elsewhere (Lomas 1962) I have attempted to show that one characteristic of the mother of our society, regarded by common consent and by psychoanalytical theory to be normal, yet in fact pathological and crippling both to herself and her child, is masochism. Psychotherapeutic investigation of mothers suffering from post-partum breakdown reveals the existence of such an urge, originating in guilt feelings and fear of envy based on unconscious fantasy (Lomas 1962). But is it possible that a fear of envy is not necessarily a neurotic one—nor confined to mothers who break down—but one based on an unhappy reality which causes her to propitiate those around her by making costly sacrifices?

Summary

My aim in writing this chapter is to suggest some ways in which the rationale of current childbirth care is open to question. In the first place, we may be so under the influence of the overt organizational–technological viewpoint that we take a rather limited look at the overall needs of mother, baby, and family. In the second place, there would appear to be hidden, underlying patterns in society which influence the way we handle childbirth. These two factors are not independent of each other. For instance, the drive to control childbirth by technical measures, a drive which seems to reach obsessive dimensions at times, may derive some of its force from unconscious feelings of antipathy towards the process of procreation.

A comparison with childbirth ritual in primitive society suggests that our own practice may contain elements, both positive and negative, the reasons for which we are largely unaware. We offer the mother a *rite de passage*, a period of respite from the demands of everyday life, during which she can effect the difficult transition of childbirth and nursing. But we do not allow her much time for this change and our means of helping her is to take her to a place where she is subjected to excessive control and where the spontaneous, loving relationship between mother and baby, so vital to the future development of both, is all too often made difficult or impossible. Indeed the degree of her subordination is so great that one wonders if the *rite de passage* serves to facilitate control in a way that is far less advantageous to the mother (at least in our own society) than the ideas of Van Gennep would suggest.

In searching for possible means for the existence of a concealed hostility to childbirth which limits our capacity to help the mother and child one could think in terms of the conflict between men and women, individual and state, or physical and spiritual. But the conflict which has, I believe, the deepest significance, is that between creativity and sterility.

Both society and the individual maintain their liveliness by a compromise between stasis and growth. It would appear that, in the forms in which we know them, growth presents them with a problem that is difficult and dangerous and from which they protect themselves with a greater or lesser degree of rigidity. To the extent that this occurs, they fear growth and change. Certainly the conservative element in society is a very powerful one and it is no doubt this fact that has led to the 'functionalist' theory of social systems, of which that of Talcott Parsons is an influential descendant. The distrust and alarm with which manifestations of creativity in art, science, or religion is met is impressive, and adults do not take easily to the spontaneous creativity and innocent penetration of the child. Is it not then to be expected that the creative event of birth will be viewed with a similar degree of anxiety? A mother and baby are very appropriate symbols of growth, and for this reason a rigid and insecure society may see the necessity to control and restrict their spontaneous joy. Just as plants will manage to grow in the cracks between paving stones, so does joy emerge in our labour wards, but this fact should not diminish our efforts to seek out whatever stands in its way.

References

Bettelheim, B. (1955). *Symbolic wounds*. Thames and Hudson, London.

Cohen, A. (1974). *Two-dimensional man*. Routledge and Kegan Paul, London.

Crawley, E. (1927). *The mystic rose* (2nd ed.). Methuen, London.

Douglas, M. (1968). 'Couvade and menstruation'. In *Implicit meanings* (ed. M. Douglas). Routledge and Kegan Paul, London.

Freud, S. (1913). 'Totem and Taboo'. In *The complete psychological works of Sigmund Freud*.

Illich, I. (1975). *Medical nemesis*. Calder and Boyars, London.

Lomas, P. (1960). 'Dread of envy as a factor in the aetiology of puerperal breakdown'. *British Journal of Medical Psychology* **33**, 105.

—— (1962). 'The concept of maternal love'. *Psychiatry* **25**, 3.

Lomas, P. (1966). 'Ritualistic elements in the management of childbirth'. *British Journal of Medical Psychology* **39**, 207.

—— (1969). 'Taboo and Illness' *British Journal of Medical Psychology* **42**, 33.

Reik, T. (1914). 'Couvade and fear of retaliation'. In *Ritual: Four Psychoanalytic Studies* (1962) New York, Grove Press.

Roth, J. *'Ritual and Magic in the control of contagion' Amer. Sociol. Review.* **22**, 310.

Van Gennep, A. (1960). *The Rites of Passage.*

J. A. MACFARLANE; D. M. SMITH, AND D. H. GARROW **12**

The relationship between mother and neonate

The study of the relationship between the mother and her baby has developed out of animal studies of bonding between mother and neonate. For the first time the ways in which the mother and baby learn about each other are being analysed and variations observed associated with the context in which the birth and immediate post-natal behaviour takes place. Longitudinal research is also being done in which they are being studied months and even years after to see if there is any association between the experience which both go through at and just following birth and subsequent interaction. Two of the basic categories of behaviour studied are those involving contact and continuity of relationship on the one hand and separation on the other.

Childbirth in hospital is much more likely than childbirth at home to mean that the mother and infant are separated from each other for at least part of the 24 hours.

This chapter examines the beginnings of the relationship between the mother and baby and some of the effects of interference in hospitals where the importance of the first days, hours, and even minutes after birth is not recognized.

This chapter is concerned with two aspects of the very early relationship between human mothers and their infants. In the first part of the chapter the extreme sensitivity of the baby to the environment, both before and after birth is described, as are the patterns of behaviours which both the mother and the child demonstrate towards one another immediately after birth. In the second part of the chapter the effect of interference with mother–infant interaction are reviewed behaviour that may occur as a result of early interruptions in the normally developing relations between mother and baby, by separation.

PART 1 J. A. MACFARLANE

Animal studies

Many of the ideas and techniques used in the research outlined in this chapter have their origins in animal work. In animals the mother's behavioural changes may begin before birth—for instance the self-licking of the ano-genital region in the pregnant rat, or the loss of hair in the rabbit, or the tendency of the domestic ewes to seek shelter indoors away from the herd as parturition approaches. There are species specific differences also during birth, such as the increase in self-licking in many species, and the rolling and rubbing in the cat: and finally there are the post-natal behaviours such as sucking, nest building, retrieving, grooming etc. (Rheingold 1963).

Adequate maternal care in animals depends on a large number of factors—many of which are little understood. In part maternal behaviour depends on the conditions under which the mother herself was reared. Monkey mothers which have been reared in a severely deprived social environment are often incapable of rearing their own offspring (Harlow and Harlow 1965).

Some of the more immediate behaviours of the mother are dependent on: (1) the preceding maternal behaviours—if a mother rat is prevented from indulging in pre-delivery ano-genital licking by means of a collar, she may either consume some of her litter or refuse to suckle them (Birch 1956); (2) the behaviour of their offspring—the maternal behaviour of female mice is 'primed' by the ultrasonic calls of the young (Noirot 1972); (3) the actual presence of the newborn after birth: in many species separation for a few hours after birth will result in considerable disturbance of mothering behaviour when the animals are reunited. The mother may fail to care for her young, she may butt them, or show no preference to them when feeding the newborn (Hersher, Richmond, and Moar 1963, Klopfer, Adams, and Klopfer 1964, Moore 1968). Rhesus monkey mothers which had been deprived of tactile contact with their babies, but allowed to see and hear them after 2 weeks, showed a rapid decrease in the amount of time that they spent viewing their offspring (Harlow, Harlow, and Hansen 1963).

There are also the hormonal aspects of maternal behaviour in animals—blood transfused from a lactating female rat into a virgin female rat increases the tendency of the latter to behave maternally (Rosenblatt 1970).

What of the behaviour of newborn? This too obviously varies from species to species, dependent in part on maturity at birth, and the environment into which it is born. In certain birds and animals there appears to be a learning process by which during the first hours and days after birth the newborn shows filial responses to the features of any object directly in its environment. This has been called 'imprinting' and is normally directed to the mother but in an artificial situation may be a wooden box, a flashing light, or anything else that is around. Over this time, in these species the responses grow more specific to the individual characters of the object on which it is becoming imprinted (Hinde 1974).

Maternal and newborn behaviour naturally vary enormously between species and it is dangerous to draw conclusions from one species about another. For instance nothing like the well-known phenomena of imprinting in birds occurs in human infants. However, the capacity of the newborn human infant to respond and discriminate and a state of heightened sensitivity in the mother after delivery make it likely that the first hours and days are important in laying the foundations of the subsequent mother–child relationship.

Human mother–infant interaction

Recent scientific observations of the newborn baby which are discussed in this chapter have confirmed the more naturalistic observations of mothers made over the many centuries, that their babies are, at birth, already extraordinarily perceptive of their environment. Because the initial care of pregnancy, delivery, and the newborn child is undertaken by those trained in 'scientific method' these observations are only now beginning to achieve recognition, and a place in the management of mothers and babies. This should mean that more respect is paid to the mother's own observations, and to her own individual needs, and to the individual needs of her baby.

There has been in our culture a marked inclination to consider a baby as a feeling and sensitive human being only at some time after birth, giving but little weight to its existence either *in utero* or immediately post-natally. Especially in the period after birth, we have tended to ignore the fact that the baby might have sensitivities comparable to, or even greater than those that we have as adults. For instance we still find it acceptable (though ever less so) to, by circumcision, remove a considerable area of extremely sensitive skin from the newborn without anaesthetic, and subject them, in special-care baby units, to procedures, which an adult could never endure without the benefit of sedation or analgesia.

We have until recently also been convinced that the baby could not see, and showed no response to sound. Part of the influence for this attitude may have come from doctors, who when developing techniques to improve the chances of survival of children, were concerned more with the long-term outcome than the more immediate effects, and therefore were happy to adopt the idea that the painful and invasive techniques which they were using did not have any effect on an 'unfeeling' baby. Although such invasive techniques are still necessary in some cases, in order to help survival, much of the research done with very small children now indicates how sensitive the newborn is to its surroundings, showing that not only does it have the ability to appreciate and react to stimulation provided by the environment immediately after it is born, but also to react to the stimulation provided by its intrauterine environment. The forms of such stimulation will be many times more varied after birth than before, none the less, tactile and auditory stimulation are available to the foetus before delivery.

The foetus' own movements will meet with increasing resistance from the uterine wall, and the uterus itself will provide periodic pressure changes by its contractions. The fluid media of the amniotic fluid does not entirely buffer the movements of the mother, her coughing, her vomiting, her changes of position, etc. In moving the foetus may touch itself, setting off such reflexes as the sucking reflex or the rooting reflex. It develops in the noisy environment (85 dB) (Walker 1975) of the blood flowing through the uterine vessels, and the rhythmicity of a similar type of sound has a marked quietening effect on the child during the first weeks after birth (Salk 1973). Other sounds, external to mother, are transmitted across the uterine wall to the baby, causing changes of activity and of heart-rate (Sontag 1936; Grimwade *et al.* 1971.). Towards the end of pregnancy, the abdominal wall and the uterine wall may be thin enough to transmit some light through to the foetus. There is also evidence to suggest that the taste of the amniotic fluid may alter the rate at which the baby swallows it, and that the emotions of the mother, such as anxiety, may alter foetal activity (Sontag 1941).

At birth these environmental sensations suddenly change in almost all their modalities, however it is reasonable to hypothesize that the closer the baby is to the mother after birth, the less extreme the changes. If the baby is held against the mother, then there will be a continuation of many of the tactile and temperature sensations, as well as the auditory one of the mother's heart-beat. If the baby is with the mother, it will also mean that perhaps the most sensitive of the baby's perceptual abilities, its vision, is directed towards the novelty of its mother's external form. At this stage, after birth, visual perception is such that the baby will not only follow a human face, but also can turn its eyes in the direction of a sound (Wertheimer 1962).

It is interesting to note that studies done to examine the newborn's preferences for different visual stimuli indicate preference for those features which are normally found in the human face; contour, contrast, three dimensions, movement, etc. (Franz 1961; Franz *et al.* 1975). Studies made of the baby's appreciation of sounds after birth also indicate that the sounds the baby responds most to are the combination of tones that are normally found in the human voice (Hutt 1973).

By the age of 5 days, smell too seems to be playing a part in the baby's preferences. If at this age they are presented with a clean breast pad on one side of their nose and a breast pad that has been up against a mother's breast for 3 hours on the other side, they tend to spend more time turned to the breast pad that had been in contact with the mother. In the same study, at 6 days of age, the babies turned more towards a breast pad which had been in contact with their mother than one which had been in contact with a strange mother (Macfarlane 1975). This appeared to be a learnt response, as it was not present when the babies were 2 days old. Similar abilities of babies, to distinguish between their own mother's face and a stranger's face, were found by Genevive Carpenter (1974), when babies were 2 weeks old. At 3 weeks of age Margaret Mills (1974) was able to show their ability to distinguish between their own mother's voice and a strange mother's voice. In a less controlled study, Hammond (1970) had shown a similar ability in babies aged a few days.

It therefore appears that over the first week after birth the baby moves from simply responding more to human beings in general (as against, to objects), to responding more specifically to their own mother in particular. This conclusion is further substantiated by the findings of Louis Sander, Strechler, Burns, and Julia (1970). They arranged for a group of babies who were going to be adopted to be looked after by one highly experienced caretaker in a rooming-in situation, for the first 10 days of life. At 10 days the care of the baby was taken over by a second highly experienced caretaker. With the new caretaker the babies showed certain very specific changes in their sleep, eating and activity patterns, as if they had already become adapted to the rhythms of the first caretaker, and had difficulty adapting to the new caretaker.

All these factors indicate that shortly after birth (if not before) the baby has at least in part adapted to a specific relationship with his or her mother. This relationship will be altered by both the quality and quantity of his or her contact with the mother.

What of the maternal side of this relationship? Much argument has gone into the question of the mother's relationship with her child whilst she is pregnant: is she capable of loving it, or feeling attached to it, in anything like the same way as she does after it is born? There are so many variables involved that there is probably no answer to these questions. In a recent unpublished survey I asked 97 mothers having their first babies the question 'When did you first feel love for your baby?'. Forty one per cent said during pregnancy, 24 per cent said at birth, 27 per cent during the first week, and 8 per cent after the first week.

When the child is born how does the mother react to it initially? Observations made in the United States (Klaus and Kennel 1970) show mothers who are given their babies nude, within 12 hours of birth, tend to go through 'an orderly and predictable pattern of behaviour' commencing with hesitant fingertip contact on the extremities and proceeding to massaging and encompassing the baby's trunk with the hands. However, from a series of observations of videotapes made in an English hospital, in the labour room, this rarely seems to occur in the clinical situation, where the baby is well wrapped up before being given to the mother—in this case (Macfarlane, unpublished) although 10 out of 12 mothers showed some finger tip touching, only 3 out of the 12 went on to stroke or massage their babies. From these videotapes it appears that some of the variance in the mother's behaviour might be explained by whether the father is present, how well the mother knows her medical attendants, and the type of analgesia used during labour, as well as many other factors.

The further analysis of these videotapes of deliveries showed that the average time for the baby to be with its mother after birth in the labour room was 6·5 minutes, with a variation between 1 minute and 15 minutes. The average time interval between the baby being born and being given to the mother was 3·5 minutes. Whilst holding their babies the mothers spend almost three-quarters of the time looking at the baby, and one-third of this time was spent in smiling or laughing. Also from these videotapes it could be observed how the parents became adapted to the sex of the child, especially where a child of the opposite sex had been strongly desired, and also how frequently the mother referred to some feature of the infant looking like its father.

Kennell *et al.* (1975) after observing both hospital and home deliveries in the United States suggested that home deliveries in a select population show 'in some aspects, a pattern of behaviour different to hospital deliveries where we observe only fragments of these behaviours'. Their findings in a home delivery were:

1 The mother is an active participant,
2 She picks up the infant immediately after birth.
3 She begins to stroke its face with her fingertips and moves to palm contact of the body and head within a few minutes.
4 A striking elevation in mood observed in association with great excitement of the other participants.
5 Everyone is drawn to look at the infant for prolonged periods.
6 The mother is groomed.
7 Breast-feeding starts within 5–6 minutes, beginning with prolonged licking by the infant.
8 The parents use a high-pitched voice when talking to the infant.

Point 4 has been observed by many people (but not as far as I know scientifically recorded), as has the fact that the baby also seems to go through a period of increased alertness immediately after birth lasting up to 2 hours. This occurs more frequently if the mother has not received narcotic medication during labour, and the baby may not have another period of alertness of such duration for several days (Wolf 1963).

That this period after birth may be one of increased sensitivity for the developing relationship between mother and baby has been suggested by Klaus, Kennell, and others (see also the next section of this chapter); Kennell also (Kennell *et al.* 1975) quotes unpublished work by N. Winters, who gave six mothers in one group their babies to suckle immediately after birth, and contrasted these with six other mothers who did not get their babies to breast-feed until approximately 16 hours later. All mothers had originally stated a desire to breast-feed and no mother stopped breast-feeding for physical reasons. At follow-up 2 months later, all six of the first group of mothers were still breast-feeding, but only one out of the six in the second group were. In another study done in a Maternity Hospital in Guatemala, Kennell (1975) reports that twelve mothers were given their babies to handle nude immediately after birth and another twelve mothers were given their babies nude to handle 12 hours after birth. At 36 hours both groups of mothers were observed with their babies to assess maternal behaviour. The mothers that had been given the early contact with their babies showed significantly more maternal behaviour using their measures than the late contact group.

Much of the research of the effects of early contrast and separation, as outlined in the next section of this chapter, is concerned with the long-term effects on both mother and baby. However it is necessary to remember that we do not live life only for the long-term outcome but also for the more immediate satisfaction and happiness of life as it happens.

PART 2 D. H. GARROW AND D. M. SMITH

Interference with mother–infant interaction

In the last part of this chapter Dr. Macfarlane described how responsive a baby is to the environment. After delivery the interaction that occurs between a mother and her infant is a reciprocal one. Successful interaction leads to a relationship with adequate mothering which through long periods of evolution must have been vital. Failure to form an adequate bond often led to infant death; nowadays, though rarely fatal, it causes much unhappiness and may present as a behaviour disorder or psychosomatic syndrome. We here review the evidence that interference with mother–infant interaction in the puerperium may disturb behaviour for months or years afterwards.

Separation

Separation is common after delivery in hospital but rare after home confinement. In a small retrospective survey of 266 deliveries in the United Kingdom (Garrow and Smith (1) 1976) there were 26 births at home, in all but one the mother held her baby in the first hour. Of the 240 hospital deliveries 74 (31 per cent) mothers had not held the baby for some hours, or even days, after birth; 34 (14 per cent) of these babies were nursed in an incubator or a special-care baby unit which frequently meant that the mother was excluded. A survey in 1970 of 1400 premature nurseries in the United States revealed that only 34 per cent allowed mothers in to handle their babies (Klaus 1975). Hospital routines in maternity departments and special-care baby units are now more permissive than this (see Chapter 14) and so they should be. Careful studies have shown that allowing mothers and their infants more than what was the usual amount of contact had a favourable effect upon subsequent maternal behaviour (Klaus, Jerauld, Kreger, McAlpine, Steffa, and Kennell 1972). In this study 14 mothers of full-term babies were given their babies naked for 1 hour soon after birth, and for 5 hours on each of the next 3 days. A control group were allowed only a glimpse of their babies at birth, followed by visits to the nursery at feed times. The results of follow-up studies of these two groups at 1 month, 1 year, and 2 years have now been reported. At 1 month the extended-contact mothers were more involved with their babies, soothed them more, and in a film of a feed showed more eye-to-eye contact and fondling than the controls. At one year they still expressed more concern for their babies at interview and were more responsive to their crying (Kennell, Jerauld, Wolfe, Chesler, Kreger, McAlpine, Steffa, and Klaus 1974). At 2 years linguistic analysis of five mothers from each group showed that those who had been given the extra contact used more descriptive terms and fewer commands and seemed to show a greater awareness of their children's interests and needs than did the controls Ringler, Kennell, Jarvella, Navojosky, and Klaus (1975). Thus, as little as 16 hours' extra contact between a mother and her full-term baby in the first 3 days of life may affect the mother's behaviour for at least 2 years.

Modifications of the routine in premature nurseries has not so far been shown to have such dramatic consequences. Leifer, Leiderman, Barnet, and Williams (1972) allowed a group of mothers to handle their premature babies in the incubators and to assist with their caretaking. This 'contact' group was compared with mothers given what was then the normal routine of only seeing their babies through the window during the first 3–12 weeks. This limited amount of contact improved self-confidence, especially of the primiparous women (Seashore, Leifer, Barnett, and Leiderman 1973) but the attachment behaviour of the two groups was not different 1 month after discharge. This is perhaps not surprising as even in the contact group there was a degree of deprivation and separation which many people would find unacceptable today, and the mothers visited their babies on average only once every 6 days during their long hospital stay. The mothers of the premature babies in both groups were also compared with 22 mothers delivered at term. One month after discharge they more often smiled at their babies and held them close to their bodies than did those who had had premature infants. Ventral contact, according to Leiderman, Leifer, Seashore, Barnett, and Grobstein (1973), is specific to primates and considered to indicate a normal mother–infant relationship. This is certainly our impression but it is not possible from the study of Leifer, Leiderman, Barnett, and Williams (1972) to distinguish the sequelae of prematurity from those of separation.

A study of women in Oxford by Whiten in 1975 suggests that it is the separation, rather than the prematurity, that is responsible for disturbed mothering. The separated babies were not premature, but had been transferred to a special-care baby unit for 'minor medical reasons'; they were compared and followed up with a control group whose babies roomed-in with their mothers. Whiten found that those who had been separated for only 2 days showed fewer 'interactional sequences' with their babies, smiled at them less often, talked less, and adopted the '*en face*' position less often than did the control mothers. By 4 months of age, however, these differences had begun to fade. This does not mean that there might not still be long-lasting effects. Broussard and Hartner (1971) have found a correlation between a mother's attitude to her baby at 1 month and the child's behaviour more than 4 years later. In this study a series of primiparous women were given questionnaires on the second and third day post-partum and 1 month later to compare their perception of their infants as better or worse than average. Children who had been rated as worse than average by their mothers at 1 month (but not at 2–3 days) were significantly more likely to require 'therapeutic intervention' at an independent clinical assessment made at $4\frac{1}{2}$ years of age. Broussard and Hartner suggest that the relationship, fluid at first, had 'set' for better or worse by 1 month. If this is true, interference with mother–infant interaction by modifying maternal attitude in the first few weeks might be expected to be followed by an increased incidence of problems in later childhood.

The authors of this review, in a retrospective study of 22 children who had been separated soon after birth, also found a greater number of psychological problems than in the control siblings (Garrow and Smith 1976). We also noticed that the tendency for a mother to reject her separated child seemed to lead to an upset in family dynamics with friction between the parents, the father tending to take over the child's mothering. Such disturbance was still more obvious in the Stanford families studied by Leifer (1972). After a period of 21 months there were six divorces between the parents of the premature babies and none amongst those with full-term infants. One of the divorces was in the group of mothers allowed into the premature nursery, the other five were in those who had been more severely separated.

Rooming-in, allows more contact and increases a mother's self-confidence (Newton and Newton 1962, Greenberg, Rosenberg, and Lind 1973). Rooming-in also helps breast-feeding to succeed; the breast-feeding rate at Duke Hospital rose from 35 per cent to 58·5 per cent when this practice was adopted (Newton and Newton 1962). A delay in contact between a mother and her baby for as little as 16 hours was found in a controlled study by Winters to reduce the success and duration of breast-feeding.

Perhaps the most florid example of disturbed mothering is found in the battered-child syndrome. A whole constellation of factors is associated with the families involved in child abuse. The incidence of low birthweight in babies who have been battered is between 20 per cent and 25 per cent, as compared with the expected incidence of between 5 per cent and 8 per cent (Klein and Stern 1971; Smith and Hanson 1974; Baldwin and Oliver 1975). Separation may well be important; such infants often have long periods in a special-care baby unit with consequent separation from the mother. Klein and Stern (1971) noted that the mean stay in hospital for the 12 low-birthweight babies in their series of 51 abused children was 41·4 days. Neonatal separation was one of the significant factors that emerged from a study of a series of battered children compared with their control siblings (Lynch 1975). In a further 50 children referred for abuse or neglect, Lynch, Roberts, and Gordon (1976) have found that concern over the mothering had often been recorded by maternity hospital staff (72 per cent of cases compared with 15 per cent of a contrast group). The relationship in these cases seemed to have set into an unfortunate pattern in the first days or weeks of life.

Medical procedures

Interaction between a mother and her newborn baby may be upset by medical procedures even before birth, for example, by the use of obstetric analgesics or anaesthetics. There is a very marked difference in the frequency with which these drugs are used in different countries. It is very low in Holland, for instance, where it is the exception for analgesics to be administered. In the United Kingdom and the United States it is by contrast exceptional for a woman not to be given an analgesic in labour. Kraemer, Korner, and Thoman (1972) quote a series of 404 vaginal deliveries at Stanford University Hospital in 1968 in which only two women had no drugs and seven no anaesthetics. It is difficult to assess the effects of drugs used in obstetrics. They tend to be given in various combinations and doses and at different times before delivery; the length and difficulty of labour are further variables to be considered (Kraemer *et al.* 1972). The side-effects of drugs on the mother are not uncommon, though frequently neglected (O'Driscoll 1975) but in an infant they persist much longer because of immature enzyme systems and inefficient detoxication. Barbiturates, for instance, make babies unresponsive and difficult to rouse for feeding for several days (Brazelton 1961). A mother may be very upset by her baby's unresponsiveness, even though he is by her side. This 'chemical separation' interferes with mother–infant interaction just as effectively as a physical separation. Brazelton (1970), in a review of the effects of drugs on the neonate, wrote that 'watching a drugged mother and a depressed infant who must make a "go" of each other should stimulate us to re-evaluate the routine use of premedication and anaesthesia in pregnancy and delivery in the light of its effect on early mother–infant interaction, as well as its lasting effect on their lives together.'

Borgsted and Rosen (1968) found that the level of 'consciousness' in the first 3 days was depressed in 29 out of 33 babies whose mothers had received medication (usually Meperidine 50–100 mg with Promethazine 25–50 mg) during labour compared with 1 out of 8 infants of unmedicated mothers. Twenty-eight out of the 33 medicated group showed EEG alterations (defined as an increase in fast-wave activity) as compared with 1 out of 8 who had not received drugs. They do not define what they mean by an increase, but the tracings were read without identification of the patient.

In a study of 20 full-term infants Stechler (1964) was able to show that the visual attentiveness at 2–4 days of age was depressed. The mothers had received one or more of the following drugs in varying dosage; Pethidine, Alphaprodine, Pentobarbitone, and Promethazine; by taking into account dosage and time of administration he was able to show that the effect was related to dose of the drugs and was more marked when they had been given within $1\frac{1}{2}$ hours of delivery. The ability to inhibit a reflex response to a repeated stimulus is considered to be an indication of cortical integrity. It is disturbing that Pethidine given in labour has been shown to affect this ability for a month or even longer (Conway and Brackbill 1970). These workers also found impaired responses to tests of muscular, visual and neural function associated with Pethidine but not with length of labour, maternal age, parity, birthweight, family income, or education.

Maternal medication influences infant feeding. This was studied in a remarkable controlled experiment by Kron, Stein, and Goddard (1966). Infants whose mothers were randomly selected without medical indications to receive 200 mg Secobarbital by intravenous infusion during labour sucked more slowly and less efficiently for 4 days than did controls given no drugs. In another study Richards (1974) found that babies whose mothers had received Pethilorfan needed more stimulation and the length of feeds and sucking bouts were reduced. There was also a long-term after-effect; the drug babies were less involved in social interchange with the mothers at 30 and 60 weeks.

There is now an increasing use of local regional anaesthesia in childbirth and it is not sufficiently realized that local anaesthetics also cross the placenta and are readily detectable in the blood-streams of the infant. Although Apgar scores at birth are usually satisfactory, behavioural assessment has demonstrated that muscle tone is lowered in the first hours of life (Scanlon, Brown, Weiss, and Alper 1974) and also at 3 days (Standley, Soule, Copans, and Duchowny 1974). The babies are alert but floppy and irritable.

Long-term side-effects have not yet been reported but Wolff has pointed out that 'congenital' differences in muscle tone, mobility, duration of alertness, vigour of sucking, frequency of smiling, and the stability of the sleep-waking cycle all contribute as much to the mother–infant relationship as does the mother's individuality. In this context obstetric medication, which affects all these characteristics will alter the early interaction of mother and infant and so affect the relationship in the long term.

The place of birth
When comparisons are made between hospital and home confinements it must not be forgotten that many of the procedures carried out in hospital are necessary and life-saving, and at the present time in the United Kingdom some 90 per cent of all women are delivered in hospital. Understandably, but regrettably, these normal women are referred to and treated as 'patients'; they expect to be given 'treatment'. Treatment in hospital is part of the ethos. Is it not a waste of a hospital bed if a woman needs no treatment? Both medical procedures and drugs tend to be used too frequently. One procedure only too often leads to another, each having repercussions on the mother, the infant, and their interaction.

We believe that the best place for a normal woman to be delivered is in her own home. Of course risk factors must be excluded. The home must be made ready and there must be back-up facilities available for unforeseen complications which will occasionally occur. Birth at home is an exciting family affair, whereas in hospital (although it may also be exciting and happy) labour is too often reduced to a series of technical procedures. Exciting events make a deep impression and so aid the attachment process.

When a mother first meets her baby her behaviour shows a characteristic pattern (Klaus, Kennell, Plumb, and Zuehlke 1970). This is modified simply by being in hospital. Rubin (1963) has shown that delay in contact, or even wrapping the baby up, may inhibit greeting behaviour and may render intercourse between mother and baby less intimate for several days. An undrugged neonate is especially alert and responsive during the first hour after delivery (Brazelton 1961). This should be the very time for a mother and baby to get to know each other. Regrettably, most hospital routines make prolonged and intimate contact during this first important hour impossible. The baby is 'whisked away' to be bathed and the mother often left to undergo the repair of an episiotomy, which is becoming a very common procedure in hospital. In the United States separation after birth is the rule, (Kennell *et al.* 1975); the mother goes to be monitored in a recovery room and the baby to a transitional care nursery. In hospital all mother–infant pairs suffer some interactional deprivation when the quality and caretaking nature of the relationship are taken into account (Barnett, Leiderman, Grobstein, and Klaus 1970). This deprivation is severe if the baby is taken to a special-care baby unit and the mother only allowed to view through the nursery window.

When a baby is rooming-in and feeding is 'on demand', there is little interference. Yet in a hospital or maternity unit a mother is not truly in charge as she is at home. She will be constrained by the needs of other mothers and babies in the ward and influenced by advice, often conflicting, from a variety of experts. Rooming-in where it is practised is often only allowed by day. Of course, mothers must rest, but many find this difficult. Without her baby near her a woman may lie awake listening for sounds from the nursery. The existence of set times for resting, sleeping, feeding, and visiting may conflict with individual needs or wishes. However homely and enlightened hospital staff may try to make their wards, some routines seem to be essential. In one study it was found that when mothers have experienced birth at home and in hospital, 80 per cent prefer birth at home (Richman and Goldthorpe 1974). Maternal preference should receive consideration and the effects of freedom of choice for the woman on her interaction with her baby should not be forgotten.

The regime in nurseries with multiple caretaking and a 4-hourly feeding schedule is thought by Sander (1969) to be stressful for babies. Infants so cared for are more restless and cry more than those rooming-in. The routine for looking after a baby in hospital is likely to become the model for care after discharge; a mother may try to imitate the hospital practices instead of developing an awareness of her own child's idiosyncrasies. A baby develops expectation of its caretaker very early; Brazelton (1975) has described video-tape studies showing how a 3-week-old baby ceased interaction and withdrew when his mother presented an impassive face. Sander is reported (Brazelton 1975) to have found that the rhythms of sleeping and feeding of 7-day-old infants were disturbed for 24 hours by the mother simply wearing a mask.

A period of post-natal depression is more common after confinement in hospital, 64 per cent of 193 cases, than after home delivery, 19 per cent of

86 cases (Cone 1971). A mother who is depressed tends to be withdrawn and unable to respond to her baby. In this situation there is what may be described as 'psychological separation'.

Conclusion

Many hospital routines and current medical practices are harmful to the early response of mother and baby to each other but continue because they are not critically examined. What ethical committee would countenance a research protocol requiring one group of mothers only to be permitted access to their newborn babies after 2–3 days and another group only to see them through the nursery window for the first 3–12 weeks? A woman is abnormally receptive after delivery not only to her baby but to her environment. Inconsiderate behaviour by her attendants, anxiety, and above all separation from her baby, whether physical, chemical, or psychological, may leave an indelible impression.

In the last 10 years paediatrics in the United Kingdom has been revolutionized by encouraging mothers to come into hospital to look after their own sick children. The introduction of this common sense and humane practice met with much resistance; there is similar resistance now against allowing mothers to be fully involved in the care even of their normal babies immediately after delivery.

We believe that there should be facilities in hospital for a mother to help look after her sick or premature baby; most up-to-date units are now taking steps to make this possible. The special-care baby unit at our own hospital at High Wycombe has been built with special facilities for mothers to be admitted straight from the labour ward to the unit with their babies. Sick and healthy mothers need to be cared for differently. Active measurements to deal with complications or illness should be available to both but normal physiology must be respected and not invaded, as it is in far too many hospitals today, by procedures appropriate only to pathology. Childbirth is not a disease.

References

Baldwin, J. A. and Oliver, J. E. (1975). 'Epidemiology and family characteristics of severely abused children'. *British Journal of Preventitive and Social Medicine* **29**, 205–21.

Barnett, C. R., Leiderman, P. H., Grobstein, R., and Klaus, M. (1970), 'Neonatal separation: the maternal side of interactional deprivation'. *Pediatrics* **45** 197–205.

Birch, H. (1956). 'Sources of order in the maternal behaviour of animals'. *American Journal of Orthopsychiatry* **26**, 279.

Borgstedt, A. D. and Rosen, M. G. (1968). 'Medication during labour correlated with behaviour and EEG of the newborn'. *American Journal of Diseases of Childhood* **115**, 21–4.

Brazelton, T. B. (1961). 'Psychophysiologic reactions in the neonate. Part II, Effects of maternal medication on the neonate and his behaviour'. *Journal of Paediatrics* **58**, 513–18.

—— (1970). 'Effect of pre-natal drugs on the behaviour of the neonate'. *American Journal of Psychiatry* **126**, 1261–6.

——, Tronick, E., Adamson, L., Als, H., and Wise, S. (1975). Early mother–infant reciprocity. In *CIBA Foundation Symposium 33; Parent–infant interaction*, pp. 137–54.

Broussard, E. R. and Hartner, M. S. S. (1971). 'Further considerations regarding maternal perception of the first born'. In *Exceptional infant 2, studies in abnormality* (ed. J. Hellmuth), p. 432. Brunner/Mazel New York; Butterworths, London.

Carpenter, G. 'Mother's face and the newborn', *New Scientist*, 21 March 1974, 742–4.

Cone, B. A. (1972). 'Puerperal depression'. *International Congress on Psychosomatic Medicine in Obstetrics and Gynaecology*, London 1971, pp. 355–7. Karger, Basel.

Conway, E. and Brackbill, Y. (1970) 'Delivery medication & infant outcome: An empirical study. The effects of obstetrical medication on foetus and infant'. Monograph of the Society for Research on Child Development **35**, 24–34.

Franz, R. L. 'The origins of form perception'. *Scientific American* **204**, 66–74.

——, *et al.* (1975). 'Early visual selectivity'. In *Infant perception: from sensation to cognition* (ed. L. B. Cohen and P. Salatpatek), Vol. 1. Academic Press, London and New York.

Garrow, D. H. and Smith, D. (1976). 'The modern practice of separating a newborn baby from its mother'. *Proceedings of the Royal Society of Medicine* **69**, 22–5.

Greenberg, M., Rosenberg, I., and Lind, J. (1973). 'First mother rooming in with their newborns; its impact upon the mother'. *American Journal of Orthopsychiatry* **43**, 783–8.

Grimwade, J. C. *et al.* (1971). 'Human foetal heartrate change and movement in response to sound and vibration'. *American Journal of Obstetrics and Gynecology* **109**, 86–90.

Hammond, J. 'Hearing and response in the newborn'. *Developmental Medicine and Child Neurology* **12**, 3–5.

Harlow, H. F. and Harlow, M. K. (1965). 'The affectional systems'. In *Behaviour of non human primates*. (ed. A. M. Sahrier, H. F. Harlow, and F. Stollnitz, Vol. 2. Academic Press, New York and London.

Harlow, H., Harlow, M., and Hansen, E. (1963). 'The maternal affectional system in rhesus monkeys'. In *Maternal behaviour in mammals* (ed. H. Rheingold). John Wiley, New York and London.

Hersher, L., Richmond, J., and Moar, A. (1963). 'Maternal behaviour in sheep and goats'. In *Maternal behaviour in mammals* (ed. H. Rheingold), John Wiley, New York and London.

Hinde, R. A. (1974). *Biological bases of human social behaviour*. McGraw Hill, New York.

Hutt, S. J. (1973). 'Auditory discrimination at birth'. In *Early human development* (ed. S. J. and C. Hutt) Clarendon Press, Oxford.

Kennell, J. H., Jerauld, R., Wolfe, H., Chesler, D., Kreger, N. C., McAlpine, W., Steffa, M., and Klaus, M. H. (1974). 'Maternal behaviour one year after early & extended post-partum contact'. *Developmental Medicine and Child Neurology* **16**, 172–9.

Kennell, J. H., Trause, M. A., and Klaus, M. H. (1975). 'Evidence for a sensitive period in the human mother'. In *Parent–infant interaction*, p. 87. CIBA Foundation Symposium 33.

Klaus, M. H., (1975). 'Parent–infant interaction', p. 303. CIBA Foundation Symposium 33.

—— and Kennell, J. (1970). 'Human maternal behaviour at first contact with her young'. *Paediatrics* **46**, 187–92.

——, and —— (1970) 'Mothers separated from their newborn infants'. *Paediatric Clinics of North America* **17**, No 4. Plumb, N., Zuehlke, S. (1970). Human maternal behaviour at the first contact with her young. Pediatrics **46**, 2, 187–92.

——, Jerauld, R., Kreger, N. C., McAlpine, W., Steffa, M., and Kennell, J. H. (1972). 'Maternal attachment. Importance of the first post-partum days'. *New England Journal of Medicine* **286**, 460–3.

Klein, M. and Stern, L. (1971). 'Low birth weight and the battered child syndrome'. *American Journal of Diseases of Childhood* **122**, 15–18.

Klopfer, P., Adams, D., and Klopfer, M. (1964). 'Maternal "imprinting" in goats'. *Proceedings of the National Academy of Science* **52**, 911.

Kraemer, H. C., Korner, A. F., and Thoman, E. B. (1972). 'Methodological considerations in evaluating the influence of drugs used during labor and delivery on the behaviour of the newborn'. *Developmental Psychology* **6**, 128–34.

Kron, R. E., Stein, M., and Goddard, K. E. (1966). 'Newborn sucking behaviour affected by obstetric sedation'. *Pediatrics* **37**, 1012–16.

Leiderman, P. H., Leifer, A. D., Seashore, M. J., Barnett, C. R., and Grobstein, R. (1973). Mother–infant interaction: effects of early deprivation, prior experience and sex of infant. *Research Publications, Association for Research in Nervous and Mental Diseases* **51**, 154–75.

Leifer, A. D., Leiderman, P. H., Barnett, C. R., and Williams, J. A. (1972). 'Effects of mother–infant separation on maternal attachment behaviour'. *Child Development* **43**, 1203–18.

Lynch, M. A. (1975). 'Ill health and child abuse'. *The Lancet* ii, 317.

——, Roberts, J., and Gordon, M. (1977). 'Early warnings of child abuse in the maternity hospital'. *Developmental Medicine and Child Neurology*. (In press.)

Macfarlane, J. A. (1975). 'Olfaction in the development of social preferences in the human neonate'. In *Parent–Infant Interaction* (Amsterdam CIBA Foundation Symposium 33, new series, ASP, 1975).

Mills, M., and Mellinish, E. 'Recognition of mother's voice in early infancy' Nature 1974, **252**, 123.

Moore, A. (1968). 'Effects of modified care in the sheep and goat'. *Early experience and behaviour* (ed. G. Newton and S. Levine), pp. 481–529. Charles C. Thomas, Springfield.

Newton, N. and Newton, M. (1962). Mothers' reactions to their newborn babies. *Journal of the American Medical Association* **181**, 122–6.

Noirot, E. (1972). The onset of maternal behaviour in rats, hampsters, and mice: a selective review. *Advances in the Study Behaviour* **4**, 107–46.

O'Driscoll, K. (1975). 'An obstetrician's view of pain'. *British Journal of Anaesthesia* **47**, 1053–9.

Rheingold, H. (ed.) (1963). *Maternal behaviour in mammals*. John Wiley, New York and London.

Richards, M. P. M. (1974). 'The one day old deprived child'. *New Scientist*, March 1974, 820–2.

Richman, J. and Goldthorp, W. O. (1974). 'Maternal attitudes to unintended home confinement, a case study of the effect of the hospital strike upon domiciliary confinement'. *Practitioner* **212**, 845.

Ringler, N. M., Kennell, J. H., Jarvella, R., Navojosky, B. J., and Klaus, M. H. (1975). 'Mother to child speech at 2 years—effects of early post-natal contact'. *Journal of Pediatrics* **86**, 141–4.

Rosenblatt, J. S. (1970). 'Views on the onset and maintenance of maternal behaviour in the rat'. In *Development and evolution of behaviour* (ed. L. R. Aronson *et al.*) Freeman, San Francisco.

Rubin, R. (1963). 'Maternal touch'. *Nursing Outlook* **11**, 828–31.

Salk, J. (1973). 'The role of the heartbeat in the relationship between mother and infant'. *Scientific American*, March.

Sander, L. W., Strechler, G., Burns, P., and Julia, H. (1970). 'Early mother–infant interaction and 24 hour patterns of activity and sleep'. *Journal of the American Academy of Child Psychiatry* **9**, 103.

Scanlon, J. W., Brown, W. U., Weiss, J. B., and Alper, M. H. (1974). 'Neurobehavioural responses of newborn infants after maternal epidural anaesthesia'. *Anaesthesiology* **40**, 121–8.

Seashore, M. J., Leifer, A. D., Barnett, C. R., and Leiderman, P. H. (1973). 'The effects of denial of early mother–infant interaction on maternal self-confidence'. *Journal of Personality and Social Psychology* **26**, 369–78.

Smith, S. M. and Hanson, R. (1974). 134 battered children: a medical and psychological study'. *British Medical Journal* iii, 666–70.

Sontag, L. W. (1936). 'Changes in the rate of the human foetal heartbeat in response to vibratory stimuli'. *American Journal of the Diseases of Childhood* **51**, 583–9.

——, (1941). 'The significance of foetal environmental differences'. *American Journal of Obstetrics and Gynecology* **42**, 996–1003.

Standley, K., Soule, A. B., Copans, S. A., and Duchowny, M. S. (1974). *Science* **186**, 634–5.

Stechler, G. (1964). 'Newborn attention as affected by medication during labour'. *Science* **144**, 315–17.

Walker, D. *et al.* (1971). 'Intrauterine noise, a component of the foetal environment'. *American Journal of Obstetrics and Gynecology* **109**, 91–5.

Wertheimer, M. (1961) 'Psychomotor coordination of auditory–visual space at birth'. *Science* **134**, 1692.

Whiten, A. (1975). In *Interactions in infancy* (ed. H. R. Shaffer). Academic Press, London.

Wolff, P. H. (1963). 'Observations on the development of smiling'. In *Determinants of Infant Behaviour* (ed. B. M. Foss). Vol. 2. Methuen, London.

BIANCA GORDON **13**

The vulnerable mother and her child

Mothers are important not only because they bear children, but also because they bring them up. This chapter focuses on the mother's psychological needs. For the baby, loss of maternal care is as important in the emotional as in the physical sphere. A mother does not necessarily have to be physically absent to be unable to enter in a loving relationship with her child. A psychotherapist discusses how to provide for women a facilitating environment in which women can give birth and become mothers.

Introduction

Workers in the caring professions tend to focus necessary attention on specific issues such as the control of pain; the presence of fathers during labour and delivery; the 'rooming-in' of babies; or induction, but unfortunately do so at the expense of a deeper examination of the overall needs of expectant and new mothers. The danger of this practice is that such issues, although important, are presented as solutions or even 'breakthroughs' in obstetric care, thus diverting attention from the continuous need to improve ongoing psychological care.

We still tend to think that pregnancy should be a state of bliss, and of childbirth as a time of fulfilment and harmony, free from stresses and inner conflicts. For incalculable numbers of women, reality falls short of such expectations. They discover that pregnancy and childbirth are times of crisis, of unexplained fears and forebodings, of self-doubt, disappointment, and depression. The expected blissful moment when the mother holds her baby for the first time is often over-shadowed by anxiety and feelings of emptiness, inadequacy, or even hostility.

Whether or not a mother's experience of childbirth is a happy one depends not only on the physical care she receives, but also on the care for emotional needs, and on the recognition of her as a unique individual. My observations are based on more than 23 years' involvement in in-service training at well-baby clinics, in paediatric and obstetric departments, and on short-term psychotherapeutic work in these settings. Mothers were seen initially because of difficulties with their babies, such as excessive crying, sleeping and feeding disturbances, or an ill-defined feeling that something was wrong with the infant. It was found that they had, almost invariably, been unable to form mutually satisfying relationships with their child.

It is inappropriate to generalize about the relative value of home or hospital confinement without considering the physical, social, and emotional condition of the mother. Whichever appears the ideal place for one mother may still fail to meet the emotional needs of another. Yet the place of birth is nearly always discussed in terms of physical suitability. Even the best-appointed home, hospital, or private clinic will be no more than a convenient place for delivery of a baby unless it provides the mother with psychological support, and enables her to experience birth as an enriching achievement. Given these conditions, it is more likely that she will be able to relate to her baby with confidence.

Psychological care in pregnancy

As long ago as 1966 a report of The Royal College of Midwives entitled 'Preparation for parenthood' highlighted the importance of a good working relationship between a mother-to-be and those taking professional care of her. It stressed that sustained antenatal care encompassing both the mental and the physical needs of the pregnant woman is crucial. That the latter are concentrated on more than the former may be because physical changes are within the competence of those entrusted with antenatal care, whereas psychological work with individuals is not. Our maternity services, both public and private, are thus very deficient. Pregnancy and childbirth are too readily seen as isolated events, rather than as milestones in the personal history of the woman. It is not sufficiently recognized that a woman's emotional background can decisively affect her personal reaction to pregnancy and to childbirth. It is also likely that it will affect her relationships with her child and her family, and may leave its mark on the future development of both herself and her infant.

Gestation and motherhood are biologically and psychologically inseparable conditions. Many hitherto dormant emotional difficulties that come to the surface at the time of birth are visible to a trained observer early on in pregnancy. Unfortunately at present they are often not noticed, or their significance not appreciated.

Every woman comes to childbirth in a very vulnerable state and clinical work suggests that the number of mothers who are at risk is much greater than is commonly recognized. This should not cause surprise if one remembers that the relationship between a mother and her infant starts in the pre-natal stage, and that during its development through to birth and beyond it is open to many influences for good and ill, both from within the mother herself and from outside. To ensure that this crucial relationship is given the best possible chance to mature healthily, it is essential that every mother's emotional needs are approached with the same skilled conscientiousness as are her physical needs.

During pregnancy the mother-to-be is anxious about what is happening in her body, and in her as a person. She worries about the changes taking place and about the even greater ones ahead of her. She is feeling a whole new orientation within herself, and in her relationship with her family: she desires answers to questions on specific matters such as breast-feeding, and feeding on demand, or whether she should have her baby induced or opt for 'natural childbirth'. These are subjects which she may have heard discussed, often inconclusively or contradictorily, by the media and by other mothers. She therefore needs to feel reasonably confident about the care she is going to receive before and after the birth. Doubts and anxieties are felt by all mothers, and not only by those who suffer from emotional difficulties. Therefore nearly all women during early pregnancy benefit from a sustained relationship with a sensitive member of the maternity team, who allows them to express these feelings, and satisfies their need for clear, unbiased information. This creates the continuity of care that is so essential to the mother, and is a source of comfort and support throughout the pregnancy.

It is as harmful to neglect the needs of women who require special help, as it is to behave in a way that is perceived as interfering and domineering by the more independent, confident woman. The latter is very loath to accept with equanimity the bullying predilections of some of the authoritarian characters to be found in a number of our maternity units.

An enlightened antenatal service will take differing needs into account when considering a woman's physical condition, and on this basis will assess the relative merits of hospital and home confinement. She can then be given advice, not only on the safest environment for the birth itself, but on the setting which will best meet the medical and personal needs of herself and her baby. For one mother this will be in hospital, for another it will be in her own home. The aim of the maternity services should be to improve the quality of total care available in both locations. What is therefore required is a supportive psychological service with staff who are skilled in recognizing the signs of emotional vulnerability; who can answer questions fully and without bias; who can discuss a mother's fears and fantasies, and can spot early indications of an impaired relationship between her and her baby. These staff in turn must be supported by psychologically trained personnel, to whom mothers at risk can be referred.

Constant demands are made for elaborate theoretical research into the emotional needs of expectant and new mothers. However, there is ample opportunity for each member of any professional care team to explore these needs in our day-to-day work by simply talking to patients. By asking mothers how they feel and what they find helpful, we are afforded the best possible chance of enriching our knowledge, not only about their attitudes, but also about the effectiveness of the services we are providing. If women are offered the opportunity to participate in the decisions that affect them psychologically and physically, it is likely that their decision will be the right one.

I am focusing here on the psychological ill-effects of a lack of choice concerning the place of birth. However, complaints by mothers cover, as they have always done, a much wider area. Those most frequently voiced in clinical work concern inconsistent information and advice, frequent changes of staff, long and sometimes stressful waiting at clinics, loneliness during labour, and above all a lack of understanding about the emotional needs of parents. The help that I am suggesting would *not* make mothers more dependent—on the contrary, it would give them the independence which they desperately want to achieve, but are at the same time afraid of taking. They need *our* help to gain the confidence that they can manage on their own. In order to achieve this, the staff must treat women as adults and not, as is so often the complaint, as if they were dependent children.

Psychological care at and after the birth

Whether or not a mother's experience of childbirth is a happy one depends not only on the physical attention she is given, but also on the care she receives for her emotional needs. I have described and discussed these in the context of antenatal care, but they are even more acute during the very period of the birth when the mother is most anxious, most dependent, and therefore most vulnerable.

Childbirth is emotionally and physically very demanding, and nearly every mother-to-be is anxious about her ability to bear a normal baby and to fulfil her maternal role competently. This is especially true of the woman giving birth to her first child. Many women cannot spontaneously 'switch on' maternal feelings the moment they are presented with their babies, and it is immensely helpful to them to know that their uncertain, initial responses do not necessarily indicate the lack of a maternal instinct.

Some mothers have very disturbing dreams in the post-partum period, unlike any they have had before. In others old conflicts with members of their immediate families are revived, and feelings and incidents which have been repressed for years are brought to the surface of consciousness. These upsurges of dormant disharmony, recrimination, and fantasy can be frightening, and are bound to disturb the mother's initial adjustment to her child.

At this early stage she is the baby's whole world, and it is absolutely dependent upon her. There is constant mutual interaction between the two, so it is impossible for the state of one to be understood without considering that of the other. The importance of therapeutic intervention at the first sign of an impaired mother–baby relationship cannot be overstressed, for any emotional damage that is ignored at this stage can develop into severe psychological problems for mother or baby.

The screening of parents suspected of potential child abuse is to be commended. However, this should be accompanied by greater attention to the underlying causes of *all* emotional 'at-risk' situations. These can be perceived early in the mother–infant relationship. Baby battering is an extreme manifestation of an impairment in this relationship. Other manifestations, often less obvious, are far more common and invariably have a long-term effect on the emotional well-being and development of the child. Children who, from the beginning of their lives have been subjected to undue emotional stress, are vulnerable. There is a need for ante- and post-natal care to concern itself with the wide range of signs of infant and maternal distress, and not just with the safety of the baby and the mother.

My clinical experience in this field, during which I have treated several hundred mothers from all walks of life, indicates that impediments in the mother–baby relationship are rarely due to conscious rejection of the baby. They tend to stem from complex problems within the parent. Unresolved emotional difficulties in the mother are often at the root of such disturbed relationships. These are frequently due to her own childhood problems with her parents, to sibling rivalries, or to the early loss of a parent or sibling, rather than to social and economic conditions. Such conflicts can remain dormant for many years, until they are revived by the birth, and fought out in the new relationship with the baby, especially during feeding, for it is principally at this time that a mother communicates to the infant her disharmonies and inner tensions.

A woman's inability to gratify her baby can stem from not having herself enjoyed a satisfying relationship with her own mother. This deprivation may make her turn eagerly to her baby for the love and protection for which she had looked in vain, and for gratification of her past longings. When a mother makes such demands on her baby, a role reversal is occurring; she is acting as an unloved child, seeking in her baby a parent. When the baby, being unable to fulfil this role, becomes unhappy or responds in a demanding manner, her past cravings are revived, accompanied by frustration, anxiety, and hate. These reactions cause her to withdraw from, to run away, shake, beat, batter, and in extreme cases kill the infant.

Unresolved sibling rivalries can also cause a mother to perceive her baby as a once-hated brother or sister, and thus make it the target of the revived hostile feelings that belong not to him, but to that disliked sibling from her own childhood. As a result she experiences again the pain, rejection, and despair of that period, and finds it hard or impossible to respond to her baby in an appropriate manner.

The experience of death of a parent or a sibling during her own childhood can also affect the mother's relationship to her baby. If the process of mourning was abnormal, unfinished, or non-existent, it can distort a mother's responses to her pregnancy and to her baby. It can contribute to later psycho-pathology, and be the cause of transient depressive reactions or breakdowns.

This happened in the case of a young mother who was referred to me because her first baby presented a screaming problem, and showed intense fear of noises and strangers. As a child the mother had suffered the loss of a baby brother from pneumonia. Her own mother had blamed herself for the illness and tragic end of the baby's life, and had lived with the belief that she had neglected him. When the surviving daughter became a mother, her attitude to her own baby was influenced by this childhood experience. Her development had been profoundly affected by the death of her baby brother and she had suffered from guilt because she had resentfully seen him as a rival. Now she feared that some malignant fate would strike her own baby in a similar manner, and her over-anxious attitude and behaviour produced various phobic reactions in her child.

Of the many predicaments which can confront a mother with her new-born, the baby's crying is the most distressing; it is also the most common. She can never be sure whether it is signalling that it is hungry, cold, wet, in pain, or whether it is simply calling for attention. She is therefore uncertain whether to comfort it or ignore it. In all cases of excessive screaming known to me, the babies were found to be physically fit, and sedatives proved to have no effect. Screaming, especially when it is felt to be accusatory rather than a signal of distress, can drive a despairing mother to batter her infant. If it is ignored, other symptoms of the impaired relationship may show in the child, such as rocking or head-banging. The symptoms may also be of a psychosomatic nature. Being outwardly less disturbing than the screaming, these may go unnoticed for some time, yet the replacement of screaming by less immediately alarming symptoms indicates the end of the baby's search for fulfilment of its needs from its mother. Instead, it is turning to its body for satisfaction. This development probably signifies a rupture of communication with the mother which is bound to impede the child's capacity to relate to the outside world, and to form satisfactory relationships in later life.

Ideally, professional contact with a mother should be established during pregnancy, but even when made immediately after the birth, it can reveal much about her capacity and her difficulties, and can provide helpful insights into any problems she is having with her baby. At this early stage, even the vaguest expressions of disapprobation towards the infant should arouse concern. At this time when a mother communicates her feelings by touching, holding and looking, a skilled observer is in a good position to gauge a great deal about her feelings by the way she holds, feeds, bathes, and talks to her baby, and by the manner in which she dresses it and changes its nappies. I recall one mother who was holding her frantically screaming baby girl rigidly at arm's length. When I enquired if she knew of any way to soothe her, she revealed the gap between her conscious understanding and her ability to act on it. She replied without hesitation, 'Yes, she will be quiet if I hold her close to me.' Yet she could not bring herself to do this.

Note should also be taken of expressions of regret or disparagement if the baby is not of the sex the mother wanted, if it is said to resemble a dis-liked relative, or of any undue delay in naming the child. In such cases it should not be assumed that the maternal instinct will automatically assert itself, and that without psychological help the mother will in due course be able to relate to her child, and come to love him.

Post-natal depression

Post-natal depression is a common phenomenon. It can be associated with unexpected developments such as a premature birth, induction, complications during delivery necessitating the use of forceps, or a Caesarian section. Some mothers who give birth while anaesthetized do not feel that they have had a baby, or that the baby is theirs. Depression can also follow the birth of a handicapped or a still-born child or from internal psychological disharmony. Whatever the cause of the depression it interferes with the mother's capacity to adjust to the new happenings in her life. Without help some mothers find it impossible to relate to, and care for their baby satisfactorily, as they passionately wish to do.

Some mothers suffer breakdowns, and because of their inability to care for their infant, have to be separated from it. These depressions cannot be fully understood in terms of recent disappointing hospital or other external experiences, though these may be significant. They have been caused by much older conflicts, which have remained dormant. It is inappropriate to try and urge a mother to 'snap out of it' or to jolly her out of her depression. On the contrary, such misguided attempts will only add to her feeling of not being understood. She will be pained if made to feel that if only she tried harder, she would radiate success and happiness at having produced a normal baby.

Most of my work in this area has been with mothers who have had their baby in hospital. However, these problems also arise among mothers who have had a baby at home. A heavy responsibility lies with the hospital which does not promptly attend to these depressions, most of which manifest themselves in an easily recognizable manner. If there is an argument in favour of hospital deliveries, I think it is that the continuous presence of professionals from different disciplines should make it easier to identify these conditions and to provide appropriate help. Instead many hospitals appear to regard post-natal emotional distress as part of the process of childbirth, which will abate in due course, almost as speedily as the physical pain of labour. It is regrettable that professionals often tend to focus on a safe and satisfactory birth, without giving sufficient thought to continued efforts towards the successful creation of a mother. Physical safety of mother and baby is thought in some quarters to be not only the overriding, but the only reason for hospital delivery. Hospital practices may even exacerbate psychological problems. It is a sad reflection of our maternity services that mothers suffering from depressive responses are discharged merely when they are considered physically fit. The following comments will illustrate how far from emotionally fit some mothers are after a hospital birth and how many hospitals fail them when they are in need of emotional help.

When I went into hospital I was relaxed and happy that the day had come, but was horrified to hear that not only could my husband not enter the ward, he even had to leave the hospital—although I sorely needed him with me. I began to feel swamped by the pain. I couldn't speak and what I found most frightening was the utter callousness of the nurses ... they could hear me gasping, trying to tell them, trying to *contact* them during this awful experience, and they remained utterly unimpressed. It wasn't only the pain, it was the way nobody around seemed to acknowledge it. It was the fact that I couldn't cope alone and in dignity or in the company of caring people with this pain I found so horrifying. I think it was being left alone for so long, very confused and totally humiliated in the way I was behaving. I could not stop crying.

Hours later when I was brought the child I knew immediately that I did not want to hold him. Throughout my stay in hospital I did not want to feed him or change him, but I did, because in a public ward and with social mores being the way they are, it is very very difficult to say 'by the way I don't seem to love this child'. Gradually over six months, with a *very* loving and understanding husband, I have grown to love this child deeply and truly, but when I am tired I still get depressed about his birth.

Mrs. C. suffered from depression which led to her referral for psycho-therapy 3 weeks after the birth of her first, much longed-for baby. Her baby's constant screaming added considerably to her distress:

I had arranged to suckle the baby while on the delivery table, but she was not offered to me to hold, touch, or suckle until 40 minutes after delivery. It was an extremely long delay after a normal delivery and she was then asleep. The post-natal care is characterized for me by a lack of continuity among the people involved in my antenatal care, and by there being no single person who was responsible for the management of us both. Every day there was a different doctor, and none of them told the nursing staff what they should do. The nursing staff changed several times a day, and each nurse had a different way of doing things, so I became confused by all the contradictory advice. I found I was out of step with the institution, and I was always off schedule no matter how hard I tried. It seemed that I was constantly being reprimanded, 'Hurry up and finish feeding the baby.' When I said I did not know how to hurry the feeding of a baby, the response would be a repeated 'Hurry up', and a quick departure, which was no help at all.

It seems natural that I should have become depressed, and then the only advice offered was an admonishing, 'Don't cry, you have nothing to cry about', or 'Crying only makes things worse.' Even my request to the paediatrician and obstetrician for a psychologically trained person to talk to did not produce such a person.

Another thing which bugged me was that after my saying day after day to the paediatrician and sister, 'Don't you think the baby should be on demand? She is never awake at feeding times, is difficult to wake and screams in between', one sister told me, 'All our babies are on demand here.' This was a sick joke because they obviously were not.

I strongly wanted my second baby at home. I still have strong reactions in remembering Jane's birth. The intensity of the feelings surprised even myself. Having a baby at home in my country is a rare event. It just isn't done so I spent months and hours on the telephone making inquiries trying to find a doctor who would do a home delivery. This wanting a home delivery was very important and central to my anxieties and when I succeeded in making arrangements, the anxieties began to resolve and things went well after this.

The total experience of labour and delivery was as close to my hopes and desires as I could ever have hoped for. I am very enthusiastic about home delivery.

These experiences not only emphasize the need for psychological help, but also bring home the point that even mothers who are vocal in asking for what they believe to be the correct management of their baby encounter difficulties in hospital. However, it may well be that this type of articulate woman is in a particularly difficult position *vis-à-vis* the staff, who may feel that their status as professionals is threatened, and dislike being challenged by a 'mere mother'.

Mrs. E. has this to say 5 years after the birth of her child, following which her post-natal depression was not treated:

When I left the hospital I had a very bad dose of post-natal depression and I have never recovered from it. With the aid of drugs and a very understanding husband, I have lived a reasonably normal life, but I am not the same person I was before the birth. Whatever I go to my doctor with, I am told to take tranquillisers— that is all I am ever offered. I have asked him if I should be referred to a psychiatrist, but he said I don't need this, and that I should accept that I am the sort of person who has to have tranquillisers. I cannot accept this though. I did not behave like this once, so why now? I have had bouts of ill-health. The doctor maintains it is tension, and when I say that I am not tense he says it is subconscious tension. Well, what can I do about that? My relationship with my little boy is not a good one. He is a difficult child. He starts school next week and I could cry when I think of his tumultuous first five years which I can never have back again to do better.

These comments show that post-natal depression is often anything but transitory. Had she received professional help at its onset, it is unlikely that she would still be suffering its effects 5 years later. Was it 'safe' for the hospital to discharge her without providing the kind of help she has been strenuously searching for ever since?

Enlightened and sympathetic management, so vital for all mothers, is imperative for those giving birth to premature, handicapped, or still-born babies. They should get sustained help in dealing with the problems which arise from these special circumstances. The following examples are un-fortunately in line with much of my experience with mothers whose needs have not been met by hospitals.

Mrs. F's baby was born with a cleft palate and hair-lip:

When I woke from the anaesthetic my husband was crying, and I had never known him to cry before. Because of this I believed my baby was dead, but then I was assured he was not. I suspected something was wrong and repeatedly asked the staff, but they refused to say anything. This further convinced me that something was wrong. My husband told me the next day that the baby had a hair-lip; in fact he also had a cleft palate. They had shown him the baby without any prior warning that anything was wrong, and he nearly fainted when he saw him. It was a terrible shock to see such a baby; he was like something out of a horror film, and of course it was impossible to breast-feed him. I was very disappointed because I had set my heart on breast-feeding. I had a rough time as each feed lasted two hours, so I was feeding twelve hours out of each day. When he was four months old he had the repair to his lip done and my incipient nervous breakdown slowly began to come to a crisis. I completely rejected my baby and wanted him to be taken from me. I do not want any more children for obvious reasons. My little boy is in a nursery as I am still unable to cope with him all day.

Mrs. G. recalls her experience when giving birth to a still-born baby and her sadness at the way this was managed by the hospital staff.

My husband was told very briefly and without expressions of sympathy by the hospital registrar. At first he was only concerned about how I would be affected mentally by the loss of the baby, but later he felt angry about the way in which my confinement had been mismanaged. Later still he felt he had failed in his duty towards me and the baby by not having brought more pressure to bear on the registrar to speed up the labour.

We would have welcomed any attempt on the part of members of the staff to show a human, sympathetic interest in our plight. Their treatment of us was detached to the point of callousness. There was an inability to identify with me, and a reluctance to become involved.

Mrs. H., the mother of a still-born baby, was in an emotionally disturbed state for a long time after the confinement. She too was saddened by the thoughtless and unfeeling treatment she and her husband received at the hospital.

It seems impossible to believe that my baby died six months ago, I have neither forgotten it nor did I get over it. I was not told the baby was dead or its sex or anything and I was fully conscious. I heard someone say it had red hair and I had to ask what it was. I was not asked whether I would like to see her, just tidied up, cleaned up and asked if a Post Mortem was O.K. and told to leave the disposal arrangements to them.

Obviously my husband realised something was wrong, but was not told until finally he guessed. Eventually someone came and told him, 'It was a little girl and she did not live. Please sign the form and go to the Registrar of Births.' At no time did anyone consider his feelings.

I was left alone far too much. There was no medical reason for my remaining in a post-natal ward at all. There is nothing worse than being woken up by the babies in the nursery, nurses being too busy to give you sleeping tablets, hearing excited fathers visiting; seeing women with their third day blues in the bathrooms and feeling like murdering them, as they have no right to be depressed.

The medical staff weren't very tactful—comments like: 'You're 26—plenty of time for a string of them.' 'We'll do a post mortem and let you know what happened.' 'Don't try again for a year, here is a supply of the Pill, etc.'

One feels at this time completely inconsolable and out of things. For a start there is the physical pain which is of course temporary. It is the mental anguish which is hardest. The medical staff do try to cure your pain but completely ignore the other aspect. Their attitude throughout was that it was of no consequence at all— but quite honestly it is not like any other sort of bereavement—it is totally shattering.

I became terribly anxious about everything and finally went to my G.P. who was terribly surprised that I was still upset. While describing my symptoms (palpitations, panic, etc.) he said that these usually happened after a bereavement and that I was treating it like a real death—but of course this is what it was to me. He was not unkind, just terribly thoughtless.

As for the caring professions and the medical staff, where are they?

These examples serve to show the urgent need for parents, particularly in the post-partum period, to have someone understanding and supportive to talk to. In relating their experiences, mothers demonstrate that the doctor most valued by them is the one who is interested in the patient as a person and not only in her physical condition. Medical services, especially in our hospitals, are deficient in their facilities for one-to-one contact. Doctors, midwives, nurses, and social workers in these settings are in key positions to avert or reduce the hazards resulting from a potentially bad experience. Too few professionals make it their business to spend time with, and listen to, the new mother, in an effort to answer her questions and deal with her preoccupations. At present this aspect is often grossly neglected, and hardly any provision is made in hospitals for rooms in which patients can be seen without constant interruptions from other staff or the telephone. Hospitals and clinics should be designed so that patients can talk in privacy. There should be more respect for the pregnant woman and the new mother, so that she can be strengthened in her regard for herself at a time when she often lacks confidence in her capacity and inner resources.

Attention to the mother's emotional difficulties shortly after birth even after considerable initial distress, can be very rewarding because at this time she feels very close to the infantile part of herself, and to the unconscious problems associated with her childhood. In addition her urgent desire to relate to her baby makes her highly motivated to use the help which preventive psychiatry can give. The baby who displays symptoms of an impaired relationship often shows startling changes in its state when work with the mother has improved her ability to relate to it. Encouragement to express herself allows the mother to bring to the surface thoughts and feelings of which she has previously been unaware. When she is helped to link these with her past, feelings which were chaotic and frightening begin to appear logical and to make sense. Even during a first session with a mother, one often notices that she becomes calmer, and that there is a striking improvement in the baby. The speed with which the baby establishes contact with his mother the moment the line of communication between them is cleared never fails to amaze me.

I feel, therefore, that there should be greater emphasis on preventive psychological work in obstetrics. When vulnerable mothers have opted for hospital delivery, this work can be carried out by the introduction of regular ward rounds. These have the purpose of giving all mothers of new-born babies an informal opportunity to discuss anything they wish about themselves, their infant, or their older children.

Special interest should be shown in cases where the infant has a mental or physical abnormality, whether or not the mother recognizes or has complained of such a handicap. The team can keep an eye on unmarried mothers and mothers who have had premature babies or still births. I have experienced the great benefits derived from such ward rounds, and have been impressed by the way most mothers find it easy to air their preoccupations on these occasions.

There is a need for very special concern for the large number of mothers from socially and economically deprived backgrounds who have opted for a hospital delivery because this gives them a respite from oppressive domestic responsibilities. Many of this group do not make use of the maternity and after-care services, but they are those most desperately in need of them. Among them are some of the most vulnerable mothers. During routine ward-rounds they can be identified without being made to feel singled out. In this way they can be reassured about the continuity of our interest in them. Unless our services succeed in establishing and maintaining contact with these women, their stay in hospital will have been no more than a convenient place for delivery providing a welcome period of absence from home, to which they return without being any better equipped to cope than they were before their admission. There is much evidence that our services have as yet failed to reach this particularly deprived section of the community. Once ward-rounds for emotional care of the kind described are conducted as a routine, they will benefit all mothers. Such a service can be expected to make a significant contribution towards overcoming the artificial dichotomy between physical and psychological care in obstetrics.

The mother's vulnerability makes it necessary for her to be in an emotionally supportive environment. For some this will be home; for others hospital. In the case of women with psychological problems which come to the fore in the post-partum period, early recognition and help are vital.

The father

In the past the father has been thought to be of little significance to the baby during the very early phase of its life. The effect he has on the baby is often only an indirect one, in that the emotional support he can give to the mother strengthens her ability to cope with the new demands being made on her. The current cultural change towards the father's greater participation in the upbringing of the infant enables both parents to be involved in the care of their child from the beginning, making it a joint venture in the responsibilities and pleasures of which they have an equal share.

The father's ability to assume a supporting paternal role depends also on his own childhood experiences, particularly on his early relationship with his mother. If he has been exposed to emotional deprivation as the result of an unsatisfactory maternal relationship, or the arrival of a brother or sister, latent feelings of insecurity may now lead him to regard the new-born as a rival for his wife's love. He may perceive the crying and the demands of the baby as competing with his own wish for fulfilment of unsatisfied longing and needs. At moments when they lose control over their unconscious fears, this erroneous perception causes some fathers to abuse their infants physically. 'I will show him who is governor in this house,' yelled a father while physically assaulting his baby son.

When psychological intervention in a family is required, a father's perceptive involvement can do much to reduce the mother's tension and enable her to make more effective use of professional help. By the same token the vulnerable father who cannot fulfil this role may contribute to the mother's and the baby's distress. My clinical experience provides few examples, apart from fathers who physically abuse their child, of a baby's distress being causally related to the father's psychopathology, and of its being overcome through the treatment of his condition. Nevertheless the significance of the father's role at this time is probably greater than has been generally appreciated. With the greater emphasis on sexual equality, more attention should now be given to his role in the early phase of infant development.

In spite of official policy favouring the father's presence at delivery, not all hospitals welcome fathers. Yet there can be no doubt that the presence of a husband who wishes to be at the confinement can only be beneficial. In his presence the mother will feel supported and reassured knowing that he is there to speak on her behalf. She may thus achieve a more relaxed mental state, and be better able to do her part at delivery. The father himself may feel that seeing his child being born gives a sound and completely necessary basis for his continuing relationship with it.

As yet it is only in a home delivery that the degree of the husband's participation does not depend on being given 'permission' to be with the wife, or to touch and hold their baby. We look forward to the day when hospitals will provide a setting where the atmosphere approximates as much as possible that of a home, and where birth can be experienced by all concerned as a significant family event.

Conclusion

Birth is an intimate, emotional, family event. Its professional management is a decisive factor in the relationship which develops between a mother and her baby. The physical benefits deriving from recent advances in obstetric technology are only of limited value to the vital relationship between parents and their baby if they are allowed to obscure the emotional implications of birth.

No one approach, or type of treatment, can possibly be appropriate for all mothers. Any decision, as for instance choosing the place of birth, should involve careful consideration of individual needs, and all the professions involved should aim at a maternity service which allows all women to make a personal choice on the place of confinement, while giving them full information and assistance.

I have outlined some emotional problems of motherhood which are especially relevant to the type of maternity service that is offered today. In an ideal service, skilled and sensitive care from early pregnancy onwards would guard against lasting emotional damage, and be the best guarantee that a mother's eventual decision in favour of hospital or home delivery will be the right one for her. Once it is accepted that every mother-to-be should have a choice about the place of birth it follows that we must strive for an improvement in the quality of physical and emotional care in the hospital as well as in the home.

There is an urgent need for the dissemination of existing knowledge about the psychological processes associated with pregnancy, birth, and early infancy. Only when this is achieved will there be a fundamental improvement in our maternity services.

Attention to the physical safety of mother and child is vital but there is a danger that the current preoccupation with safety may absorb the energies of our services and overlook the emotional problems faced by women throughout pregnancy, confinement, and the early months of motherhood. The effectiveness of otherwise excellent medical care is reduced because a mother who is under stress cannot benefit fully from it. At present, psychological training is sadly lacking in the majority of our medical and nursing schools, where it is still widely assumed that the skills concerning human relations develop of their own accord. Such training and the change of attitude that will accompany it would enable staff to care for the woman who is apprehensive about her condition, and about whether she will acquit herself well. Continuity is a most important component of total obstetric care; without this even the most efficient technical service will fail to meet the mother's needs and make her confident about the care she is receiving.

Stress should be dealt with when it first reveals itself. Antenatal services in maternity departments and family health clinics are in an ideal position to screen women throughout the 9 months of pregnancy and identify those liable to suffer emotionally. Sustained contact with psychologically trained personnel would enable mothers to express and discuss their fears and fantasies long before they face the stresses of labour and confinement.

I have tried to show how the failure of a mother to establish a satisfactory relationship with her baby is often caused by her own unresolved family conflicts. Such failure is frequently damaging to the child's future development. Short-term psychotherapy with the emotionally vulnerable mother can help her to understand and resolve those conflicts which bear directly on her relationship with her infant.

The demands of mothers themselves will in future make it increasingly difficult for the professions to ignore the emotional problems associated with childbearing. Already much more is known about the emotional needs of women during pregnancy and childbirth than is acted upon. Further psychological studies in this field should therefore not be undertaken without a concurrent investigation of the reasons for our failure to develop maternity services more closely related to what is already known about the emotional concomitants of pregnancy and birth. The current economic crisis might prove a blessing in disguise if it results in a reassessment of priorities, and the allocation of a greater proportion of our limited resources to preventive care for mothers and babies, in hospital as well as in the home.

References

Gordon, W. D. (1966). 'Preparation for parenthood'. Royal College of Midwives.

Gordon, B. (1970). *A psycho-analytic contribution to paediatric practice*. Psycho-analytic study of the child, Vol. 25. International Universities Press.

—— (1974). 'An inter-disciplinary approach to the dying child and his family'. In *Care for the child facing death* (ed. L. Burton). Routledge and Kegan Paul, London.

—— *An approach to the problems of mothers and babies*. Baillièrè Tindall, London. (In press.)

The family and neonatal intensive care

Babies at risk should be born in hospital, and not only in a hospital but in one with a special care-baby unit attached. When babies need intensive care, the emotional needs of the family should be given careful consideration. The environment can either reject or support the parents. In this chapter a neonatologist and a midwife consider the organization of intensive neonatal care so that it supports the family unit.

The case for neonatal intensive care

In recent years most developed countries have recorded a persistent fall in perinatal mortality rates (Department of Health and Social Security 1976; Davis 1976). It is difficult to identify the many factors involved in bringing about these changes but undoubtedly improvements in socio-economic standards have been of great importance. This is exemplified by the persistence of differences in perinatal mortality-rates within a single society between the various socio-economic groups (Chamberlain, Chamberlain, Howlett, and Claireaux 1970). However detailed analyses of perinatal mortality statistics from individual hospitals strongly suggest that modern obstetrics and neonatal intensive care do have an important effect over and above those resulting from changes in society (Davis and Stewart 1975). It is among the infants of the lowest birthweight group (less than 1·500 kg) that the most marked improvements in survival rates have been reported (Davis and Stewart 1975).

It is essential to know that these surviving small infants will grow into healthy children free from physical and mental handicaps. The evidence from numerous follow-up studies is that associated with increased rates of survival there has been a decline in physical and mental handicaps (Davis and Stewart 1975).

This is the case for the intensive care of the small, sick, pre-term infant. In the remainder of this chapter we shall discuss some of the effects on the family when an infant undergoes intensive care in a special-care baby unit.

The families at risk

Some families know before conception that the foetus will be in danger and require early delivery with the prospect for the baby of prolonged intensive care. These families include hypertensive mothers, mothers with previous bad obstetric histories, and mothers who have had infants severely affected by rhesus isoimmunization. These families should be given the opportunity for a full discussion of the risks involved when a new pregnancy is contemplated.

For other families it becomes apparent during the antenatal period that the foetus is at risk; for example a mother in her first pregnancy developing severe toxaemia. In such cases there is time to acclimatize the family to the idea that the foetus will need to be delivered early to give him the maximum chance of survival while minimizing the risk to the mother's own health. Similarly, mothers with twins, triplets, and higher multiple births have an increased chance of pre-term delivery. These families must adjust to the idea of the mother spending prolonged periods at rest in hospital antenatally which may be followed by the baby's prolonged admission to the special-care baby unit.

For these groups of mothers it is essential that their antenatal care is supervised at a hospital with special facilities for foetal monitoring and intensive care of the baby. Antenatal preparation should include a visit to the special-care baby unit so that the family can become familiar with the unit and the staff who will look after the baby.

However, about a third of mothers who deliver prematurely do so unexpectedly (Rush, Keirse, Howat, Baum, Anderson, and Turnbull 1976). For these families, and for the family whose baby suffers severe birth asphyxia or becomes unwell in the neonatal period, there can be no antenatal adjustment to the idea of separate admission of the baby to a special-care baby unit. Such unexpected problems may mean that the baby is delivered at a place where there are no facilities for neonatal intensive care and as a result the baby may require urgent transfer to a distant hospital.

Birth, resuscitation, and separation

Immediately after birth a normal baby can be held by the mother and the father and the mother may hold the baby to feed at her breast. This is not possible for low-birthweight and asphyxiated infants who may require resuscitation including endotracheal intubation and artificial ventilation. Severely asphyxiated babies may also require insertion of an umbilical venous catheter and the administration of alkali.

Nevertheless, we have found that it is often possible to allow the mother and father to hold their baby for a few moments following resuscitation. This has even been the case when there is an umbilical catheter in place. We believe this involves no additional risk to the infant; and it gives the mother and father a chance to see, hold, and recognize their baby momentarily prior to his admission to the special-care baby unit. Although this period of contact is brief we believe it is of the greatest importance; we base this belief both on published studies (Klaus and Kennell 1976), and also on our own experience of the parents of babies admitted to the unit.

The criteria for admission to the special-care baby unit

It is essential for certain infants to be admitted to a special-care baby unit if their safe survival is to be ensured. This is mandatory for the very low-birthweight infant born many weeks before term who is at risk of many disorders associated with immaturity, in particular respiratory failure. It is also essential for infants who have suffered severe birth asphyxia to be admitted for intensive care since these infants may require intravenous fluids, assisted ventilation, or sedation for some time after birth. Other infants born before 36 weeks of gestation have poor coordination of sucking and swallowing and are admitted to the unit for tube feeding which requires skilled nursing care. In addition there are infants with major congenital malformations who are admitted to a special-care baby unit for feeding, assessment, and sometimes surgical treatment.

Some infants need additional attention and observation in the newborn period but do not require admission to a special-care baby unit. These infants can be cared for on the post-natal maternity wards provided that there is adequate nursing staff and that the mothers themselves are allowed to help with observation and care of their infants. Examples of such infants are those who have suffered lesser degrees of birth asphyxia, infants born by the breech, those delivered by Caesarean section, infants of diabetic mothers, and certain low-birthweight infants who require additional feeding and screening for hypoglycaemia.

Some infants on ordinary post-natal maternity wards may develop problems which require some additional attention but do not justify the admission of the baby to a special-care baby unit. The commonest example of this is the infant developing physiological jaundice in the first few days after birth. With adequate organization it is possible to measure the baby's plasma bilirubin level daily and to start treatment with phototherapy without removing the baby from the mother's bedside. Over the last 3 years we have changed our criteria for the admission of these borderline cases to the special-care baby unit in Oxford. We have found that the post-natal maternity nursing staff and the mothers have been able to manage these infants. This has resulted in a fall in the number of admissions to the unit and a change in the pattern of admissions (Fig. 14.1). Fewer term infants are initially admitted to the unit for observation; fewer infants are brought from the post-natal maternity wards to the unit for the management of jaundice; at the same time rather more low-birthweight infants have been born in this hospital who have required admission to the unit. This change in attitude—where possible trying to keep babies out of the special-care baby unit—has produced a similar fall in the admission numbers to special-care baby units in other parts of the country, notably in Cambridge (Richards and Roberton 1977).

The families of babies admitted to the special-care baby unit
The initial hours and days after the baby's admission to the unit are naturally a period of great anxiety for the family. At this stage it is desirable that the mother and father visit the baby if at all possible and that the medical and nursing staff make them welcome. At the time of this first visit, as on

Plate 14.1 A scene from the special care baby unit illustrating the equipment involved which is likely to bewilder the unprepared parents. See p. 219

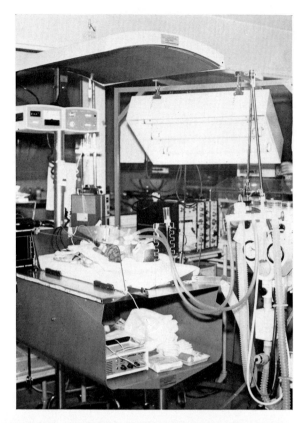

Plate 14.2 A polaroid photograph being taken, which is to be given to the mother of a newborn infant in the special care baby unit. See p. 220

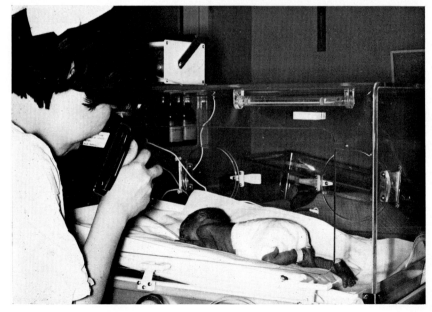

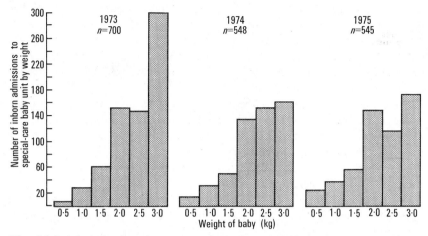

Fig. 14.1 Admissions to the special care baby unit in Oxford over the last three years. Fewer term infants are admitted following difficult births; fewer infants are brought from the post-natal maternity wards for the managment of jaundice; at the same time an increased number of low-birthweight babies have been born in this hospital and required admission to the unit.

subsequent visits, it is important that the medical and nursing staff spend sufficient time with the parents to explain to them what is happening. In order to do this we try to ensure that the maternity staff notify the special-care baby unit when the baby's father and mother are coming to the unit so that they can be met at the entrance. Alternatively, if the parents arrive unannounced on this or subsequent occasions they ring a bell at the nursery entrance. This enables one of the medical or nursing staff to show them how to put on gowns before entering the unit, to say a word about hand washing before touching the baby or his incubator and then to bring them in. This procedure is not only designed to welcome them to what may be seen as a hostile environment; it also provides a safeguard against untimely arrival. For example it would be undesirable if the parents arrived without any prior warning at the baby's bedside to find him undergoing some emergency procedure.

For some families, especially for those whose premature delivery was unexpected, this is a time of great bewilderment; their baby may be surrounded by and attached to tubes, electrical leads, ventilators, lights, recording equipment and the baby may be underneath a radiant heater (Plate 14.1).

At the time of this first visit the parents are likely to be preoccupied with the baby's chance of survival and of his being brain-damaged. In order to avoid conflicting information relating to these difficult questions one member of the medical staff is made responsible for each family. At this first meeting and subsequently (as far as possible) this doctor provides the family with information and progress reports. If the mother is unwell immediately after delivery and unable to visit the unit the doctor reports to the mother regularly with news of her baby. In order to support the mother's feelings about her baby at this early stage we arrange to take a polaroid photograph of the newborn infant for the mother (Plate 14.2). We believe this is particularly important when the mother is at a different hospital, distant from the special-care baby unit.

Following the anxieties of the first visit to the unit continued contact between the parents and their baby creates different problems. The mother may have recovered and be ready to go home a day or two after delivery with the prospect of her baby remaining in the unit for many weeks. Preservation of the unity of the family group then becomes a matter of stamina.

We have tried to measure the feelings of a group of mothers during the time when their babies were in the unit. Using a visual analogue scale

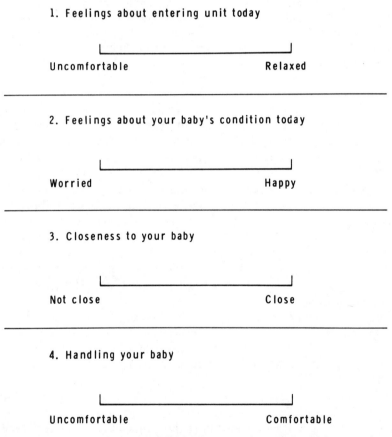

1. Feelings about entering unit today

Uncomfortable   Relaxed

2. Feelings about your baby's condition today

Worried   Happy

3. Closeness to your baby

Not close   Close

4. Handling your baby

Uncomfortable   Comfortable

Fig. 14.2 The four questions and visual analogue scales used in assessing the mothers' levels of anxiety about their babies in the unit when they visited their baby.

each mother was asked by one of us (P.H.) to try and assess her feelings about her baby by marking a position on a 10 cm line corresponding to each of four questions (Fig. 14.2). For each question a high score represents a lesser degree of maternal anxiety. The total score from these questions, expressed as a percentage, was looked at against the post-natal age of the baby. The period of maximum anxiety was in the early days after birth; subsequently the degree of anxiety fluctuated widely, generally tending towards optimism (a high score) at the time of taking the baby home. An individual example of this graphical expression of the mother's feelings is shown in Fig. 14.3.

During the time after the mother's discharge from hospital attempts

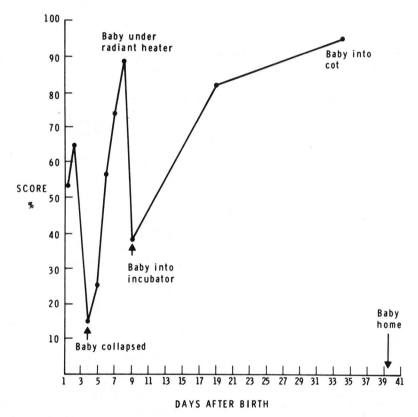

Fig. 14.3 An example of a mother's feelings about her baby as 'measured' using the linea analogue scale.

The mother's anxiety increased at a time when the baby collapsed; she became more confident over the next few days until he was transferred from the radiant heater to an incubator (a step of improvement from the point of view of the medical staff but viewed with alarm by the mother); thereafter the mother grew in confidence as the baby continued to improve until the time of discharge.

are made to maintain daily contact with the family. They are encouraged to telephone daily and to visit daily when possible. It is important that the medical and nursing staff know each family very well especially concerning such details as the financial stresses imposed by visiting and problems of finding babysitters for siblings. We have seen families with infants under intensive care in the unit caught up in a self-imposed ritual of daily or twice daily visiting with evident feelings of guilt if they miss a single visit. For other families, especially those visiting from a distance, each day's travel can be exhausting. It becomes important for the doctor responsible for a particular family, in consultation with the senior nursing staff, the hospital medical social worker, and the family's general practitioner (G.P.), to steer the family through this difficult period. Occasionally it is advisable for the parents to take a weekend off without visiting. We believe that such breaks are very important for parents who may have to wait 80 or 90 days before taking their baby home from hospital.

Other members of the immediate family may also be interested to see the baby. Grandparents, aunts, and uncles and other members of the family are welcome to view the baby from an observation corridor. Once the threat to the baby's immediate survival is passed we generally encourage parents to bring older siblings with them on visits. In this way brothers and sisters are able to share in the reality of having a new baby in the family. However, we do not usually allow these siblings to enter the unit and touch the baby until the day of discharge.

The role of the nurse on the special-care baby unit
Neonatal intensive care has resulted in a change in the traditional role of the clinical nurse. During the time of the baby's acute illness the nurse is acting as a highly skilled technician playing a central role in maintaining the baby's life support system. During periods of intense work it is difficult for even the most experienced nurse to avoid feelings that visits from the parents are an intrusion. Over the days of intensive care many nurses become attached to their patients; this adds to the problems of preserving for the parents their feelings that the baby belongs to them and not to the special-care baby unit and its staff. Providing such problems are recognized we believe they can effectively be dealt with by discussion among the staff and by including the whole of the family group as being in need of intensive care.

The role of the hospital medical social worker in the special-care baby unit
We have a part-time social worker fully occupied in our unit dealing with the emotional problems and anxieties of all the parents whose babies are admitted to the unit. Most of her work is centred on the family crises surrounding the baby's admission to the unit and the support offered to the

parents is limited to the duration of the baby's stay. However, about 10 per cent of the families whose babies are admitted to the special-care baby unit have serious social and emotional problems and require a more involved and long term contact with the medical social worker.

In the 12-month period June 1975–June 1976 there were 450 admissions to the special-care baby unit in Oxford. Fifty-two of these families were considered to have serious social or emotional problems requiring additional help from the hospital medical social worker. In 16 cases the mothers were known to have suffered emotional disturbances in their own childhood and were known to social services as having psychiatric problems. Twelve families were known to have severe marital problems including physical aggression; some of these families were on the confidential 'at-risk' register in view of violence towards, or neglect of previous children. A further 24 mothers were noted to have been unusually depressed, apathetic, or disturbed in their attitude towards their baby, either antenatally or post-natally and to warrant closer attention by the medical social worker. Where the emotional problems or psychiatric disturbances of the family are considered to be severe further help is obtained from the local children's psychiatric hospital. This may result in the transfer of the baby together with his parents to the family unit in the human development research unit at the Park Hospital For Children following the baby's discharge from the special-care baby unit. When support can more appropriately be given in the community, referral is made to the relevant team of community social workers.

The family and the baby's future development

During the early post-natal days, corresponding to the most critical time of the infant's illness, most parents are worried largely about the life and death of their baby. Once this period is over, usually when a small infant is able to breathe without the assistance of an artificial ventilator, the emphasis of the parents' concern changes to the possibility of physical or mental handicap. Recent follow-up studies of very low birthweight infants have provided us with optimistic information with which to counsel the families of such infants (Davis and Stewart 1975). The outlook for infants who have suffered severe birth asphyxia is less certain. Nevertheless the immense powers of recovery of the newborn infants who survive birth asphyxia do, on the whole, justify an optimistic outlook (Scott 1976). It is important that statements about the baby's future development are made to the parents by the doctor who has come to know them best; in this way the parents can be assured of consistent information which they can understand from someone they have come to know well.

When the infant is seriously ill it is important not to over-protect the family. The parents must know if the baby is in a critical state or dying. The mother and father may require additional lengthy discussions with the medical staff and with the medical social worker. We enlist the support of the family doctor and his health visitor who can frequently offer additional emotional support for the family in their home.

For some infants the outlook is bad: for example infants who have suffered severe episodes of hypoxia perhaps associated with convulsions and infants with serious congenital malformations. It is perhaps in these situations that the communication skills of the medical and nursing staff are most severely tested. In a series of interviews the family must be given some idea of what the future holds in store and be assisted in making the appropriate preparations. However, we do not as a rule try to look too far into the future but rely upon out-patient follow up visits to one of the senior members of the paediatric staff to deal with the problems as they arise.

The family and infant feeding

During the time when the infant is very ill it may be necessary to provide fluids by intravenous infusion. As the infant recovers and grows, intravenous infusions are replaced by intragastric milk feeds. At this stage the mother, or less frequently the father, may learn to give feeds via a feeding tube into the stomach. In this way in addition to visiting, sitting, watching, touching, and speaking to the baby, the parents have an opportunity of being involved in the actual care of their growing infant. However, not all parents feel capable of performing such tasks and it requires sensitivity and experience on behalf of the senior nursing staff to judge which parents to involve in this way.

We believe that human milk is the most appropriate form of nutrition for the low-birthweight and sick newborn infant. Unfortunately the smaller and sicker the infant the more remote is the possibility of the baby being able to feed at the breast and sustain the mother's lactation. Nevertheless, it has proved possible in some cases for the mother to sustain lactation by manual expression of her breasts and by the use of a hand or, more effectively, an electrical breast pump.

In order to assess how successful mothers of babies entering the special-care unit in Oxford have been in establishing and sustaining lactation we recently conducted a small survey. Over a period of 12 months 70 letters were sent out to mothers of babies admitted to the unit who were known to have wanted to breast-feed. This does not represent all the mothers wishing to breast-feed over this period of time since many mothers whose babies were only on the unit for a few days were omitted from the study, and mothers whose babies died were excluded. Of the 70 mothers sent questionaires 52 replied. Twenty took their babies home fully breast-feeding; 17 took their babies home entirely bottle-feeding; 15 took their babies home on the breast with bottle supplements, of whom 7 eventually established complete breast-feeding. Thus 27 out of the 52 mothers were successful in fully breast-feeding their babies. In general the mothers' chances of fully breast-feeding their babies were poorer the longer the baby stayed in the unit, the shorter the gestational age of the baby at birth, the lower the birthweight of the baby, and other related factors.

The mothers who answered the questionaire offered many comments on how they might have been better supported in their efforts to sustain lactation. Their suggestions included: better availability of the electrical breast pumps; more time spent with experienced midwifery staff gaining assistance in milk expression; and the provision of a comfortable private room on the unit for early attempts at breast feeding once the baby was well enough to feed at the breast. In general the mothers agreed that the overriding problem was that of determination and stamina and that they depended very much on the encouragement and support of the nursing staff. It may be that future attention to these details will allow a larger proportion of the mothers of very small infants to be successful in establishing and maintaining lactation.

The baby's experiences in the special-care baby unit
It is sometimes difficult for medical and technical staff to remain constantly aware that the very small, sick, newborn infants with their disordered biochemistry and physiology are conscious and feeling human beings. The

Table 14.1 The scoring sheet used for 'measuring' the babies' unpleasant experiences on the special-care baby unit

Procedure	Score
Passage of naso or orogastric tube	1
Face mask over baby's face	1
Endotracheal or nasotracheal intubation	3
Endotracheal or nasotracheal suction	4†
Umbilical catheter inserted or removed	1
Oropharyngeal or nasopharyngeal suction	1†
Eye drops instilled	1†
X-ray taken	1
Heel prick	1
Peripheral vein puncture	1
Intramuscular injection	1
Lumbar puncture	3
Insertion of chest drain	3
Removal of elastoplast (etc.) including urine bags	1
Temperature in incubator over 34 °C	1†
Baby's rectal temperature less than 36 °C	1†
Artificial ventilation	4†
Phototherapy	2†

† Maximum score for this item for 24 hours

physical discomfort of these patients is presumably substantial. We have made an attempt to measure the degree of trauma to which an average infant is subjected during intensive care. We took two groups of 20 infants during the first week of their admission to the unit: Group A represented 20 infants undergoing intensive care; and Group B 20 infants undergoing simple supportive care in the unit. We drew up a scoring system indicating the number of unpleasant experiences to which such infants might be subjected in a day. This system of scoring must not be taken too seriously since it is unreasonable to equate the unpleasantness of a heel prick, for example, with the unpleasantness of the background noise of a ventilator. The scoring system is shown in Table 14.1.

Each time a procedure was carried out on a baby the nurses noted it on the tabulation sheet. At the end of the first 7 days a total score was calculated. For the babies under intensive care the mean score for the week was 144 compared with 38 for the babies receiving routine nursery care. If one takes the attitude that even the smallest infant is aware of trauma and pain, then one builds up a picture of the overall discomfort which the baby suffers during intensive care.

At an older age one might expect that such a prolonged unpleasant experience would be followed by emotional and behavioural disorders. Perhaps some of the difficulties which mothers experience with their babies on taking them home from the special-care baby unit represent 'neurotic behaviour' by the baby resulting from his traumatic post-natal experiences. We have no idea whether such experiences have any lasting effects on our patients.

Family reunion

After a prolonged stay in the special-care baby unit it is often difficult for the medical and nursing staff to appreciate the emotional significance and practical repercussions on the family of the baby's discharge from hospital. The parents feelings must be coloured by reservations and anxieties about the future health of their baby. Nevertheless many parents pass through a phase of euphoria when they first take their baby home which may last several weeks. In many cases this is followed by a period of exhaustion, depression, and anxiety largely related to irregularities in the baby's sleeping and feeding pattern. Then sooner or later these problems resolve as routines are established and confidence restored as the baby is seen to be growing and developing normally (Blake, Stewart, and Turcan 1975). We try to talk to the parents about these problems before they take the baby home. We also try to ensure that the mother is confident in the practical aspects of caring for her baby before discharge from hospital. In many cases the mother lives in the hospital for 24 hours during which time she takes full responsibility for the baby's care. However, not all mothers have taken advantage of this facility and we are uncertain how important this is. Those hospitals with specially built mother and baby rooms report an enthusiastic response from the parents (Rubissow and Brimblecombe 1977)

When the time comes for the baby to go home it is important to ensure that arrangements have been made for continued support for the family if this is indicated. It is essential that the G.P. and the health visitor are informed before the baby is actually discharged from the unit. In addition the G.P. must be given a detailed account of the baby's medical problems and any additional specific problems relating to the parents.

We try to avoid making out-patient follow up visits to the hospital a routine for all babies who have been on the special-care baby unit. Such visits are of course important when there are specific indications. However, in many cases the baby's development is followed by the G.P. who, provided he has an interest in the care of babies and infants, is better situated to view the whole of the family scene than the hospital-based doctor.

There are some families for whom we have found it useful to offer an additional kind of support. Parents who have had babies with particular problems and who have seen them progress through all their difficulties over the first year or two provide a valuable source of encouragement for parents currently concerned about their babies on the unit. This has particularly been valuable for mothers with very low-birthweight infants and infants with specific malformations such as cleft palate. We bring these parents together for a talk and have found this kind of self-help meeting to be greatly appreciated by the families concerned.

The family which is not reunited

Some infants die on the special-care baby unit. In other cases the babies survive but are seriously malformed or are recognized to have sustained severe neurological damage. Such babies may require further protracted or even permanent hospital care. For the families of these babies we believe it is important to arrange an after-care service. These families will have been under intense strain while the baby has been on the unit. They will have suffered the emotional ups and downs but at the end of it all do not have a baby to bring home. There is then the danger that there will be no routine visits from the health visitor and an absence of all the activity that is usually associated with the homecoming of a newborn baby. If the baby dies well wishers tend to keep away and unless special provisions are made the family may be isolated in their grief, exhausted, and bewildered. The situation is not unlike that of the family whose baby has been still born (Lewis 1976). We believe that the intensity of their mourning is generally under-estimated. Through our hospital medical social worker we have tried to make arrangements for meetings with these families, talking over the experiences of the pregnancy, the child's birth, the admission to the unit, and the child's eventual death or permanent disability. Some parents have indicated that they did not really need nor want any further contact with the hospital. Other parents however, have welcomed contact with the hospital doctors, nurses, and social worker and there have been instances where parents have requested repeated meetings for periods up to a year after the death of their baby.

Conclusions

Modern methods of intensive care of the newborn have resulted in a reduction in neonatal mortality and at the same time a reduction in handicap among the survivors. These results are the over-riding concern of those working in this field. Intensive care of the newborn is an exacting task demanding devotion and great technical skill of both the nursing and medical staff. However, this need not be to the exclusion of attention to the psychological and social problems of the family. This is not just a humanitarian exercise since the parents attitude towards their baby is the foundation on which the aftercare of the baby is based once he is discharged from hospital.

References

Blake, A., Stewart, A., and Turcan, D. (1975). 'Parents of babies of very low birth weight: Long term follow up'. In *Parent–infant interaction*, p. 271. Ciba Foundation Symposium 33 (new series). Elsevier, North Holland.

Chamberlain, R., Chamberlain, G., Howlett, B., and Claireaux, A. (1970). *British births 1970*, p. 17. William Heinemann Medical Books, London.

Davis, P. A. (1976). 'Infants of very low birth weight'. In *Recent advances in paediatrics* (ed. D. Hull), p. 89. Churchill Livingstone, Edinburgh.

—— and Stewart, A. L. (1975). 'Low birth-weight infant: neurological sequelae and later intelligence'. *British Medical Bulletin* 31, 85.

Department of Health & Social Security (1976). 'Health Services development: report of the working party on the prevention of early neonatal mortality and morbidity'. Health Circular, HC (76) 40.

Klaus, M. H. and Kennell, J. H. (1976). 'Parent-to-infant attachment'. In *Recent advances in paediatrics* (ed. D. Hull), p. 129. Churchill Livingstone, Edinburgh.

Lewis, E. (1976). 'The management of stillbirth: coping with an uncertainty'. *The Lancet* ii, 619.

Orme, R. C. L'E. and Buxall, J. F. (1977) 'Organization of the Exeter special care baby unit related to mother/child contact'. In *Early separation and special care nurseries* (ed. M. P. M. Richards and F. W. Brimblecombe). Clinics in Developmental Medicine (SIMP) and Heinemann Medical Books. (In press.)

Richards, M. P. M. and Roberton, N. R. C. (1977). 'Admission and discharge policies for special care baby units'. In *Early separation and special care nurseries* (ed. F. S. W. Brimblecombe and M. P. M. Richards). Clinics in Developmental Medicine (SIMP) and Heinemann Medical Books. (In press.)

Rush, R. W., Keirse, M. J. N. C., Howat, P., Baum, J. D., Anderson, A. B. M., and Turnbull, A. C. (1976). 'Contribution of preterm delivery to perinatal mortality'. *British Medical Journal* ii, 965.

Scott, H. (1976). 'Outcome of very severe birth asphyxia'. *Archives of Disease in Childhood* 51, 712.

Obstetric practice:
past, present, and future

Obstetric practice involves not only medical but social judgments, and in coming to conclusions about the medicine we want we also have to decide the kind of society for which we are striving, and the relations between men and women, doctors and patients, and experts and lay people.

In this chapter an obstetrician, who was largely responsible for introducing modern monitoring and other techniques into obstetrics in Britain, puts maternity care and reproductive medicine today in a historical context, criticizes present practice, and looks forward into the future.

Society is gradually recognizing that women can play a unique dual role, and that they should be able to exercise one or both, and contribute to the community without regard to their sex, and/or be mothers. It is only recently that some women have been able to enjoy their sexuality—as men have always done—independently of the reproductive consequences. But real options and choices for women cannot exist until such time as the means to choose are available to all. Such means include: equal opportunities with men for education, employment, status, and representation; protection of employment during childbearing and motherhood; support for one-parent families; facilities for the day-care of children; flexible working hours; recognition that motherhood is an experience of life equivalent to uninterrupted employment; ready access to contraception and safe abortion; and the provision of appropriate maternity and gynaecological care.

I find no inconsistency or paradox in striving to improve conditions for childbearing women and their children, and in my support of the freedom of women to choose whether or not pregnancy should continue (Huntingford 1976), and where the birth of their child should take place. To my mind the State has no right to decide whether pregnancy should continue, or where babies should be born. To offer people a real choice is to promote understanding, whereas to deny choice is to deprive people of responsibility, and of the stimulus to increase their knowledge. I would argue that the *sine qua non* of happiness and satisfaction in childbearing is that the child is wanted and that it is born where the mother feels secure. As this happens more and more it is not surprising that parents are increasingly aware of what they want from the maternity services. In this chapter I shall endeavour to set in perspective the reasons for the present dissatisfaction with the care of women during pregnancy and labour.

The development of maternity services in Britain

Antenatal care

Modern maternity care began in Britain with 'A plea for a pro-maternity hospital' by Dr. J. W. Ballantyne of Edinburgh (1901), which was followed by the setting up of antenatal clinics and the provision of beds for the care of pregnant women distinct from those available for their confinement.

The Maternity and Child Welfare Act (1918) permitted local authorities to establish antenatal clinics, educational classes, dental treatment, and home visiting for expectant mothers. The number of antenatal clinics increased from 120 in 1918 to 891 in 1929 and to 1931 in 1944. The proportion of women whose pregnancies were supervised by local authorities and general practitioners rose from 41 per cent in 1933 to 76 per cent in 1944. By 1946, it was estimated that 99 per cent of women had some sort of antenatal care (Royal College of Obstetricians and Gynaecologists and Population Investigation Committee 1948).

Before the National Health Service was set up in 1948, a pregnant woman might be cared for by any of the following either alone or in combination: a midwife, a general practitioner (G.P.), a private specialist obstetrician, a local authority clinic, or the maternity clinic of a voluntary or local authority hospital. She might be delivered at home, in a voluntary or local authority hospital, or in a private nursing home.

With the introduction of the National Health Service all persons resident in Britain became eligible for medical and nursing care in their homes or in hospital. At first the pattern of providing antenatal care did not change very much. But by 1958 only 0·6 per cent of the population had no antenatal care, 64 per cent of the population were seen 10 or more times during pregnancy, and 48 per cent had attended for antenatal care before the sixteenth week of pregnancy (Butler and Bonham 1963). The responsibility

Table 15.1 Those responsible for providing antenatal care in 1958 (From Butler and Bonham 1963)

	Per cent
Hospital only	20·2
Hospital in part	28·5
Local Authority clinic	19·4
GP only	11·1
GP and midwife	18·7
Midwife only	0·5
None	0·6
No information	0·6

for antenatal care in 1958 was shared by a great number and variety of people (Table 15.1) but now is virtually limited to hospitals and general practitioners.

Having examined the pattern and quality of antenatal care in detail, the first report of the 1958 British perinatal mortality survey concluded that 'there was a need for better selection of women for hospital prenatal care and confinement, earlier recognition and treatment of toxaemia in pregnancy, greater recognition of the importance of the length of gestation and above all, unification and extension of the maternity services.'

The place of birth

The policy of institutional confinement was developed from 1924 by the Ministry of Health (Campbell 1924). The Local Government Act (1929) allowed local authorities to provide new maternity units and to improve those taken over in Poor Law hospitals. In 1944, the Royal College of Obstetricians and Gynaecologists in a report on a national maternity service recommended that provision should be made for 70 per cent of births to take place in hospital under a single administrative authority. The proportion of women delivered in institutions gradually increased from 15 per cent of live births in England and Wales in 1927 to 54 per cent in 1946.

By 1958, the proportion of women delivered in hospital had reached 64 per cent. The Cranbrook Committee (Ministry of Health 1959) recommended that 'provision should be made over the country as a whole of a sufficient number of maternity beds to allow an average of 70 per cent institutional confinements ...' It took 15 years for the Government to take the advice of the Royal College of Obstetricians and Gynaecologists. The target was actually reached six years later in 1965.

By 1970, when the Sub-Committee of the Standing Maternity and Midwifery Advisory Committee of the Central Health Services Council on domiciliary midwifery and maternity bed needs under the chairmanship of Sir John Peel reported (Department of Health and Social Security 1970), 86 per cent of women were having their babies in National Health Service hospitals or in a private institution. The Peel Committee recommended that the greater safety of hospital confinement for mother and child justified providing sufficient facilities to allow 100 per cent hospital delivery. This target has almost been achieved. In 1974, 95·6 per cent of all babies were born in an institution. Three national maternity surveys (Table 15.2) allow us to compare the changes that have occurred in the place of birth in 12-year intervals between 1946 and 1970 (Chamberlain, Chamberlain, Howlett, and Claireaux 1975). The major change between 1946 and 1958 was a shift from the private sector to the National Health Service. In 1958 the increasing influence of consultants was apparent despite the establishment of general practitioner units (GPUs).

The Cranbrook Committee (Ministry of Health 1959) recommended that 'general practitioner maternity beds are best situated within, or very close

Table 15.2 The place of birth in 1946, 1958, and 1970
(From Chamberlain *et al.*, 1975)

Place of delivery	Percentage of mothers		
	1946	1958	1970
Home	42·4	36·1	12·4
Consultant bed	40·6	48·5	66·3
GP bed/unit		12·4	18·5
Private	13·1	2·9	1·2
Born unattended	4·0	0·1	0·7

to, consultant maternity hospitals or general hospitals with maternity departments. A consultant should have overall responsibility of general practitioner maternity beds.' With this recommendation the independence of GPs in maternity care ceased. By 1970, the majority of women were delivered in consultant beds, and virtually all GP beds were under the direct control of consultants. The rise in the proportion of women delivered in a GP bed or GPU between 1958 and 1970 from 12·4 per cent to 18·5 per cent is, therefore, deceptive. Consultant control was increasing at the same time as the concept was developing of GP maternity beds within a consultant unit. The Peel Committee (Department of Health and Social Security 1970) favoured the replacement of small isolated obstetric units by larger combined consultant and GP units in general hospitals.

Who delivers the baby?
A comparison of those undertaking the delivery of babies in 1946, 1958, and 1970 (Chamberlain *et al.* 1975) shows that despite 40 000 less births, 86 per cent of deliveries in hospital, 3000 more midwives notifying their intention to practice, and at least a 20 per cent increase in medically qualified obstetric personnel, the number of mothers delivered by a qualified person of experience actually declined (Table 15.3).

Between 1946 and 1970, the proportion of women delivered by a medically qualified person remained at 19 per cent. More women were delivered by young doctors and there was a decline of 15 per cent in the number of women delivered by a trained midwife. Although more trained staff were available to look after less women in 1970 compared with 1946, the proportion of women delivered by a person in training increased from less than 20 per cent to more than 33 per cent.

Table 15.3 The person undertaking delivery in 1946, 1958, and 1970
(From Chamberlain *et al.*, 1975)

Person undertaking the delivery	Percentage		
	1946	1958	1970
Consultant	1·5	2·8	2·6
Registrar	6·8	3·1	7·7
House officer		3·4	6·0
GP	10·7	4·4	2·8
Medical student	4·8	3·9	3·9
Midwife	60·5	52·6	44·7
Pupil midwife	10·8	27·6	31·4
No trained person	4·9	2·1	0·7

Doctors

The General Medical Council was founded in 1858 for the registration of doctors and the control of their training. In 1886, it became compulsory for a medical student to pass an examination in midwifery and gynaecology before he or she could register a medical qualification. Ever since 1933, the Royal College of Obstetricians and Gynaecologists has awarded a diploma based on postgraduate hospital experience for those intending to provide maternity care in general practice.

The Cranbrook Committee (Ministry of Health 1959) concluded that 'under present day conditions the practice of obstetrics requires the exercise of special skill beyond the competence of general practitioners and a degree of experience that, with the present high institutional confinement rate, the average family doctor is unlikely to be able to maintain.' In 1961, local obstetric committees were required to approve a practitioner's obstetric experience. The Royal Commission on Medical Education (1969) recommended that trainees for general practice should spend 6 months in a hospital appointment in obstetrics and gynaecology. However, they also observed that 'as domiciliary confinement is becoming less common, most maternity work will be concentrated in in-patient facilities.'

The Peel Committee (Department of Health and Social Security 1970) dealt the final blow to domiciliary midwifery in a whole series of recommendations. GPs were also effectively excluded from maternity care, and supreme control was given to consultant obstetricians. These recommendations became effective with the reorganization of the NHS in 1974 (Secretary of State for Social Services 1972).

The training of consultant obstetricians is controlled and supervised by the Royal College of Obstetricians and Gynaecologists. The combined specialty is surgically orientated, and experience is acquired in hospital appointments exclusively. The higher specialist qualification, Membership of the Royal College of Obstetricians and Gynaecologists (M.R.C.O.G.), is obtained by examination generally 4–5 years after medical qualification, having completed the pre-registration year and 3 years in approved specialist appointments. Further clinical experience, up to 4–6 years, is acquired as a registrar and senior registrar, before a specialist gains independence as a consultant obstetrician and gynaecologist.

Midwives

In 1902, the Central Midwives Board was founded to direct the training, certification, and supervision through local authorities of midwives. It became an offence for an unqualified person to call herself a midwife or to attend women in childbirth. The Central Midwives Board maintains the roll of certified midwives. The second Midwives Act (1918) made it compulsory for a midwife to summon medical aid in an emergency. As from 1936, local authorities were able to introduce a whole-time salaried service of domiciliary midwives. Assistant medical officers of health carried out the antenatal care of mothers booked both for home confinement by local authority midwives, and for confinement in local authority hospitals. Consultant obstetricians advised local authorities and provided consultations for women referred by clinic doctors or by GPs.

In 1947, a Working Party (Ministry of Health 1949) was set up to examine the recruitment and training of midwives, and their proper duties. This report drew attention to the problems of doctors taking over the whole of antenatal care and relegating midwives to the status of maternity nurses. These problems were not solved and have increased as not only midwives, but also GPs have been increasingly displaced from playing an active part in maternity care.

Until 1967, the training of midwives was in two parts. In the first part, lasting 6 months, pupil midwives had theoretical and practical training in a maternity hospital. The second part of training also lasted 6 months, at least 3 months of which was spent in domiciliary practice. There were variations in the pattern and length of training according to the previous experience of the pupil midwife. From 1968, two-part midwifery training has gradually been phased out in favour of an integrated course lasting 1 year, based on hospital-centred maternity services, although 3 months of the training is still spent in the community.

Emergency obstetric services

According to Stallworthy (1963) the first obstetric 'flying squad' served Lanarkshire. Later, emergency obstetric services were modelled on the one founded by Farquhar Murray (1938) in 1935 for Newcastle (Stabler 1947). By 1957, over 150 flying squads operated from maternity hospitals in England and Wales, receiving about 3000 calls a year. It was estimated that they were called to between 1 and 2 per cent of home deliveries. The emergency obstetric services have gradually fallen into disuse. The last published report on confidential enquiries into maternal deaths in England and Wales, for 1970–2 (Department of Health and Social Security 1975) observed: 'Failure of a consultant unit to provide flying squad service was assessed as an avoidable factor in one case of (fatal) post-partum haemorrhage. Now that more than 90 per cent of women are delivered in hospital, the need for a flying squad has diminished but is still present. However, because of the decreased frequency of calls for service, it becomes increasingly difficult to maintain a flying squad in a state of readiness. To surmount this problem it might not be inappropriate to organize practice calls.'

Neonatal care

The care of new-born infants has developed along parallel lines with the maternity services (Department of Health and Social Security 1971). With the establishment of the Central Midwives Board, the care of the newborn baby was included in the training syllabus of midwives. In 1931, a unit for the care of premature babies was opened in the Sorrento Maternity Hospital, Birmingham, which later served as a model throughout Britain.

In 1961, recommendations were made for the prevention of prematurity and the care of premature infants (Ministry of Health 1961), including: regular and thorough supervision for all pregnant women; adequate provision of hospital antenatal beds; careful selection of women for hospital confinement; and the establishment of special-care nurseries for new-born babies. Throughout this decade the concept of specialized paediatric care for new-born babies was developed, together with foetal medicine (Huntingford 1971). Emergency resuscitation teams for the new-born were established (Barrie 1971).

The report of the Expert Group on Special Care for Babies (Department of Health and Social Security 1971) followed the increasing trend towards the centralization of specialist services by recommending two tiers of neonatal care: special-care nurseries in district hospitals and combined special-care and intensive-care nurseries at regional level.

Maternal mortality

Maternal mortality rates per 1000 total births have been published annually for England and Wales by the Registrar General since 1863. The rate remained almost constant at 4–5 per 1000 total births until 1935, when it began to fall (Fig. 15.1). From 1952, the Ministry of Health with the support of the Royal College of Obstetricians and Gynaecologists conducted 'confidential enquiries into maternal deaths in England and Wales'. Seven reports have been published so far, each covering the maternal deaths notified in consecutive periods of 3 years. The latest report (Department of Health and Social Security 1975) is for the years 1970–2.

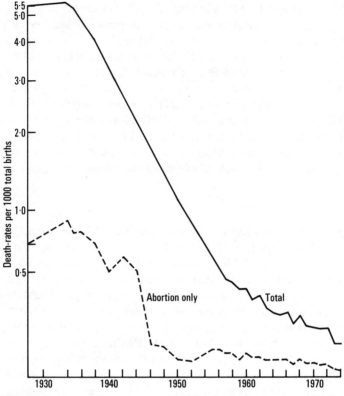

Fig. 15.1 Maternal deaths per 1000 births in England and Wales.

The main causes of maternal deaths have changed in order of importance over the years. Until 1937, infection accounted for more maternal deaths than any other single cause. By 1938, puerperal infection had dropped into third place, and by 1952 it accounted for only about 4 per cent of maternal deaths following delivery. Since 1952 (Table 15.4), the four commonest causes of maternal deaths have been toxaemia, abortion, haemorrhage, and pulmonary embolus. Toxaemia was the commonest cause from 1937 until 1958, when its place was taken by abortion. Pulmonary embolus rose to second place in 1955, displacing haemorrhage, which now occupies sixth place as a cause of maternal death.

The confidential enquiries into maternal deaths have assessed in each case whether or not an avoidable factor was present (Table 15.5). In the latest enquiry for 1970–2 (Department of Health and Social Security 1975), 57·4 per cent of the avoidable factors occurred during the antenatal period, 26·2 per cent during labour or an operation, and 16·4 per cent in the puerperium. Responsibility for the avoidable factors was apportioned as follows: hospital obstetric staff 42·1 per cent; the patient 30·5 per cent; the

Table 15.4 The main causes of maternal deaths due to pregnancy and childbirth in England and Wales from 1952 to 1972, expressed as a percentage of the total maternal deaths in each 3 year period. (From Reports on Confidential Enquiries into Maternal Deaths)

Cause	1952/54	1955/57	1958/60	1961/63	1964/66	1967/69	1970/72
Toxaemia of pregnancy	22·5	19·9	15·9	15·0	11·6	11·6	13·2
Haemorrhage	17·2	16·0	17·5	13·3	11·7	9·0	7·6
Pulmonary embolus	12·6	18·2	17·8	18·6	15·7	16·5	17·2
Abortion—total	14·0	16·4	18·2	20·1	23·0	25·7	22·8
illegal	9·9	10·6	11·1	11·1	16·9	16·3	10·7
spontaneous	3·9	5·8	7·0	8·2	4·3	5·5	1·7
legal	0·2	—	0·1	0·8	1·8	3·9	10·4
Sepsis—total	14·5	18·4	16·7	16·0	21·2	19·3	19·7
with abortion	8·3	9·5	10·4	10·7	11·4	13·6	10·7
puerperal	3·8	5·3	3·2	2·6	4·8	2·6	4·2
with surgery	2·4	3·6	3·1	2·7	5·0	3·1	4·8
Cardiac disease	11·1	11·8	8·9	9·8	7·4	7·5	9·3
Ectopic pregnancy	5·4	4·9	3·8	6·1	7·3	7·0	9·6

Table 15.5 Maternal deaths with avoidable factors as a percentage of the total maternal deaths in each 3-year period in England and Wales from 1952 to 1972 (From Reports on Confidential Enquiries into Maternal Deaths)

Cause	1952/54	1955/57	1958/60	1961/63	1964/66	1967/69	1970/72
Deaths directly due to pregnancy and child-birth	43·1	41·0	42·5	37·9	44·6	56·0	53·8
Deaths directly due to pregnancy and child-birth excluding abortion and ectopic pregnancy	40·0	37·3	38·9	34·4	34·9	49·0	33·8
Deaths associated with pregnancy and child-birth	16·8	16·8	17·7	13·9	13·1	14·8	19·5

GP 16·6 per cent; the anaesthetist 8·4 per cent; the midwife 2 per cent; and administration 0·3 per cent.

The decline in maternal mortality is often and all too easily accounted for by the shift from domiciliary to hospital confinement, by advances in obstetric technology, and by the displacement of midwives and GPs by specialists. Thus, the Royal College of Obstetricians and Gynaecologists in their report on a 'national maternity service' (1944) expressed the opinion that 'the incidence of maternal mortality and morbidity is primarily a matter of obstetric personnel—of the individual skill of midwives, general practitioners, and consultants, with the proviso that all must be supported by first rate maternity institutions and equipment.' The arguments for alternative explanations, which hold today, were clearly put by the Working Party on Midwives (Ministry of Health 1949):

... some of the largest and most gratifying reductions in mortality (including maternal mortality) occurred during the last three years of the recent war. This was, in fact, precisely the period when midwives, general practitioners, consultants and maternity beds were scarcest and working under the most intense pressure. It would not have been surprising if, in these difficult circumstances, more mothers had died in childbirth.

We are not justified, therefore, in attributing the improvement in the maternal mortality rate solely, or even primarily, to a better midwifery service during the past decade. Other factors must have contributed to this improvement, their influence varying both in time and place. Treatment by sulphonamides and penicillin has undoubtedly pulled down the sepsis rate; the national blood transfusion service together with the development of the flying squad have helped. There may have been less instrumental interference. As the risks of death are controlled, to some extent, by the age of the mother, the number of previous pregnancies and the interval between pregnancies, any changes since 1935 in the respective influence of these factors, such as fewer sixth or subsequent births to elderly worn-out mothers, could well reduce the overall death rate. On the other hand, if there were an increased proportion of first confinements, the rate would be higher. Similarly, a reduction in the incidence of abortion, spontaneous or induced, together with the fact that the sulphonamides have made abortion safer, could also lower the rate.

More important still, however, a larger proportion of mothers who have had babies in the past few years may have been, physically, better mothers; they themselves may have had a better start in life 20 to 25 years ago.

Pursuing a similar argument Wrigley (1963) observed that

The decline in the number of maternal deaths from sepsis is too often ascribed to the discovery and use of 'sulpha' drugs and subsequently to the antibiotics. Prontosil was certainly not available for general use before 1937, by which year the number of (maternal) deaths from sepsis had fallen from 800 (1934) to half that figure—347. Penicillin, similarly, was not available in Great Britain before 1946, by which year the number of deaths from sepsis had dropped to a mere 53 per annum. The initial and major decrease in maternal death from sepsis must be due to a sudden and unexplained diminution of the pathogenecity of the haemolytic streptococcus.

Wrigley, far from contradicting the Working Party on Midwives, reinforces their arguments by presenting yet another explanation other than that of technological advances to account for falling death-rates.

Perinatal mortality

In Britain we are fortunate to have not only accurate data on maternal deaths, but also in England and Wales since 1906 for neonatal deaths, and since 1927 for still births. We have national data on the quality and achievement of the maternity services from three surveys conducted in 1946, 1958, and 1970: *Maternity in Great Britain*: a survey of social and economic aspects of pregnancy and childbirth in 1946 was undertaken by a Joint Committee of the Royal College of Obstetricians and Gynaecologists and the Population Investigation Committee (1948); the 1958 British perinatal mortality survey was conducted under the auspices of the National Birthday Trust Fund (Butler and Bonham 1963; Butler and Alberman 1969); and *British births 1970*, the most recent survey, was under the joint auspices of the National Birthday Trust Fund and the Royal College of Obstetricians and Gynaecologists (Chamberlain *et al.* 1975).

Perinatal mortality rates (still births plus first week neonatal deaths per 1000 total births) began to fall in 1936, but at a much slower rate than maternal mortality (Fig. 15.2). The rate of fall in perinatal mortality accelerated from 1940 to 1946. In 1954 the rate of fall again accelerated, but

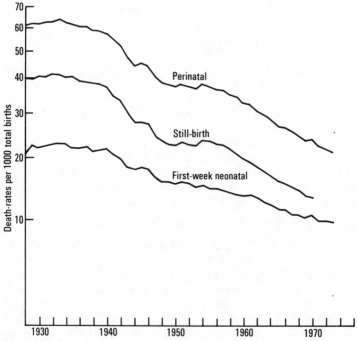

Fig. 15.2 Perinatal mortality, still-birth, and first-week neonatal death-rates for England and Wales 1928–75.

then remained constant. Until 1958, the still-birth and neonatal death-rates were parallel, since when the still-birth rate has fallen faster than the neonatal death-rate. The still-birth rate fell by 39 per cent between 1958 and 1970, compared with a drop of 14 per cent in the first-week neonatal death-rate.

The main causes of perinatal death are still births with intra-uterine asphyxia (26·3 per cent); congenital malformations in both still-born and live-born infants (21·5 per cent); still births without an anatomical lesion (14·9 per cent); the respiratory distress syndrome in the first week of life (13·7 per cent); first-week deaths following intra-uterine anoxia (7·6 per cent); and immaturity (6·8 per cent).

Between 1958 and 1970 the main improvements in perinatal mortality included a reduction in the incidence of pneumonia from 1·3 to 0·1 per 1000 deliveries; birth trauma from 3·0 to 0·4 per 1000 deliveries; massive pulmonary haemorrhage from 0·9 to 0·2 per 1000 deliveries; and haemolytic disease from 1·3 to 0·6 per 1000 deliveries.

Immaturity (infants weighing less than 1·000 kg at birth and with no other cause for death demonstrated) accounted for 15 per cent of first-week deaths in 1970. The underlying cause of death was prematurity (birthweight less than 2·500 kg) in 68 per cent of babies dying in the first week of life.

Changes in obstetric practice

Important technical advances which have been made in obstetric practice, particularly in the last 15 years, have increased our knowledge, making childbearing safer, and more comfortable. The most important advances include: the ability to prevent rhesus haemolytic disease and better methods for the treatment of the condition when it does occur; the refinement and development of safe ways for resuscitating new-born infants; the application of new methods of diagnosis and investigation, such as amniocentesis, pulsed ultrasound, foetal blood sampling, and blood-gas analysis, continuous foetal heart monitoring and placental function tests; the synthesis of oxytocin and improvements in the control of its administration for the induction and augmentation of labour; and the availability of potent local anaesthetics to provide prolonged and efficient epidural analgesia.

Perhaps the most striking and controversial change in obstetric practice has been the very rapid increase in the induction of labour from 13 per cent of deliveries in 1958, to 40 per cent in 1974. In some hospitals induction rates of 60 per cent are acknowledged. The three most common reasons for inducing labour today are prolonged pregnancy, a rise in blood pressure, and suspected impairment of foetal growth. No one would dispute that there are good medical reasons for inducing labour in about 10 per cent of women having babies. But, in the remainder the indications are doubtful and can certainly be contested. The benefits of a high rate of induction to the baby have not been demonstrated and there is also reason to suspect, that it might be harmful. In many women, probably up to 30 per cent, the duration of pregnancy is not known with certainty. Single recordings of an elevated blood pressure are often used as an indication to induce labour, when in fact they may not represent a danger to the baby, but merely reflect a passing moment of maternal anxiety or stress often provoked by the obstetric environment. In spite of advances in diagnostic methods these are still too imprecise to distinguish with certainty between small healthy babies, poor foetal growth, and mistaken dates. There can be little doubt that induction of labour merely for convenience cannot be supported by epidemiological data.

In 1958, Butler and Bonham recorded that 15·9 per cent of women having first babies were in labour for 24 hours or more, and 2·7 per cent for 48 hours or more. Few labours now last as long as 24 hours, and many obstetricians regard 12 hours as the upper limit of normal labour even with a first baby. Without precise knowledge of either the benefits or the hazards intravenous oxytocin is being used to accelerate labour in an unknown, but increasing, number of women.

It is since 1970 that induction and acceleration of labour have been used on such a wide scale, mainly because the techniques have become available not only to a few obstetricians concerned with research but also to maternity units everywhere. The greater use of epidural analgesia has made it possible to increase the speed of labour, and instruments for making continuous records of uterine contractions and of the foetal heart-rate have provided early warning if danger threatens either the mother or the baby. Often without enquiring whether or not mothers wished to have labour induced or accelerated, or knowing whether or not the results were worthwhile, obstetricians and midwives have succumbed to the temptation to use available technology in an unselective way.

Concurrently with these advances the rate of obstetric interference has also increased in other ways (Table 15.6). Between 1958 and 1970, the national

Table 15.6 Method of delivery (percentages) for singleton births in 1958 and 1970 as a percentage of total births (From Chamberlain et al., 1975)

Method of delivery	1958	1970
Spontaneous	88·2	83·7
Breech	2·3	2·5
Forceps	4·7	7·9
Vacuum extraction	—	0·7
Caesarean section	2·7	4·5
No trained person	2·1	0·7

rate for delivery by Caesarean section almost doubled. By 1973, it had increased still further so that 5·2 per cent of all women having babies were delivered by Caesarean section (Department of Health and Social Security 1976). Delivery by forceps has also doubled since 1958; in 1973, 11·9 per cent of women were delivered by forceps. In many hospitals the rates for operative delivery are still higher: Caesarean section being used to deliver up to 10 per cent, and forceps for 20 per cent of women. These increases can be accounted for mainly by the anxiety of obstetricians to shorten labour at all costs, the failure to invariably induce labour, too rapid acceleration of labour, misinterpretation of continuous records of foetal heart-rate, and to the use of epidural analgesia or heavy sedation.

In 1958, episiotomy was performed in 12·5 per cent of all women having a first baby, and in 3·5 per cent of those having a second or subsequent baby. In many hospitals the use of episiotomy has become almost routine so that it is now most unusual to find any woman who has had a first baby without also having had an episiotomy. As the presence of an episiotomy scar is also regarded as an indication for repeating it in the next pregnancy by many obstetricians and midwives, the possibility of episiotomy being done in all women is coming near to reality. This trend is a consequence of those already described, and also of obstetric anxiety to limit the time for delivery by the clock rather than by the state of the mother and the baby, and to prevent foetal death by treating all women in the same way rather than endeavouring to seek out more precisely those whose babies are really in danger.

An assessment of the present state and the probable future of obstetric practice

The practice of obstetrics and the organization of our maternity services has undoubtedly been to the benefit of the vast majority of mothers and babies in this country. There is no doubt, too, that childbearing is safer today, both for mothers and babies, than ever previously, and that further improvements can be expected. But these two statements do not necessarily mean that they are cause and effect, nor that our maternity services could not be improved still further not only to the benefit, but also to the satisfaction of parents.

A review of the official reports concerned with the development of the maternity services sadly shows how concern for the comfort and wishes of individuals has been sacrificed gradually for the sake of bureaucratic and professional interests and organization. First the midwife and then the GP have been demoted in obstetric care. Secondly, institutional delivery has replaced home confinement. And, thirdly, technology has been allowed to take precedence over the needs of individuals.

Many of those responsible for providing maternity services will regard the publication of this book as irresponsible and against the interests of women. Our critics will argue that for the past three decades the maternity services have been developed to provide maximum safety for mothers and their children. No-one doubts the sincerity of these intentions, but a great deal has been sacrificed in the achievement of this objective. Those of us contributing to the book wish to point out that not all technological advance results in acceptable improvements, and especially not if it is applied arbitrarily, without selection, without evaluation, without reference to consumers, and by depriving them of choice. But this is exactly what is happening.

Most of the fall in maternal and perinatal mortality rates (Figs 15.1 and 15.2) has been attributed to scientific advance and to the concentration of maternity care in the hands of specialists working in relatively few centres. However, the improvements in obstetric performance could equally well be accounted for by social changes, such as: more women bearing children at a safer age (i.e., fewer very young or old women having babies); an overall improvement in standards of living, especially amongst those least well off; a reduction in the number of mothers of very large families; a general increase in the standards of nutrition and stature of women; general improvement in maternal and child care because more people are better informed; the more widespread use of contraception and to the Abortion Act (1967) that has allowed many more women to bear only those children that they really want. Such a view is supported by data from the perinatal mortality survey (Butler and Bonham 1963; Butler and Alberman 1969), and from the British births survey (Chamberlain et al. 1975).

It has already been shown in this chapter that even in 1949 there was doubt as to whether falling maternal mortality rates were due to advances in technology as some would claim, or due to a combination of factors including social change. In 1960 Sir Dugald Baird also pointed out that more had been achieved to improve maternity care by raising social standards than by advances in medical practice. I believe that this is still true today, since affluence continues to reduce the number and size of risks caused by malnourishment, large family size, pre-term delivery, and ignorance. Baird and Thomson (1969) felt that 'it would be difficult to estimate the influence of demographic changes alone upon perinatal mortality rate, but it has undoubtedly been beneficial. It may well be that the current rapid fall in perinatal mortality rates is due in large measure to the cumulative effect of 25 years relative economic prosperity.... Such changes may be at least as important as improvements in the scope and quality of the maternity services.'

At a time of financial crisis with inflation adding to the problems of cut-backs in expenditure in maintaining the NHS, it is vital that what money is available should be spent wisely. Already hospitals, including those with maternity beds, are closing, and further closures are threatened. Maternity beds that are closed tend to be GPUs and those that are separate from general hospitals. Such maternity beds have often provided local service on a personal basis. No wonder then that there is such an outcry when their closure is threatened or takes place. In terms of financial priorities it may well be right that isolated maternity beds are closed. It may also be correct from a theoretical consideration of the medical and obstetric points of view. But, the people who are affected both fear the loss of personal local services, and resent the removal of choice.

Strategic plans for the NHS in the 1980s are now being prepared. Preliminary drafts do not even contemplate babies being born at home. Indeed, if the draft plans are realized babies will only be born in a relatively few centralized units staffed by specialists providing a uniform service. If the service to be provided were of a uniform high standard, taking account of whole people and their emotional needs as well as their physical safety, we would be happier. But, in the present and foreseeable times of financial stringency the services are certain to be restricted and in determining priorities physical safety will take precedence at the expense of emotional satisfaction. Such an approach is likely to be counter-productive, because however safe a system may be people will not use it as designed if they do not like it. Analyses of maternal deaths place the responsibility for a proportion of avoidable deaths on the women themselves. Usually, such situations are described with incredulity. The writers seem to have little insight as to why women sometimes reject advice and care; certainly, the question of why they did so is seldom asked. No thought is given to the idea that the services themselves and the way in which they were offered may have been so unacceptable that the women preferred instead to risk their own lives. Even if the women were wrong, a system that ignores such eloquent pleading and denies any responsibility is so insensitive to certain psycho-logical needs that we can expect dissatisfaction with almost every aspect of the services that it offers. We do not wish to turn the clock back; we wish to move forwards into the future. But into a future that takes more and more account of individuals not less and less.

A further consequence of present financial constraints is not only the loss of buildings, but more important still a reduction in the number of midwives and doctors available to maintain the maternity service. The abandonment of domiciliary midwifery services and the loss of the intimate involvement of GPs in maternity care means that not only has the choice of place been reduced, but also the choice that women have of the people to look after them during pregnancy and childbirth. Furthermore, each member of staff has less time to spend with individuals, because of the combination of a reduced number of staff attempting to cope with a greater load in those maternity units that remain. One of the reactions to such a situation is for the staff to seek ways and means to reduce their work load by resorting to the mechanization and automation of maternity care.

It is a matter of concern that consumers feel compelled to find ways in which, from their point of view, childbearing can be made not only safe but also satisfying. What has happened in the last few years to make men and women feel so strongly that their interests no longer receive prime attention in the conduct of childbearing? Why do those having babies no longer feel that their voices are being heard? Why do a few women go to such extremes to have their babies in their own homes? In spite of technical advances why do those having babies not feel more grateful to those who look after them? Why do we have extensive press, radio, and television coverage of these topics, and why are books published, such as this and others that are critical of obstetric practice: e.g., *A season to be born* and *Immaculate deception* by Suzanne Arms; *Birth without violence* by Frederick Leboyer; and *Naturebirth* by Danaë Brook? It is safer than ever before for women to bear children. Fewer babies die as a result of complications during pregnancy and labour. More babies survive with less and fewer crippling handicaps. Pain can be relieved more effectively and in a greater variety of ways; agonizing prolonged labour is a thing of the past. Labour itself has been made so short, and can be arranged to order so that the once uncertain process of giving birth, need no longer be surrounded by anxiety and fear of the unknown. What then is all the fuss about? I believe that at the heart of it all is public dissatisfaction with the attitudes of those attending women during pregnancy and labour.

Compare the attitude of 1924 (Campbell) when local authorities were advised to provide self-contained maternity homes of 15–20 beds within easy reach of women, and so that local practitioners would be able to look after them with the final recommendations of the Peel Committee (Department of Health and Social Security 1970): 'The changes in professional thought and the administrative action which, it is recommended in this report, should flow from it, must be associated with a change of community attitudes towards midwifery and maternity matters. To a great extent we look upon this educational responsibility as being one for the professions concerned. The obstetric team, which we have indicated as necessary for the service itself should include among its reponsibilities the education of the community to the desirability and benefits of the reorganization.'

The Working Party on Midwives (Ministry of Health 1949) and the Cranbrook Committee (1959) both took evidence from interested parties, including consumers, but so far as the Peel Committee is concerned the report does not mention evidence from these sources. Since 1974, when the NHS was reorganized, Community Health Councils have slowly defined their roles and developed their strength. Instead of using them as partners and allies in the development of the maternity services, the Royal College of Obstetricians and Gynaecologists has chosen to regard them as thorns in the flesh. Fellows and Members were recently advised not to respond to requests from Community Health Councils for information concerning the treatment of individuals. Organizations concerned with the improvement of maternity services, such as the Patients' Association, the Association for the Improvement of Maternity Services, and the National Childbirth Trust have always been regarded by the Royal College of Obstetricians and Gynaecologists as a nuisance and slightly odd, rather than as helpful and sharing the same objectives. Even if the premises on which the maternity services have been developed in this country were correct and not open to question, the arrogance of the professionals in riding roughshod over those they are meant to serve is hardly the best way of changing community attitudes. Far from taking educational responsibility the professions concerned stand in need of education and of having their own attitudes changed.

The professionals have taken control and dismantled the domiciliary service. The justification at a time when we are increasingly more able to make precise diagnoses is that childbearing is unpredictable. Now we have reached the situation when few doctors and midwives are left who have experience to enable them to deliver women in their homes. GPs who wish to continue with domiciliary midwifery, and at the same time satisfy those women who ask to have their babies at home, are condemned by the medical establishment as being out-of-touch (the most charitable view of the establishment), or irresponsible.

For a while the public were beguiled into thinking that all was well, for the policy documents were associated with the building of smart custom-built maternity units. But, who were the customers? The women who were to be delivered or the obstetricians? The new maternity units were designed by obstetricians for obstetricians. Few women, if any, who had had babies and who were not specialists, had any part to play in their design or use.

Likewise few women, if any at all, are consulted about the details of maternity care. All patients are people, and still more, mothers having babies are not only people, they are not patients. As such they are individuals with varied needs. Much obstetric dogma has been formulated at the expense of individuals. A few mothers die in childbirth from avoidable causes each year, therefore, all must have their babies in hospital. Prolonged pregnancy and labour cause problems for some mothers and their babies: therefore, planned labour and delivery for the majority must be beneficial. Women suffer pain in labour and complain about it, therefore, all women require maximum pain relief. Women in pregnancy and during the distress of labour are not entirely responsible, normal, discerning, well-informed, aware of dangers—this patronizing attitude to women, fostered by men, justifies all sorts of arbitrary management, including ignoring the feelings, reasonable questions, and demands of women having babies. Is it really necessary, for example, to make all women who are having a baby have a pubic shave, an enema, and a hot bath? The list of attitudes revealed by current obstetric practice that ought to be challenged continues with episiotomy, position during delivery, guarding the perineum, the dismissal of the father during obstetric procedures, breast-feeding *vs.* bottle-feeding, demand feeding, and the removal of babies from their mothers after delivery into special care. It is assumed that everyone desires maximum safety in physical terms with the least discomfort even at the expense of sacrificing some personal satisfaction and pleasure. Safety and comfort are not absolutes. Why then should they be thrust upon all women, who are expected to accept them without question, without being consulted, without being offered choice, and without being offered back the responsibility that is rightfully theirs?

The state in which we find the maternity services today is only in a minor way due to a shortage of funds and personnel. More important have been mistakes in planning based on false assumptions concerning cause and effect, and, therefore, the means required to solve the problems. The mistakes in planning have been compounded by neglecting the needs of individuals, and neglecting the need to consult with the consumers in building a service, because the professions concerned have been reluctant to listen to and be questioned by those for whom they provide a service.

I do not want that either women or babies should die unnecessarily, or that women should suffer during labour. But I am not convinced that to save mothers and babies, they must all be subjected to the same treatment during pregnancy and labour. Neither am I convinced that planned rapid delivery and childbirth in total oblivion removes suffering. Why are we unable to be more rather than less selective? I doubt very much whether many more than 10 per cent of women having babies, if that many, would wish to have them at home. But, if they do, why should this not be possible? And for those women having their babies in hospital either out of medical need, or choice, it should surely be possible to make hospital a little more like home, to relax the regulations, to break some rules, and to behave like adults who care about each other. We should weigh very carefully in a scientific way the advantages and disadvantages of inducing and accelerating labour. The public is perfectly capable of understanding facts clearly stated, and so they should be informed of the results of such investigations and involved with policy decisions that affect them. Few mothers wish to have their babies by operation, and none would wish to have stitches and a sore perineum, if they could be avoided. Are episitomies, sometimes made with blunt scissors and without anaesthesia, preferable to the small tears that they replace in a large number of women? There must be a balance between the amount of obstetric interference that is positively beneficial to both mother and baby, and an amount that ceases to reduce mortality and morbidity and may even increase it. I believe that this balance has been lost.

Needlessly heavy sedation and sensory deprivation during labour does not always aid the birth process, but it may reduce maternal satisfaction whilst adversely affecting the baby and interfering with the establishment of mother–child relationships. Obstetricians and midwives should deal with their own anxieties by means that do not confine mothers to bed during the first stage of labour, attached to complicated monitoring equipment. Birth attendants should realize that obsession with time in labour presents an intimidating barrier for women to what they want to achieve even more than those looking after them. Why should mothers not be allowed to deliver themselves in the position in which they are most comfortable? This is unlikely to be on a hard, high bed, flat on their backs. Why does the perineum need to be guarded at all? Women are more likely to control the delivery of the baby themselves if they can be guided by their own internal sensations without the distraction of pressure from insensitive hands and unsympathetic voices.

In the future, I look forward to further technological advance that is made to serve the needs of childbearing women, that increases their individuality rather than diminishing it, and that gives back responsibility by providing an opportunity for an informed choice. New techniques should release us so that we can spend more time with individuals, they should not become barriers or increase the distance between obstetricians, midwives, and mothers. I hope that specialists will gain respect by listening to complaints, demands, and needs; that they will respond by continuing consultation with those they serve: by giving them responsibility (which is the greatest responsibility of all, as parents will know) and by building an ideal maternity service based on consumer rather than professional satisfaction. I hope that in a time of stringency and social change what is good of the past can be melded with what is of proven value in the present to create something better for the future: the right of well-informed people to take responsibility for themselves in having their children in safety, comfort, and with satisfaction.

References

Arms, S. (1973). *A season to be born*. Harper Colophon Books, New York.
—— (1975). *Immaculate deception*. Houghton Miflin Company, Boston.
Baird, D. (1960). 'The evolution of modern obstetrics'. *The Lancet* ii, 557–64, 609–14.
—— and Thomson, A. M. (1969). 'General factors underlying perinatal mortality rates'. In *Perinatal problems* (ed. N. R. Butler and E. D. Alberman). Livingstone, Edinburgh.
Ballantyne, J. W. (1901). 'A plea for a pro-maternity hospital'. *British Medical Journal* i, 813.
Barrie, H. (1971). 'A mobile neonatal care unit'. In *Perinatal medicine* (ed. P. J. Huntingford, *et al.*). Karger, Basel.
Brook, D. (1976). *Naturebirth*. Heinemann, London.
Butler, N. R. and Bonham, D. G. (1963). *Perinatal mortality*. Livingstone, Edinburgh.
—— and Alberman, E. D. (1969). *Perinatal problems*. Livingstone, Edinburgh.
Campbell, J. M. (1924). *Reports on public health and medical subjects* No. 25. H.M.S.O. London.
Chamberlain, R., Chamberlain, G., Howlett, B., and Claireaux, A. (1975). *British Births 1970*. Vol. 1: 'The first week of life'. William Heinemann Medical Books, London.
Department of Health and Social Security (1970). *Domiciliary midwifery and maternity bed needs*. H.M.S.O. London.
—— (1971). *Report of the expert group on special care for babies*. H.M.S.O. London.
—— (1975). *Confidential enquiries into maternal deaths in England and Wales 1970–1972*. H.M.S.O. London.
—— (1976). *On the state of the public health*. Report of the Chief Medical Officer for 1974. H.M.S.O. London.
Huntingford, P. J. (1971). 'Past, present and future'. In *Perinatal medicine* (ed. P. J. Huntingford, *et al.*). Karger, Basel.

Huntingford, P. J. (1976). 'Women and their health: is there a conflict?' In *Health care in a changing setting: UK experience.* Ciba Foundation Symposium 43. Elsevier, Excerpta Medica, North Holland.

Leboyer, F. (1975). *Birth without violence.* Wildwood House Limited, London.

Ministry of Health (1949). *Report of the working party on midwives.* H.M.S.O. London.

—— (1959). *Report of the Maternity Services Committee.* H.M.S.O. London.

—— (1961). *Report of the Sub-Committee on the Prevention of Prematurity and the Care of Premature Infants.* H.M.S.O. London.

Murray, E. F. (1938). 'The obstetrical "flying squad" '. *British Medical Journal* ii, 654.

Royal College of Obstetricians and Gynaecologists (1944). *Report on a national maternity service.* London.

—— and the Population Investigation Committee (1948). *Maternity in Great Britain.* Oxford University Press, London.

Royal Commission on Medical Education 1965–1968 (1969). *Report.* H.M.S.O. London.

Secretary of State for Social Services (1972). *Re-organisation of the National Health Service.* H.M.S.O. London.

Stabler, F. (1947). 'The Newcastle upon Tyne Obstetric Emergency Service'. *British Medical Journal* ii, 878.

Stallworthy, J. (1963). Shock in obstetrics. In *British obstetric and gynaecological practice: obstetrics* (ed. A. Claye and A. Bourne, 3rd edn. William Heinemann Medical Books, London.

Wrigley, A. J. (1963). 'Observations on maternal mortality'. In *Modern trends in obstetrics* (ed. R. J. Kellar), Vol. 3. Butterworths, London.

About the contributors

John Ashford, M.A., Ph.D., F.B.C.S.

Professor Ashford came to Exeter in 1963 from the National Coal Board's Pneumo-coniosis Field Research, where he was Deputy Chief Scientist, and was previously employed as Principal Scientific Officer in the Industrial Power Reactors Division of the Research Group of the Atomic Energy Authority. He is currently Professor of Statistics, Head of the Department of Mathematical Statistics and Operational Research and Dean of the Faculty of Science at the University of Exeter.

Professor Ashford's published work covers a variety of fields, including mathematical statistics, computation, epidemiology, applied physics, and medicine. His current research interests include health and planning, maternity care, statistical epidemiology, dental care, joint action of mixtures of drugs, process control, and mathematical modelling.

Publications relevant to this book

'Epidemiological and biometric issues in infant mortality', Chapter in *Key issues in infant mortality*, Report of a Conference, Washington, D.C., April 1969 (ed. F. Falkner). National Institutes of Child Health and Human Development, Bethesda, Maryland (1970).

'International perinatal studies: statistical problems and opportunities'. In *Proceedings of the Ninth Conference of the Biometrics Society*. Boston, August (1976).

With Fryer, J. G., 'Perinatal mortality, birthweight and place of confinement in England and Wales 1956–65'. Chapter 6 of *In the beginning (studies of maternity services)* (eds. G. McLachlan and R. F. A. Shegog). Oxford University Press for the Nuffield Provincial Hospitals Trust (1970).

With Brimblecombe, F. S. W. and Fryer, J. G. 'Birthweight and perinatal mortality in England and Wales 1956–65'. Chapter 1 of *Problems and progress in medical care*, Third series (ed. G. McLachlan). Oxford University Press for the Nuffield Provincial Hospitals Trust (1968).

With Fryer, J. G. and Brimblecombe, F. S. W. 'Secular trends in late foetal deaths, neonatal mortality and birthweight in England and Wales 1956–65', *British Journal of Preventive and Social Medicine* 23, 154–62 (1969).

In *Measuring for management: quantitative methods in health service management* (ed. G. McLachlan). Oxford University Press for the Nuffield Provincial Hospitals Trust (1975).

With Brimblecombe, F. S. W. and Fryer, J. G. 'Significance of low birthweight in perinatal mortality—a study of variations within England and Wales'. *British Journal of Preventive and Social Medicine* 22, 27–35 (1968).

With Fryer, J. G. 'Trends in perinatal and neonatal mortality in England and Wales, 1960–69'. *British Journal of Preventive and Social Medicine* 26, 1–9 (1972).

With Pethybridge, R. J. and Fryer, J. G. 'Some features of the distribution of birthweight of human infants'. *British Journal of Preventive and Social Medicine* 28, 10–18 (1974).

John David Baum, M.A., M.Sc., F.R.C.P., D.C.H., M.D.

Dr. Baum qualified at Birmingham University Medical School in 1963. He held appointments at the Hammersmith Hospital and the University of London, researching on intensive care of the newborn, and at the University of Colorado Medical Centre, Denver. He is now Clinical Reader and Honorary Consultant in Paediatrics, University of Oxford, and a Fellow of St. Catherine's College. His current research interests include intensive care of the newborn, the biology of lactation, and diabetes in older children.

Publications relevant to this book

The newborn baby. Consumers' Association (1972).

With Jones, R. W. A. and Rochefort, M. J. 'Increased insensible water loss in newborn infants nursed under radiant heaters'. *British Medical Journal* ii (1976).

With Rush, R. W., Keirse, M. J. N., Howat, P., Anderson, A. B. M., and Turnbull, A. C. Contribution of pre-term delivery to perinatal mortality'. *British Medical Journal* ii, 965 (1976).

With Scopes, J. W. 'The silver swaddler—a device for prevention of hypothermia in the New-born'. *Lancet* i, 672 (1968).

With Roberton, N. R. C. 'Experience with the use of Distending Pressure in Infants with R.D.S.' *Archives of Disease in Childhood* **49**, 771 (1974).

With Roberton, N. R. C. 'Immediate effects of alkali infusion in Infants with respiratory distress syndrome'. *The Journal of Paediatrics* **87**, 255 (1975).

With Tizard, J. P. M. 'Retrolental fibroplasia. Management of oxygen therapy'. *British Medical Bulletin* **26**, 171 (1970).

With Sloper, K. and McKean, L. 'Factors influencing breast-feeding'. *Archives of Disease in Childhood* **50**, 165 (1975).

With Weller, P. H., Barr, P. A., Gupta, J., Chung, C., and Jenkins, P. A. 'Lecithin/sphingamyelin ratios in pharyngeal aspirate from newborn infants'. In *Intensive care of the newborn*. Masson, New York (1977).

Iain Chalmers, M.B., B.S.(Lond.), M.Sc.(Lond.), D.C.H., M.R.C.O.G.

After house appointments at The Middlesex Hospital, the Welsh National School of Medicine, and Raigmore Hospital, Inverness, during 1967 and 1968, Dr. Chalmers spent two years working for the United Nations Relief and Works Agency for Palestinian Refugees in a maternal and child health programme in the Gaza Strip. He returned to the Department of Obstetrics and Gynaecology, Welsh National School of Medicine in 1971 and was admitted to membership of the Royal College of Obstetricians and Gynaecologists in 1973. Awarded a Department of Health and Social Security bursary in 1973 to attend the joint London School of Hygiene/London School of Economics course leading to a Masters degree in Social Medicine in 1975, he is currently Medical Research Council Fellow, Department of Medical Statistics, Welsh National School of Medicine, and also a member of Statistics Committee of the Royal College of Obstetricians and Gynaecologists. Dr. Chalmers's research interests are concerned with the uses of epidemiology in the planning and evaluation of maternal and child health services.

John A. Davis, M.B., B.S., M.Sc., F.R.C.P.

Professor Davis has held the positions of Senior Registrar in charge of St. Mary's Hospital (Paddington) Home Care Scheme and Senior Assistant Resident, Children's Medical Centre, Boston, and Harvard Teaching Fellow. He then became Reader in

Paediatrics at the Institute of Child Health, Neonatal Unit, Hammersmith Hospital and Nuffield Fellow at the Nuffield Institute, Oxford. He has also been the Chairman of the Academic Board of the British Psychiatric Association and World Paediatric Association Representative with the World Psychiatric Association European Society for Paediatric Research, and a member of the Neonatal Society of the French Paediatric Society. Professor Davis is currently Professor of Paediatrics and Child Health and Director of the Department of Child Health in the University of Manchester. His interests are perinatal medicine, developmental psychiatry, the organization of medical services, and medical education.

Publications relevant to this book

'The first breath and development of lung tissue'. In *Scientific foundations of obstetrics and gynaecology*. Heinemann, London (1970).

'The effects of early environment on later development'. *Developmental medicine and child neurology* **12**, 98–107 (1970).

'Immediate problems at birth'. *British Medical Journal* iv, 164–6 (1971).

'Teratogenic and subtler effects of drugs in pregnancy'. In *Prevention of handicap through antenatal care*. Review of Research and Practice No. 18. Institute for Research into Mental and Multiple Handicap, London (1975).

'Childbirth—the facilitating environment'. Mabel Liddiard Memorial Lecture, 2 May 1974. *Midwives' Chronicle and Nursing Notes* July issue (1975).

'The G.P. and the care of the newborn'. Leader. *Journal of Maternal and Child Health* June issue, pp. 4–7 (1976).

With Dobbing, J. (eds). *Scientific foundations of paediatrics*. Chapters written by Davis: 'The beginning and fruition of self', and 'The pharmacology of the fetus, baby, and growing child'. Heinemann Medical Books, London (1974).

Chloe Fisher, N.N.E.B., S.R.N., S.C.M., M.T.D.

Miss Fisher is now Nursing Officer for Community Midwives in Central Oxford. She trained as a nursery nurse before undertaking her general training at Guy's Hospital, then as a midwife, in Cambridge and Oxford. Since becoming a midwife in 1956 she has practised solely in the domiciliary field. She obtained her Midwife Teachers' Diploma in 1968.

Her special interests are the management of labour and helping with and teaching about breast-feeding.

Donald Garrow

Dr. Garrow was educated at Trinity College, Oxford, and The London Hospital. He has held appointments at hospitals in London and Oxford, and was Senior Registrar at the Victoria Hospital for Children, Tite Street, his work being in the fields of epidemiology and diagnosis of respiratory infections, the problem of adeno-tonsillectomy, and the psychological effects of hospitalization in young children. He is at present Consultant Paediatrician at Amersham, High Wycombe, and Stoke Mandeville Hospitals. With a grant from the Oxford Regional Hospital Board he has studied cardiac and respiratory rhythms in newborn babies, and the effect of neonatal separation, and at present has an M.R.C. grant to study the clinical manifestations and diagnosis of toxocariasis. He at present has a further grant from the Oxford Regional Hospital Association to study mother–infant interaction.

Publications relevant to this book

With Smith, D. 'The modern practice of separating a newborn baby from its mother'. *Proceedings of the Royal Society of Medicine* **1**, 22–5 (1976).

W. O. Goldthorp M.B., Ch.B., D.Obst., F.R.C.O.G. and Joel Richman M.A.

Dr. Goldthorp is a Consultant Gynaecologist at Tameside General Hospital, Ashton-under-Lyne. He is engaged, with Mr. Richman of Manchester Polytechnic, in investigating sociological aspects of gynaecological practice, including a study of women requesting sterilization, and a follow-up on a survey of women who had their hospital confinement cancelled in 1973, to see if attitudes have altered. They are also working on patients' pre-conception of illness, and are conducting an investigation into vasectomy patients.

Publications relevant to this book

'Intestinal obstruction during pregnancy and the puerperium'. *British Journal of Clinical Practice* **20**, 367 (1966).
'A decade in the management of prolapse and presentation of the umbilical cord'. *British Journal of Clinical Practice* **21**, 21 (1967).
With Fitzgerald, T. B. 'The treatment of advanced abdominal pregnancy'. *British Journal of Clinical Practice* **22**, 487 (1963).
With Dawson, D. and Spencer, D. 'Parenteral iron therapy in pregnancy'. *Journal of Obstetrics and Gynaecology of the British Commonwealth* **72**, 89 (1965).

Joel Richman

Joel Richman is head of the School of Sociology at Manchester Polytechnic. Past research has included studies on the political structure of the Mexican Ejido and aspects of street behaviour. His present interests range over urban ethnography, deviance, and cross-cultural medicine. Since 1973 he has collaborated with W. O. Goldthorp in researching, from the medical sociological perspective, gynaecology, and obstetrics.

Joint publications by Joel Richman and W. O. Goldthorp relevant to this book

'Re-organization of the maternity services—a comment on domiciliary confinements in view of the experience of the hospital strike, 1973'. *Midwife and Health Visitor* **10**, 265 (1974).
'Maternal attitudes to unintended home confinement'. *The Practitioner* **212**, 845 (1974).
'When was your last period? Temporal aspects of gynaecological diagnosis.' Paper presented at the Manchester Meeting, April 1976, of the British Sociological Association. In *Health care and health knowledge* (ed. M. Stacey *et al.*). Croom-Helm (1977).
With Bedford, J. 'The sociologist's role in clinical medicine. Inter-disciplinary research'. *British Clinical Journal* **1**, 24 (1973).
With Bedford, J. 'The gynaecologist: friend or foe?' *New Society* **30**, 474 (1974).
With Hallam, W. 'Misunderstanding gynaecological terminology'. *British Journal of Sexual Medicine* **2** (1975) and **3** (1976).
With Simmons, C. 'Fathers in labour'. *New Society* **34**, 143 (1975).

Bianca Gordon

Mrs. Gordon studied Social Science at Birmingham University, and worked during the war for the National Association for Mental Health with ex-service personnel discharged from the Forces on psychiatric grounds. After further study at the London School of Economics, she was Psychiatric Social Worker in the Child Guidance Department of St. George's Hospital for six years. There her approach to child psychiatry was greatly influenced by the late Dr. Emanuel Miller, father of the child guidance movement in this country.

Her interest in the emotional needs of children and parents led her to further studies in child and adult psychoanalysis. Qualifying in these fields in 1953 and 1963 respectively, she has been associated, since its inception, with the Hampstead Child Therapy Clinic, founded and directed by Miss Anna Freud. From 1958 she has been involved in teaching, supervision and research.

In addition to her analytic practice, Bianca Gordon has for the past 23 years been pursuing the application of the principles of dynamic psychology to health work in community, as well as in hospital, settings. In this context she has developed her particular speciality of short-term psychotherapy with mothers in the antenatal and neonatal period, and is consulted by professional workers in the maternal and child health services. She teaches and lectures widely in this country and abroad.

Publications relevant to this book

'A psycho-analytic contribution to paediatric practice'. *Psychoanalytic study of the child*, Vol. 25. International Universities Press.
'A psychological approach to problems of mothers and babies'. In *The Family* (ed. H. Hirsch). Fourth International Congress of Obstetrics and Gynaecology, Tel Aviv (1974).
'An inter-disciplinary approach to the dying child and his family'. In *Care of the child facing death*. Routledge and Kegan Paul, London (1974).
An approach to problems of mothers and babies. Balliere-Tindall, London (1977).

Pamela Howat, R.C.N., S.C.M.

Miss Howat qualified at the Edinburgh Royal Infirmary in 1963. She trained as a midwife at Aberdeen and St. Andrews and held appointments at the Royal Victoria Hospital in Montreal, in the Intensive Care Newborn Service, and as Nursing Sister in the Neonatal Intensive Care Unit, John Radcliffe Hospital, Oxford. She is now Research Nurse in the Neonatal Unit at the John Radcliffe Hospital, studying neurological problems in infants undergoing intensive care, follow-up studies of infants who have been through the Intensive Care Unit, and other studies on the newborn.

Peter Huntingford, M.D., B.S., F.R.C.O.G.

Before 1971 Professor Peter Huntingford was Professor of Obstetrics and Gynae-cology at St. Mary's Hospital Medical School. He has been closely associated with the National Childbirth Trust almost since its foundation, supporting its objectives and activities, and has been President of the Obstetric Association of Chartered Physiotherapists. He was a pioneer in the United Kingdom of modern techniques to study the foetus. From 1971 to 1974, he worked with the World Health Organ-ization in South-East Asia in maternal and child health and family-planning pro-grammes, especially in Thailand and Indonesia. Professor Huntingford is currently responsible for teaching obstetrics and gynaecology in the University of London at The London Hospital and St. Bartholomew's Hospital Medical Colleges. His present interests include the welfare of mothers and babies in maternity hospitals, family-planning, abortion, and women's rights. He is particularly concerned about doctor–patient relationships, and the provision of maternity and gynaecological services, which are acceptable to the consumers as well as being appropriate to their health needs.

Publications relevant to this book

'Factors influencing pain in labour'. *Nursing Mirror* 412–13, 416 (1960).

'Pain in labour—and the Lamaze technique'. *Nursing Mirror* 1387–8 (1961).

'The obstetrician's contribution to prevention'. *Developmental Medicine and Child Neurology* 4, 547–8 (1962).

'Influence of anaesthesia on the incidence of maternal morbidity, Neonatal Asphyxia and Perinatal Mortality'. *British Medical Journal* 1, 1195–9 (1963).

'A direct approach to the study of the foetus'. *Lancet* i, 95–6 (1964).

'Focus on the foetus' (Sir William Power Memorial Lecture). *Midwives' Chronicle and Nursing Notes* 423–6 (1965).

'The midwives of the future' (Olive Haydon Memorial Lecture). *Midwives' Chronicle and Nursing Notes* 422–4, 444 (1966).

'Advances in obstetrics and gynaecology'. *The Practitioner* 429–38 (1967).

'Teaching the Teachers'. In *Report of a Symposium on Preparation for Parenthood*. Royal College of Midwives, London (1967).

'Past, present and future'. In *Perinatal medicine*. Karger, Basel (1972).

'Women and their health: is there a conflict?' In *UK health needs in a changing setting*. CIBA Symposium 43 December (1975).

'Attitudes'. *St. Bartholomew's Hospital Journal*. November (1976).

Sheila Kitzinger, B.Litt.

Mrs. Kitzinger is a social anthropologist specializing in comparative aspects of child-bearing and is also a childbirth educator. She did postgraduate research work in social anthropology at St. Hugh's College, Oxford, where she received her B.Litt. degree, and also research and teaching at the University of Edinburgh.

Since 1958 she has been developing her psychosexual method of preparation for birth and parenthood and has lectured widely in North and South America, Europe, and South Africa. She is on the Panel of Advisors of the National Childbirth Trust and is an antenatal teacher and tutor for the Trust. She is also a member of the Board of Consultants of the International Childbirth Education Association. From 1971–3 she held the Joost de Blank Award and did research on the problems facing West Indian mothers in Britain.

Publications relevant to this book

The experience of childbirth. Gollancz (1962); Penguin, England (1967); Taplinger U.S.A. (1972); Penguin U.S.A. (1972). (Now in 5th Pelican edition (1977).)

Giving birth—the parents' emotions in childbirth. Gollancz, England (1971); Taplinger U.S.A. (1972); Sphere, England (1972).

Education and counselling for childbirth. Bailliere Tindall (1977). 'Communicating with immigrant mothers'. In *Caring for children* (ed. M. L. Kellmer-Pringle). Longmans (1969).

'The woman on the delivery table'. In *Woman on woman* (ed. Margaret Laing). Sidgwick & Jackson, London (1971).

'An anthropological approach to education for childbirth with the underprivileged'. In *Psychosomatic medicine in obstetrics and gynaecology* (ed. Norman Morris). Karger, Basle (1972).

'Touch relaxation'. In *The family* (ed. Professor H. Hirsch). Karger, Basle (1976).

'Image and body fantasy in preparation for birth: an anthropological view'. In *The Family* (ed. Professor H. Hirsch). Karger, Basle (1976).

Episiotomy—physical and emotional aspects (ed.). Also author of chapter 'Emotional aspects of episiotomy and postnatal sexual adjustment'. National Childbirth Trust, London (1972).

Articles in: *Medical World, Nursing Mirror, Midwife and Health Visitor, Group Analysis, Marriage Guidance, British Journal of Sexual Medicine, CIBA Review, The Practitioner, General Practitioner, Journal of Maternal and Child Health, Mother, Mother and Baby*, and *New Society*.

G. J. Kloosterman, F.R.C.O.G.

Professor Kloosterman was director of the Training School for Midwives in Amsterdam from 1947 to 1957 and was chairman of the State Committee on Abortion 1970–2, and is Chairman of 'Concilium Gynaecologicum' 1968–77. He is now Professor of Obstetrics and Gynaecology in the University of Amsterdam, and Director of the Department of Obstetrics and Gynecology of the University Clinic. He is a Fellow of the Royal College of Obstetricians and Gynaecologists and an Honorary Fellow of the American College of Obstetricians and Gynecologists.

He has written four books, including a textbook of obstetrics and gynaecology. He has published widely in Dutch, and his publications in English and French include the following.

Publications relevant to this book

The avoidance of prematurity. *4th European Congress on Perinatal Medicine*, Prague (ed. E. A. Sternbera), pp. 194–200. Thieme, Stuttgart (1974).

On intra-uterine growth (the significance of prenatal care. *International Journal of Obstetrics and Gynecology* **8**, 895–911 (1970).

Zur Förderung der Mutter–Kind–Bindung in der moderne Geburtshilfe. Die Welt des Neugeborenen. *Monatsschrift für Kinderheilk* **124**, 563–9 (1976).

Michael Lee-Jones, M.B., B.S.; M.R.C.P.; M.R.C.G.P.; D.R.C.O.G.

Qualified at Middlesex Hospital Medical School, 1960, Dr. Lee-Jones entered general practice in 1962, then returned to hospital medicine, including two years in the United States. He joined a group practice in Wallingford, Oxfordshire, in 1971. Wallingford Community Hospital is an experimental general practitioner unit with facilities for maternity, general, and long-stay care. Dr. Lee-Jones's recent research and publications have been related to the role and function of the community hospital.

Peter Lomas, M.R.C.Psychiat.

Dr. Lomas is a Freudian-trained psychoanalyst. He was a general practitioner for six years, followed by work in mental hospitals, a Child Guidance Clinic, and the Cassel Hospital, Richmond, at which he did two years' research on post-partum breakdown. He also made a study on childbirth and the family, with his wife Diana, under the auspices of the Institute of Psychoanalysis. Since 1966 he has practised, taught, and written independently as a psychotherapist in Sussex. During this time he has developed a method of psychotherapy which focuses on the elemental features of a helping relationship as distinct from the exercise of technical expertise.

Publications relevant to this book

'The husband–wife relationship in cases of puerperal breakdown'. *British Journal of Medical Psychology* **32**, 117 (1959).

'Dread of envy as a factor in the aetiology of puerperal breakdown'. *British Journal of Medical Psychology* **33**, 105 (1960).

'Puerperal breakdown and defensive organisation'. *British Journal of Medical Psychology* **33**, 61 (1960).

'Observations on the psychotherapy of puerperal breakdown'. *British Journal of Medical Psychology* **34**, 345 (1961).

'The concept of maternal love'. *Psychiatry* **25**, 256 (1962).

'Ritualistic elements in the management of childbirth'. *British Journal of Medical Psychology* **39**, 207 (1967).

Introductory chapter and 'The significance of post-partum breakdown'. In *The predicament of the family* (ed. P. Lomas). Hogarth, London (1967).
'True and false experience'. Allen Lane (1973).

Aidan Macfarlane, M.A., M.B., B.Chir., M.R.C.P.

Dr. Macfarlane qualified at Cambridge in 1964. He held appointments at Hillingdon Hospital, Paddington Green Children's Hospital, Harvard Medical School, Radcliffe College and Boston Children's Hospital, Massachusetts, St. Bartholomew's Hospital, The Department of Experimental Psychology, and the Park Hospital, Oxford. He is now working in paediatrics at the Radcliffe Infirmary, Oxford. He has worked on the effects of analgesics and other drugs given during labour on newborn behaviour; early mother–child interaction; the role of olfaction in neonatal behaviour; auditory and visual responses in the neonate, and effects of induction on mothers' feelings in the first two months post-partem. He has also worked with a 'threatened to batter' group of mothers and children.

Publications relevant to this book

With Harris, P. 'The growth of the effective visual field from birth to seven weeks'. *Journal of Experimental Child Psychology* **18**, 340–8 (1974).
'The first hours, and the smile'. In *Child alive* (ed. Roger Lewin). Temple Smith (1975).
Olfaction in the development of social preferences in the human neonate. CIBA Foundation Symposium 33 (new series). Associated Scientific Publishers, Holland (1975).
'Central and peripheral vision in early infancy'. *Journal of Experimental Child Psychology* **21**, 532–8 (1976).
'Auditory localisation in the newborn infant and the effects of pethidine'. *Developmental Medicine and Child Neurology.* (In press.)
Psychology of childbirth. Fontana Open Books, England. Harvard Press, U.S.A. (1977).

Lewis Mehl, M.D.

Dr. Mehl is Director of Research at the Institute for Studies of Childbirth, Human Development, and the Family, Wisconsin. Currently he is studying the impact of birth upon family dynamics and family interaction patterns and is also examining the relation of these family interaction processes to the development of psychopathology. He has also been involved in a psychoanalytic/systems theory investigation of relationships in an obstetric ward. He is a Fellow of the American College of Home Obstetrics and a Member of the Boards of Consultants of the Association for Childbirth at Home, and the American Foundation for Maternal and Child Health.

Publications relevant to this book

'Home Birth Statistics'. In *Immaculate deception* (ed. S. Arms), pp. 214–15. San Francisco Books (1975).
'Comments on physiologic obstetrics'. *Child and Family*, May (1976).
'Current status of statistical outcomes of home delivery'. In *Safe alternatives in childbirth* (ed. D. Stewart and L. Stewart). NAPSAC Press, London (1976).
'Home Births'. *Proceedings of the 1976 International Childbirth Education Association.* ICEA Press, Seattle, Washington (1976).
With Peterson, G. H. 'Management of the complications of home delivery'. In *Childbirth at home* (ed. M. Sousa). Prentice-Hall; Englewood-Cliffs, New Jersey (1976).
With Peterson, G. H., Shaw, N. S., and Creevy, D. C. 'Complications of home birth: report

of a series of 287 deliveries from Santa Cruz country, California'. *Birth and the Family Journal* **2**, 123–35 (1975).
With Sokolosky, W. and Whitt, M. C. 'Outcomes of early discharge from the hospital after uneventful labor and delivery'. *Birth and the Family Journal* (1976). (In press.)
With Peterson, G. H., Whitt, M. C., and Creevy, D. C. 'Outcomes of elective home delivery: comparisons with similarly selected hospital delivery'. *Journal of Reproductive Medicine* (1977). (In press.)
With Shaw, N. S. and Peterson, G. H. 'The home birth trend'. *The Atlantic Monthly* (1977). (In press.)

W. M. O. Moore, F.R.C.O.G.

Dr Moore graduated M.B. from Cork in 1954 and spent a couple of years in general practice. After resident posts in obstetrics and gynaecology at Hammersmith Hospital and the Radcliffe Infirmary, Oxford, he was Registrar at St. Luke's Hospital, Bradford, Research Assistant and Senior Registrar at Hammersmith Hospital, and Research Fellow at Johns Hopkins Hospital during tenure of N.I.H. postdoctoral fellowship. From 1965 to 1967 he was Senior Lecturer in University of East Africa and Consultant to Mulago Hospital, Kampala. Since 1967 Dr. Moore has been Reader in Obstetrics and Gynaecology, University of Manchester, and Consultant Obstetrician and Gynaecologist to St. Mary's Hospital, Manchester. His research is concerned with the role of the placenta in the determination of foetal size, and the influence of foetal growth patterns on child growth and development.

Publications relevant to this book

'The conduct of the second stage'. In *Benefits and Hazards of the New Obstetrics*, ed. Chard, T. and Richards, M. P. M., London, S.I.M.P. with Heinemann, 116–25 (1977).
With Ward, B. S. 'Placental membrane permeability to creatinine and urea'. *American Journal of Obstetrics and Gynecology* **108**, 635 (1970).
With Murphy, P. J. and Davis, J. A. 'Creatinine content of amniotic fluid in cases of retarded fetal growth'. *American Journal of Obstetrics and Gynecology* **110**, 908 (1971).
With Ward, B. S. and Gordon, C. 'Human placental transfer of glucagon'. *Clinical Science and Molecular Medicine* **46**, 125 (1974).
With Jones, V. P. and Ward, B. S. 'Fetal growth retardation in the second trimester'. *European Journal of Obstetrics, Gynecology and Reproductive Biology* **6**, 121 (1976).
With Bamford, F. N., Jones, V. P., and Ward, B. S. 'Three case reports of second trimester fetal growth retardation: two year follow up'. *European Journal of Obstetrics, Gynecology and Reproductive Biology* **7**, 301 (1977).

Martin Richards

Dr. Richards is a zoology graduate. Since 1968 he has worked on problems of human development in the Medical Psychology Unit at Cambridge and is the University Lecturer in Social Psychology. He has edited a volume of essays on social aspects of development, *The integration of a child into a social world* (Cambridge University Press, 1972) and currently is completing a polemic on medical services, 'Towards a national illness service'. His recent research has concentrated on the consequences of early separation of baby and parent and policies for special neonatal care. The results of this work will be published in a monograph he is editing with Dr. F. S. W. Brimblecombe and Dr. N. R. C. Roberton which is to be published as one of the series Clinics in Developmental Medicine.

Diana Smith

Dr Smith graduated from and then obtained a Ph.D. at Cambridge in 1956. In 1972 she became research assistant to Dr. Donald Garrow at Amersham Hospital, studying the relationship between cardiac and respiratory rhythms in newborn babies. She died before publication of this book.

Publications relevant to this book

With Garrow, D. 'The modern practice of separating a newborn baby from its mother'. *Proceedings of the Royal Society of Medicine* 1, 22–5 (1976).

Marjorie Tew, M.A.

Mrs Tew was engaged after graduation in social research at Glasgow University, before joining in 1942 the Programmes and Statistics section of the war-time Ministry of Aircraft Production as assistant to A. K. (now Sir Alec) Cairncross. She taught economics at Adelaide University for three years and published *Work and welfare in Australia* (1951, Melbourne University Press). After looking after her family for 20 years, she resumed her professional career in 1970 and as research associate in the newly founded Department of Community Health at Nottingham University was concerned mainly with analysing published statistics.

Publications relevant to this book

'Where to be born?' *New Society* Vol. 39 (1977).

L. I. Zander, D.C.H., D.Obst.R.C.O.G., M.R.C.G.P.

Dr. Zander qualified in 1960 from St. Mary's Hospital, following which he spent five years in hospital work before entering general practice. In 1965 he went to Edinburgh to join the first academic Department of General Practice to be established in a medical school, and in 1970 became Senior Lecturer in the newly developing General Practice Teaching Unit of St. Thomas' Hospital. His principal academic activities have been concerned with developing teaching programmes for under-graduates. In the field of research a major interest has been that of record-keeping in general practice. He is author of a number of articles on a range of subjects including the management of insomnia, the problem of confidentiality in general primary care, and various aspects of the management of childbirth. He has been involved in many aspects of the organization of medical care delivery, and since the reorganization of the N.H.S. in 1974 has been the general practitioner representative on a District Management Team. He has been active in the Royal College of General Practitioners and in 1975/76 was the Secretary of the General Practice Section of the Royal Society of Medicine. He is on the panel of advisers of the National Childbirth Trust.

Index